HUNGER

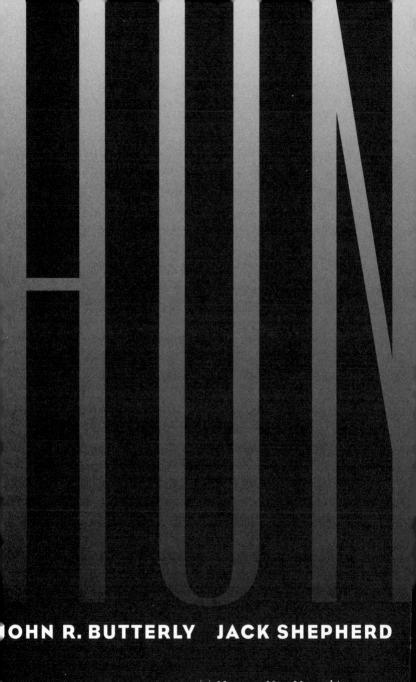

HUN

JOHN R. BUTTERLY   JACK SHEPHERD

DARTMOUTH COLLEGE PRESS [ ] Hanover, New Hampshire

Published by University Press of New England [ ] Hanover & London

GER

GER

The Biology
and Politics
Starvation

DARTMOUTH COLLEGE PRESS

Published by University Press of New England

www.upne.com

© 2010 John R. Butterly and Jack Shepherd

All rights reserved

Manufactured in the United States of America

Designed by Eric M. Brooks

Typeset in Dante, Eagle, and Empire by

Passumpsic Publishing

Library of Congress Cataloging-in-Publication Data

Butterly, John R.

Hunger: the biology and politics of starvation /
John R. Butterly, Jack Shepherd.

    p.; cm.

Includes bibliographical references and index.

ISBN 978-1-58465-926-6 (cloth: alk. paper)

1. Famines. 2. Hunger. 3. Malnutrition. 4. Starvation.
I. Shepherd, Jack, 1937– II. Title.

[DNLM: 1. Hunger. 2. Environment. 3. Human Rights.
4. Politics. 5. Socioeconomic Factors. 6. Starvation. WD 100]

HC79.F3B88   2010

363.8—dc22   2010028574

5 4 3 2 1

To **Hannah Lerner Kessel,**
who gave me hope,
to **Lynn Axel Butterly,**
who fulfilled it,
and to **Ruth Kessel Butterly,**
who taught me how things
ought to be.

To **Kathleen Kessler Shepherd**
for sharing with me every day
the joys and blessings of Africa and her people.
"Mungu Ibariki Afrika,
Wabariki Watu wote wa Afrika."
(God bless Africa,
Bless all the people of Africa.)

Contents

Acknowledgments

A book of this size and complexity is the work of many people. We want to thank some of them here. The origins of this book are found in a course we taught together with Lee Witters, MD, for four years at Dartmouth College. It was Lee's creativity and enthusiasm that enriched our efforts in that course and his deeply felt commitment to its core topic that sustained us here.

We also greatly appreciate the support and encouragement of Professor Andrew Friedland, chair (2000–2011) of the Environmental Studies Program at Dartmouth College, and the Environmental Studies faculty and staff. The department provided office and meeting space for us and for our research assistants, Amy Linn and Zoë Shtasel-Gottlieb. Various members of the department also cheered us on during our writing.

Special thanks to Ken Yalowitz, director of the Dickey Center for International Understanding at Dartmouth College, whose enthusiasm and financial support helped get this project off the ground. Ken and the Dickey Center made our research and this book possible, for which we are deeply grateful.

Amy Linn, Dartmouth Class of 2007, labored for more than eight months with patience, intelligence, and humor as our research assistant. She relentlessly pursued a long list of complex research questions and often worked weekends, taking breaks only to buy a new bicycle and go off on impressively long bike workouts. Her efforts for us filled six filing-cabinet drawers with original documents and her own unique and valued analyses. Her outstanding work was underwritten by generous contributions from the John Sloan Dickey Center for International Understanding at Dartmouth.

And just as Amy climbed on her new bicycle to pedal across the United States for Bike-and-Build, Zoë Shtasel-Gottlieb, Dartmouth Class of 2010, took over Amy's old office and spent her sophomore summer chasing down all of the remaining research. Zoë proved that determination will find anything, and her dependable and insightful research soon filled its own files alongside Amy's. Then Zoë climbed on an airplane and went off to southern Africa for her autumn term, leaving us with but one alternative: start writing this book.

John Butterly gratefully acknowledges Donald St. Germain, MD, for his mentoring and guidance that helped to start this journey on its way.

We would also like to thank Cheryl A. Wheelock, access services supervisor for the Matthews-Fuller Health Sciences Library at Dartmouth, for her friendly help and expertise in tracking down some of the older, more obscure references we wished to include. We would like to acknowledge Daniel Butterly for his advice and explanation regarding Abraham Maslow's theory on the hierarchy of human motivation; Joel Butterly for his advice in pointing out Edward Said's work on the historical political manifestations of our species' tendency to recognize other cultures as inferior; and Nancy Bagley, MD, for her discussions on "The Tragedy of the Commons."

We are indebted to Kathleen Butterly Nigro, PhD, assistant director and teaching professor of the Institute for Women's and Gender Studies at the University of Missouri—St. Louis for her careful review of this manuscript and her excellent insights and suggestions.

PART I

Platform of Understanding

Prologue **"Peasants Always Starve"**

In the middle of February 1973, a tattered band of about 1500 Ethiopian peasants appeared on the outskirts of Addis Ababa, the country's capital. Police halted them there and demanded an explanation. The peasant-farmers described drought and poor harvests around their villages in Wollo Province, some 200 miles north of Addis. They told of the repeated failure of seasonal rains; how they couldn't plant seeds for the harvests; how their plow oxen weakened and starved; and how, in desperation, they ate their seed grains instead of planting them. Those who owned land sold it for a few Ethiopian dollars. Others bartered their animals, their tools, the wood from their huts, even their clothes. And when the hunger continued sweeping through whole villages and districts, those men still able to walk left their women and children and began the desperate search for food.

Word of their arrival filtered up to the minister of the interior, who asked the governor-general of Wollo to explain the presence of these threadbare peasants outside their capital city. The governor-general, Solomon Abraham, an elderly aristocrat and political appointee, assured the Imperial Government of Ethiopia that, while there was some "problem of drought" in Wollo, there was little cause for concern. And when the Imperial Government sent an official inspection team to Wollo and Tigre provinces to investigate, the team returned to reassure everyone that only these 1500 peasants were "affected by a shortage of food." The word *starvation* was not mentioned.

After all, the Imperial Government reasoned, hadn't Ethiopia's peasants always starved? In 1958–1959, for example, perhaps 100,000 of them had quietly died in the northern and central provinces from lack of food. Few Imperial Government officials or international relief workers had worried about them. According to tradition, Ethiopian peasants bowed before their Orthodox Church, their Imperial Government, and their venerated Emperor Haile Selassie I, revered speaker at the League of Nations, defender of their land against an invading Italian army, His Imperial Majesty, Conquering Lion of the Tribe of Judah, King of Kings of Ethiopia, and Elect of God. In Ethiopia, before the harvests, peasants always quietly starved.[1]

In 1973, however, these Ethiopian peasants signaled a warning: 2000 years of Ethiopia's empire were ending; a feudal society was collapsing. Their small protest, unnoticed beyond the capital at the time, also marked the beginning of what historians call "a gateway event." Their march set in motion a new paradigm at a pivotal moment in starvation's dark global history: it came more than 125 years after the Great Irish Famine, fifty years from the time when starvation swept across the new Soviet Union, forty years since Stalin starved millions of landed peasants in Ukraine, thirty years following the Bengali Famine of 1943, and just fifteen years beyond the Great Leap Forward famine that may have killed as many as 25 million in China. In 1973–1974, the hunger that scythed across the dry savannah of West Africa's Sahel to the mountains of Ethiopia triggered a series of events that fundamentally altered our understanding of starvation, how it is defined, who suffers, when and where it occurs, and how we respond. Out of Ethiopia's peril emerged new ways of measuring and replying to starvation that shifted international policies. From that moment in hunger's history came a new paradigm of the biology and politics of starvation.

The peasants' simple protest shattered our innocence: no longer could we say we didn't know when others were hurt, diseased, or starving. It aroused humanitarian concern globally for the plight of people in developing states. It shifted the accepted theories about the causes of starvation and famine and thus reformed policies and reshaped responses. It heightened international alarm over global food availability and starvation, and it brought together donors, UN and government officials at the first World Food Conference. This in turn initiated significant global schemes to anticipate human suffering and to respond to it: for example, new and modern satellite measurements of agricultural production along with the time-honored stockpiling of food reserves against hard times. Chapter 1 discusses this paradigm shift and its important historic record and connects it to the current debate about poverty reduction and human rights—especially the right to food. But most important, from this peasant march on, we knew.

The Problem

We have chosen hunger as the focus of this book. But the ultimate problem that underlies hunger and other unacceptable social inequities is poverty. Hunger is poverty made manifest.

As we write, 1.02 billion people are suffering chronic hunger, one in six persons. For the first time in history, we have crossed the 1 billion mark: a relentless increase from 781 million in 1989 to 915 million in 2008 to more than a billion in 2010.[2]

Hunger is also causing the death worldwide of some 3.5 million children every year: almost 10,000 kids a day.[3] That number climbs to 10 million children worldwide when we add together hunger with its associated, preventable diseases.[4] That is, according to the United Nations World Food Programme (WFP), a child dies every three seconds "of hunger."[5] The statistics of global hunger, when stitched together, form a stark tapestry of population growth, increasing food demands, poverty, and risks to health. For example:

- World population is growing steadily, and more than 90 percent of that growth is in the developing world.
- Although there is enough food produced globally to feed all of us, the U.N. Food and Agriculture Organization reports that in any given season one in every six countries faces severe food shortages. For example as of this writing, one person out of every four in southern Asia, and one out of every two in Central Africa suffer from chronic hunger.
- Although the vast majority of the hungry are living in developing countries,[6] some 49 million people in the United States—almost 15 percent of all U.S. households—do not have enough to eat daily and suffer from recurring hunger, the highest rate of food insecurity in the United States since 1995.[7]
- Chronic hunger is the leading cause of death globally. It or its agents kill an estimated 9 million people every year—more than HIV/AIDS, tuberculosis, and malaria combined.[8]
- Almost all of these statistics are caused by poverty that itself is creating "a nutritional crisis." The number of humans living in poverty, earning less than US$1 a day, may range between 1 billion to 1.8 billion.[9] These are the poorest of the poor. (The World Bank estimated that by 2010 this population was increasing at the rate of 89 million people annually.[10]) Most of them are not short of food because of a sudden emergency. Rather, they suffer from chronic, long-term poverty. Another 2 billion struggle on less than US$2.50 a day.[11] (The World Bank also estimated that by 2010 people in this category were increasing by 120 million annually.[12]) These 3 billion cannot afford food that may be readily available in their markets. They are vulnerable to rising food prices, climate change that creates drought and flood, armed conflict that disrupts their planting and harvests, capricious or corrupt governments, and opportunistic diseases. They form what we call "the silent emergency" (detailed in chapter 1).

These poor must undertake daily what are called "coping strategies." "Those living on less than US$1 a day have cut out protein and vegetables from their diet," warns Josette Sheeran, the executive director of WFP. "Those living on less than US$0.50 a day have cut out whole meals, and sometimes go days without meals."[13]

The result, she concludes, is "a nutritional crisis." It is this crisis, the result primarily of poverty, which makes hunger their daily condition and renders them vulnerable to a spectrum of diseases and to starvation and famine. More than 50,000 people die daily—30 percent of all human deaths annually—from such poverty-related causes. These conditions, the result of deprivation, could be prevented easily and cheaply: 884 million people lack safe drinking water; 2.6 billion lack adequate sanitation; 2 billion lack access to essential drugs, vaccines or other medicines, or nutritious food or vitamins; 924 million lack adequate shelter.[14] For the bottom billion of the global population, this "nutritional crisis"—the result of their poverty—is defining.

Why is this problem of hunger, disease, and poverty important? Why should we care? For one thing, as mentioned, hunger affects one in six of us; it kills almost 10,000 children a day. Second, we have the economic and technical means to eradicate hunger and many of its attendant diseases, but responses to this are encumbered by what the WFP calls "a fragile world food system in urgent need of reform." Moreover, the WFP reports, "there is less food aid than we have seen in living memory."[15] Third, eliminating hunger, poverty, and disease is not only an urgent humanitarian and medical goal, it is also "a matter of national security, peace and stability," says Sheeran. "Without food, people revolt, migrate or die. This is the emergency issue of our generation, and we stand at a critical crossroads."[16]

The Framework

We frame these issues around a social science and scientific investigation. We seek to identify and analyze the scientific, medical, and human characteristics of historic and modern-day hunger, and the science that supports and underlies this condition. We use comparative analyses and case studies to build our arguments.

To begin to address these purposes, we ask several underlying questions:

○ What has caused malnutrition, chronic hunger, disease, and poverty, and why do they persist?
○ Why do they continue despite the combined efforts of well-meaning public and private, national and international agencies and people?
○ How does the human body function? How does it react to hunger, malnutrition, starvation, and the attendant diseases?

It is crucial that this investigation be framed not by the narrow issue of starvation or famine being resolved by donations of food or money but, rather, by the wider investigation of emergency and long-term assistance, of hunger, disease and their links to poverty, and the discomforting questions about our willingness to act. We therefore also seek to give voice to the voiceless, to raise a moral awareness.

Who or what has denied these 2 billion people "the right to a standard of living adequate to [their] health and well-being"?

Is it because we cannot avoid it, or because we allow the situation to continue? In 1996 Nigel Dower, the ethicist and philosopher, asked: Why in our modern world, knowing as we do when and where extreme hunger exists, able to communicate this globally and instantly, with food surpluses and advanced transportation systems, do we "not seem to be able to replicate the practices of past smaller societies of at least trying to ensure that everyone has enough of the one crucial thing it is in the power of others to provide—namely food"?[17] Reflecting on St. Augustine's question about God and the existence of evil, and on the high numbers of chronically hungry people, Dower again troubles us when he asks: "Will it [chronic hunger] exist because we *cannot* prevent it, or because we *will* not prevent it?"[18]

Case Studies

Three principal case studies will help us to discuss these conditions and to create a platform for our investigation.

Ethiopia in 1973–1974 and again in 1982–1986 gives us a complex series of events over two decades. These include bizarre changes in governments, one of the earliest global relief aid responses, shifting policy decisions, and an excellent example of a country pleading for help while the donor community debates the issue of national sovereignty. Should national sovereignty be violated to feed starving people?

The Great Irish Famine (1845–1850) holds up a distant mirror to modern hunger and starvation. It is considered Europe's last large-scale famine where between 800,000 and 3 million Irish peasants died.[19] The parallels with more recent events are striking. The Great Famine is an early example of the "poorest of the poor," or the more recent phrase, the "bottom billion," left behind by those who can emigrate or otherwise obtain food. The Famine offers an early example of humanitarian responses by religious groups operating soup lines and kitchens (complete with special recipes). These were early precursors to today's emergency relief agencies, many of which are also operated by religious organizations (Catholic Relief Services, Lutheran World Federation, Church World Service, the American Friends Service Committee). Third, the Great Irish Famine was strongly shaped by the application of a popular economic theory (*laissez-faire*, French for "leave alone") that was not unlike the present-day "free market" theory. When rigidly applied to Ireland in 1845–1850, *laissez-faire* was thought to have exacerbated the starvation and the abbreviated relief responses to it.

We follow this economic theme in our third case study: Malawi, a country in southern Africa, during 2001–2002. One of the echoes of the Great Famine found in Malawi's case is the ill-fated economic theory called "Economic Structural Adjustment Program" (ESAP), part of the wider "free market" theory so popular before the economic collapse of 2008. Also, whereas Ireland exported food during its famine, the government of Malawi sold off most of the country's grain reserves. In both cases impoverished Irish and Malawians got priced out of the food market—and starved.

Malawi thus offers a modern-day reflection on the Great Irish Famine and the economic systems and theories that drive the politics of starvation. We next match it with a study of Niger and Mali in 2005 when both faced starvation, but only Mali "escaped." This gives us the opportunity to further compare economic theories and their impacts and to discuss and analyze the history and questions about grain reserves. These, for example, have a long history and were referred to as "ever-ready granaries" in eighteenth-century China or "the moral economy" in modern sub-Saharan Africa. These were and are today a basic understanding between government and citizen, peasant producer and ruler or chief, that during times of surplus some grains would be set aside against times of adversity. As we discuss in chapter 1, these reserves are now seen as part of local efforts to alleviate poverty by smoothing out price fluctuations.

Finally, comparing the Great Irish Famine with modern developing states serves as a cautionary reminder that chronic hunger, starvation, disease, and poverty are conditions common to people regardless of nationality, religion, or ethnicity. No one has cornered poverty or racism. The Irish were vilified in the British press as being ignorant and subhuman; British commentators linked Irish and Africans, and cartoonists drew them as monkeys. The Irish were seized and sent from Ireland as slaves to the West Indies—creating a verb, to be "barbado'ed" (after their West Indies destination). Their plight emphasizes the unfortunate durability and universal character of affliction and prejudice. We discuss these commonalities fully in our special sections on the Great Irish Famine.

Plan of the Book

The book is sectioned into five parts. Part 1 discusses the fundamental problems of hunger, disease, and poverty, the scale and structure of what we call "the silent emergency," and the various theories and definitions that have informed policy decisions regarding these problems. We also further investigate the Ethiopian famines of the 1970s and 1980s and discuss them as "gateway," historical events. Part 2 considers the anatomical and physiological aspects of nutrition (and, hence, malnutrition and hunger). It traces the social evolution of nutrition and responses to it. Part 3 analyzes the various responses to hunger, from individuals at the household level through government and international agency policies and responses. Here are placed our case studies of Malawi, Niger, and Mali. In part 4, both authors interrogate the reasons some people starve and others do not. Who dies, and who does not? Why is this important, medically and in political and policy terms? Part 5 explores two important questions. Is there a "right" to food with a parallel "obligation" to feed the hungry? What are some of the "best practices" already being deployed against hunger, disease, and poverty? This includes a brief discussion of genetically modified food and its "promise" to create a new Green Revolution to combat hunger.

At the end of each of the first four parts are found the narratives and analyses of the Great Irish Famine. We call them "Lessons from the Great Irish Famine." They allow us to reflect on that famine and more recent events and to highlight connections with developing states today. Rather than containing them in one chapter, we have separated these accounts into four "lessons," so that we may pull together specific material from preceding chapters and discuss it in terms of this unique event. The result is not so much "lessons learned" as investigations of conditions repeated today (such as "poorest of the poor"). In effect these sections may also be considered lessons not yet learned.

Throughout, the book places the objectivity of science—especially medical science—against the evolving background of social science. Science is objective and tells us what is. Social science is more subjective and explores what should be. In this volume, we write as scientist and social scientist. We deliberately write in different styles; we draw information and analysis from other disciplines and fields.

Along with the politics of starvation, therefore, we examine its biology; that is, the biology of nutrition, malnutrition, and the consequences of chronic, inadequate nutrition. It is a basic precept of medicine that in order to fix something you must first understand it. We believe, therefore, that an issue of this magnitude is best explored by a complete, in-depth understanding of the biology of human nutrition, malnutrition (both macro- and micronutrient), the associated health-related factors (for the most part, preventable infectious diseases), the theories of inadequate nutrition and famine, the historical political behaviors that have led to famine in the past, and the current political behaviors that cause chronic hunger and malnutrition to remain as major health problems today. How would you treat pneumonia without knowing about the germ theory of disease, the mechanisms of normal respiration, the importance of an intact immune system, or the mechanism of action of certain antibiotics? How would you correctly set a broken bone without understanding the normal anatomy, the mechanisms of bone growth, and the time required before the cast may safely be removed?

Beginning in chapters 3 and 4, we review the basic science of bioenergetics along with the biochemistry, anatomy, and physiology of nutrition. We come to understand that the human body is able to ingest, digest, absorb, and convert nutrients into usable energy with far greater efficiency than any theoretical engine. Of the carbohydrates, proteins, and fats delivered to our digestive systems, 95 percent are absorbed, and 85 percent of this ingested energy is converted to usable energy (called metabolizable energy intake or MEI).[20] With the understanding of how humans (and other life forms) have evolved to be so exquisitely efficient in the intake and utilization of energy sources, we can begin to understand the biology of starvation: how crucial nutrition is to our survival, why it is the first element in the "hierarchy of our needs," and why it is unacceptable that even one human being, much less billions of human beings, have inadequate access to basic nutrition. A central concluding point to this book is that we commonly consider our biological processes, especially our physical ones, as completely detached from our social and political ones— including, to a large extent, our mental/behavioral processes. This is an error, which we address in chapter 11.

The Fundamental Question

Our analysis of the biology and politics of starvation starts with a simple question. This question emerges after reading Article 25 of the United Nations' *Universal Declaration of Human Rights*, written in 1948. Article 25, discussed fully in chapter 1, declares a person's "right to a standard of living adequate for the health and well-being of himself and of his family, including food, clothing, housing, and medical care."[21] Although not a binding international legal instrument, the UN *Declaration* is widely considered a watershed document, the common ground of all subsequent human rights agreements, covenants, and laws since the mid-twentieth century. This *Declaration*, including its language and intent, therefore, is both the point of departure and central reference of our work. Yet the goals of the *Declaration of Human Rights* continue to elude us. After more than a half-century, Article 25 remains "a promise diluted."[22]

We ask: "Why?"

The Silent Emergency

The march of starving Ethiopian peasants on their capital in 1973 set off a series of connected events. What emerged was a new paradigm of the biology and politics of starvation. Five core characteristics of those events help to define that paradigm; they continue to reverberate today.

Five Central Events

First, Ethiopia's famine of 1973–1974 shattered our innocence. It marked the end of a time when we could honestly say we did not know starvation was occurring in some distant place, among some unknown people. Ethiopia in the mid-1970s became synonymous with "starvation." Its plight was quickly and widely shown to the well-fed, largely because television journalists like BBC-TV's Jonathan Dimbleby hiked into the mountains of Wollo and Tigre provinces and filmed the starving peasants. (Television had a small initiatory part in publicizing the Biafran starvation in eastern Nigeria, 1967–1969.) The result was a delayed but, finally, robust response: by the end of 1974 more than forty relief organizations including the United Nations Children's Fund (UNICEF), Lutheran World Relief, and Catholic Relief Services were active in the country, along with Ethiopia's own humanitarian services; some 80,000 starving peasants were in emergency camps in Wollo alone.[1] After the peasants marched that February, therefore, we knew.

A decade later television again played a central role in Ethiopia during the famine of 1983–1986. Telecasts from the relief camps brought images of emaciated Ethiopian babies into our homes. Although television may not have directly comforted the afflicted, it certainly afflicted the comfortable. Emergency responses included simultaneous "Live Aid" rock concerts in more than fifteen locations around the world that raised the largest amount of money in the history of emergency relief funding to that time. Once it started, the outpouring of emergency aid was unprecedented. (The two Ethiopian famines are further discussed in chapters 6 and 7.)

Second, two off-continent events were later identified that may have exacerbated conditions in the Sahel and Ethiopia during 1973–1974. One was the possibility that pollutants from the industrial North may have been a factor in causing the drought that swept from West Africa to the Horn, resulting in the starvation of more than 500,000 Africans. The other was the significant impact on global grain prices and their availability by a large-scale purchaser (the Soviet Union) that entered the international grain market precisely as the number of starving Africans was rapidly increasing. The Soviet purchase overlapped with relief agency demands for emergency grain supplies for Africa. For the first time donors saw supplies of emergency grains falling far short of demand. Declines in food production and rises in food prices—and the Soviet purchases—"had a dramatic effect on food aid levels." U.S. emergency food aid exports, for example, fell from 19 million metric tons in 1962 to 3.3 million metric tons in late 1974.[2] (Both events are detailed and analyzed in chapter 9.)

Third, Ethiopia in 1973–1974 also marked the beginning of a fundamental shift away from the theories, popular at the time, of starvation's causes and effects. This shift continues today. In 1798 Thomas Malthus had published *An Essay on the Principle of Population* in which he argued that population growth increases exponentially and soon overtakes food production, which grows arithmetically, thus resulting in starvation. And starvation and famine, he suggested, were (and are) "positive checks" on human overbreeding. Malthus revised his thinking and later wrote *Principles of Political Economy* in which he sought to tie population growth not only to food supplies but also to opportunities for employment. Thus, he argued, economic growth could also benefit the poor, as long as they were not lazy and wasteful.

Despite his revised writings Malthus and his principal theory have been widely used to define starvation and our responses to it: if starvation is caused by overpopulation and subsequent food availability deficits, then our response should be to provide the means to decrease population and increase food availability. This theory was readily applied to the condition of the Irish peasant in 1845–1850, where Malthus (and *laissez-faire* or free-market economics) had a strong influence. Thus, Malthus is remembered primarily for the perception that his theories blamed the victim: starvation is the fault of the poor. The "positive check" theory remains today an important component of discussions about the causes of and responses to starvation and poverty.

With the Ethiopian and Sahel starvations of the mid-1970s as a point of reference, however, Amartya Sen and Jean Drèze, and later Alexander de Waal, Stephen Devereux, and other scholars, began generating a more contemporary and robust framework of analysis. Their theoretical contributions also continue today. Sen won the Nobel Prize in Economics in 1998 for his seminal work that redirected our focus from Malthusian food availability (supply-side economics) to food entitlement (demand-side economics). In brief, Sen argues that people starve because they are poor and cannot access food. (The theories of Sen and Malthus are discussed in detail in chapter 2.)

Sen's work refocused the developed world's analysis and responses to chronic hunger, starvation, and famine from one of emergency, short-term food relief (that is essential and continues) to one engaging long-term development aid directed toward poverty alleviation. Why is this important? For one thing, the new direction addresses the core humanitarian crisis. The alleviation of poverty will require that the more wealthy nations recognize the plight of billions of impoverished others—and act. It will also require unique resolve as well as a deeper and longer commitment from governments, donors, and international financial institutions. Wealthy nations will have to unite to shift funding from expanding their military forces to assure their security to more humanitarian programs. This will require a redistribution of monies that will be seen as risky and without guarantees for success. It might also rejuvenate questions about the "lazy poor." The Ethiopian peasants' long walk to beg for food in 1973, we argue here, can therefore be said to mark the beginning of a new challenge to famine theory and response.

Fourth, Africa's Sahel and Horn starvations gave special urgency to the first World Food Conference, which was convened in November, 1974 in Rome. From that Conference came some of the policies and instruments that today help international agencies determine that starvation is occurring in a region.

The starvation spreading at that time across the Sahel and Horn, and in India and Bangladesh, had heightened international alarm over global food production, supply, and prices. The two previous decades had witnessed steady annual increases in food supplies and surpluses, but by 1972 falling food availability and rising prices, plus severe food shortages in parts of the developing world, had alerted donors to possible future global shortfalls. The World Food Conference, therefore, met amid "reports of critical food shortages, famine, and persistent drought in some developing countries,"[3] and at a time when grain supplies available for emergency relief were shrinking rapidly while starvation was accelerating in Africa and South Asia.

Malthus' theory appeared to be coming true. Along with the peril of food shortages, expanding global population also alarmed the World Food Conference members. As a 10-year review later reported, world population increased 25 percent between 1970 and 1982, and that growth came predominately within the developing world.[4] Moreover, the *rate* of that population growth was especially worrisome in sub-Saharan Africa: Kenya, for example, reached 4 percent annually—"close to its theoretical maximum"—with a population doubling time of just 18 years.[5] In Asia, it was the *size* of the population base, especially in China, that concerned the 1974 Conference. Neo-Malthusian warnings about global population growth and world food supplies and prices appeared both real and imminently at hand.

The World Food Conference urged action. Its delegates issued warnings and challenged donors to take steps that would reduce chronic hunger, end starvation, and alleviate poverty. The Conference produced a list of relief strategies, many still discussed or in practice today. One called for stockpiling food reserves among the most vulnerable states in the developing world. Such strategic food reserves could be used for emergencies and for balancing market inequalities; detractors opposed these reserves on the grounds of possible corruption, such as the illegal sale of the reserve, or the potential for looting. (We discuss these strategies in chapter 7.)

The World Food Conference also proposed a global early warning system to monitor planting, harvests, and food production on the world's arable land. The outcomes were the Food Early Warning System (FEWS) and Global Information Early Warning System (GIEWS), among others. Today, these food early warning systems generate real-time satellite images and monitor weather assessments, insect migrations, animal and plant diseases, crop production, stocks, food aid, and grain export prices. This creates a database incorporating global, regional, national, and subnational information. GIEWS is primarily a food assessment and information-sharing resource; it is used by 115 governments and 61 non-governmental organizations (NGOS), research centers, and trade and media organizations. The FEWS gathers global information by satellites every 10 days.

In some ways the first World Food Conference was itself an early warning. While its delegates raised alarms over population growth, persistent food shortages, rising food prices, and starvation, they also challenged the wealthy donor countries to take immediate steps to end all hunger and alleviate poverty. U.S. Secretary of State Henry Kissinger's call to action in November 1974 became, verbatim, the Conference's Resolution I: ". . . that within a decade no child will go to bed hungry, that no family will fear for its next day's bread, and that no human being's future and capabilities will be stunted by malnutrition." As a review of the Conference said a decade later, however, "that goal is still far from realization."[6] This is, unfortunately, true even today.

Fifth, events in Ethiopia in 1973–1974 and the first World Food Conference awakened humanitarian concerns about the "right to food" of impoverished peoples in developing states. In 1976, for example, "legislators, development experts, and religious leaders," stirred by wide-scale starvation across Africa, India, and Bangladesh, testified in support of House Concurrent Resolution 737. This nonbinding Right to Food Resolution passed the House on September 21, 1976, and the Senate just one week later. It declared that "Every person throughout the world has a right to a nutritionally adequate diet and that the United States should increase substantially its assistance for self-help development among the world's poorest people."[7]

Following on the alarms of the World Food Conference, HR 737 gave voice to a rising awareness of deprivation, poverty, chronic hunger and disease that was becoming the accepted norm of life in the developing world. Among its sponsors was Bread for the World, founded in the spring of 1974 during the famines in Africa and South Asia. From this movement also sprouted Food First/Institute for Food and Development Policy. Both NGOs joined a small but widening phalanx of humanitarian agencies (including medical NGOs such as Doctors Without Borders / Médecins Sans Frontières) that began linking "food" and "justice" as principles "to insist that the human right to food, not transnational corporations, guide U.S. food and development assistance and influence food programs at home." From the peasant march on Addis Ababa to the halls of the U.S. Congress, at least for that moment, food and justice became "the basis of democratic citizen action."[8]

An examination of the 1970s, therefore, reveals these and other early signs of a paradigm shift away from simple emergency food-relief responses to a more complex, rights-based approach. That shift links our increasing knowledge and concern about chronic hunger, disease, and starvation with human rights and demands for poverty alleviation. It fundamentally shifts the argument from Malthus to Sen.

Universal Declaration of Human Rights

By the second decade of the twenty-first century we find a large cluster of UN agencies and international NGOs refocusing their work to include rights to food and health, sustainable development, and to the "growing understanding that poverty reduction and human rights are inextricable."[9] They are, in effect, giving a new reading and articulation to the UN *Universal Declaration of Human Rights*. This paradigm shift may yet turn out to be the most powerful long-term legacy of those desperate Ethiopian peasant farmers.

The introduction of human rights into the issues of starvation and famine — an acknowledgment of the right to food — can be traced back to its origins. This is a simple, but sad, undertaking, for in that tracing we also measure the ebb and flow of suffering on millions of fellow human beings.

The tracing is simple because its fundamental document is well known and widely discussed. On December 10, 1948 the United Nations General Assembly adopted the *Universal Declaration of Human Rights*. Its designers intended the *Declaration* to create the foundation for a single human rights covenant "that would make the principles of the *Declaration* binding on ratifying states."[10] Here, just three years after the end of the horrors of World War II, was the first postwar voice for ethical human behavior. Article 1, for example, states that all people are born free and are equal in terms of dignity and rights "and that everyone is endowed with reason and conscience and should act toward one another in a spirit of brotherhood."[11] Thus, the *Declaration's* focus on economic, social, and cultural rights was critical to the well-being and dignity of humans as groups and individuals. The General Assembly asked all member states to display, read, and disseminate the text "in schools and other educational institutions, without distinction based on the political status of countries or territories."[12]

Article 25 declares a person's "right to a standard of living adequate for the health and well-being of himself and of his family, including food, clothing, housing, and medical care."[13] Although not a binding international legal instrument, the UN *Declaration* is widely considered a watershed document, the common ground of all subsequent human rights agreements, covenants, and laws. In addition to its fundamental articulation of the human right to food, the *Declaration* sets forth responsibilities to fulfill and protect a range of human rights, especially through establishing social institutions that alleviate chronic and severe poverty. It is thus both the purveyor of rights and the proponent of ethical behavior; it requires us to go beyond self-interest to understanding and acting toward one another with reason and conscience and "in a spirit of brotherhood."[14] In this context, the *Declaration* further illuminates a core argument of our work: that the end of hunger, chronic malnutrition, starvation, and disease can come only with the alleviation of poverty.

Yet, Article 25 of the *Declaration* also identifies the most abused human rights to date. The right to food and the alleviation of poverty, the promise of dignity, equality, and "freedom from fear and want," remain unfulfilled today. Despite the rapid advance of science and technology, of continuous humanitarian efforts, extensive bilateral and multilateral agreements, and multiple covenants and pledges, inadequate nutrition, chronic hunger, and starvation remain major economic and social problems and are primary risks to health worldwide.

Thus, the intentions and goals of the *Universal Declaration of Human Rights* continue to elude us. Dr. Thomas Pogge, a philosopher and ethicist at Yale University, calls Article 25 of the UN *Declaration* "the most under-fulfilled human right" on record.[15]

Trends in the First Decade of the New Century

During the last 25 years of the twentieth century, humanitarian responses to starvation and famine appeared to be winning. World hunger seemed to be waning and with it large-scale starvation. From 1980 to 1997, the number of starving people fell from 959 million to 791 million. This came primarily as China and India decreased the number of undernourished and poor in those countries. Certainly men, women, and children in the developing world (and in pockets of the rich North) continued suffering from chronic hunger and its attendant diseases. But by the early 1990s, according to the UN's Food and Agriculture Organization (FAO), the number of people who were hungry or starving decreased by 20 million. Therefore one trend during the 1990s appeared to be the easing of chronic hunger and starvation in some developing states, especially in West Africa, Southeast Asia, and South America.

But by 2000 the number of hungry people in developing states started to rise again, at first by about 4 million annually. Early in the twenty-first century, according to the UN World Food Programme (WFP), spending on agriculture decreased, and (as we will discuss in further detail) crops and cropland were diverted to fuel, causing a price spike. The number of global hungry started accelerating: from that baseline of 781 million in 1989, to 915 million by 2008, then crossing the 1 billion mark for the first time in 2010. Among forty-seven countries, most of them in Africa below the Sahara, the number of chronically hungry was growing by 96 million persons annually.[16]

The "Bottom Billion"

By 2010 these human beings had fallen into an intractable "bottom billion," most of them in the developing world, afflicted with severe hunger, vulnerable to its attendant diseases, unable to move out of poverty, untouched by any declarations of rights to food or freedom from disease.[17] The United Nations warned that the "bottom billion" could trigger global social unrest. "Hungry people," UN Secretary-General Ban Ki-moon declared, are angry people, and their anger and hunger could breed "social disintegration, ill health and economic decline."[18]

Addressing this need will be difficult. To stave off starvation for these billion people, according to the UN FAO, global food production will have to increase by 50 percent by 2030. But other trends of the new century are working against this. In chapters 5 and 9, we discuss, along with continuing population growth, a parallel increasing urbanization of the developing world. This is combining with rising incomes to cause a major shift in diets—a "nutritional transition"—from direct grain consumption to processed foods and meat requiring far larger amounts of the same grains to produce. This "nutritional transition" is itself increasing demand and prices for grains, placing them out of reach for the "bottom billion."

This trend highlights an important distinction. There are now actually two "nutritional" crises occurring simultaneously: one is the result of global poverty; the second the outcome of widening incomes. WFP's Josette Sheeran speaks of a "nutritional crisis" caused by increasing poverty among those "bottom billion." Diametrically opposite is another crisis, the "nutritional transition" generated by rising incomes and expanding wealth that are altering diets and food demands. We focus here primarily on the "nutritional crisis" among the "bottom billion," but we will also analyze the "nutritional transition" caused by urbanization and rising incomes, primarily in terms of China, in chapter 9. Both trends are influenced by grain prices and grain (and water) availability. Demand for grains (usually in the form of meat and beverages such as beer) is increasing among those whose incomes are rising; this and other factors, discussed next, are placing grains beyond the reach of more and more impoverished people.

The disparity of poverty and wealth was further heightened when in 2007 fuel shortages, perhaps driven by market speculation, intersected with increasing demand for biofuels, a process in which grains, sugar, and palm oil are diverted to fuel for vehicles. This caused "perhaps the most aggressive pattern of global price increases ever for food commodities," wrote researchers at the International Food Policy Research Institute.[19] The winners were the wealthy; the losers were the poor.

These economic occurrences, known as "food spikes," have occurred globally three times since the mid-twentieth century. The first followed World War II, before Europe and Japan had recovered from the devastation of war, and before the Marshall Plan, itself an early humanitarian landmark, had taken effect. The second came during the 1970s, the result of a sharp rise in the cost of petroleum (and hence, increased costs for fertilizer and fuel to transport food and other goods), weather (drought), and international market demand (starvation in Africa and South Asia, and the Soviet grain purchases of 1973 and 1974). The third spike started in June 2007, as petroleum prices again escalated and demand for biofuels increased.[20] The first spike was the result of global war, the second bad weather and government errors, and the third "structural imbalances in the world food chain."[21]

During 2007–2008, the rising fuel costs and the transfer of food crops to biofuels created a severe scarcity of staple grains. It also shifted croplands to fuel production and attracted trade speculation of biofuels, agricultural land, and grains in the global markets. The WFP, for one example, saw the cost of buying basic foods for its programs increase 50 percent between 2002 and 2007 and then another 50 percent from June 2007 to February 2008.[22] The price of corn alone rose 43 percent in 2007[23] and 70 percent in 2008.[24] As a result, the World Bank estimated that about 100 million people were "pushed deeper into poverty by the high food prices," thus accelerating that trend. The WFP called the rising costs of food "a silent tsunami" overwhelming the bottom billion and causing "the biggest challenge" in the agency's 45-year history.[25]

Josette Sheeran, WFP's executive director, identified three phases in the fuel-food prices clash: the first in 2004 when climbing prices caused a drawdown of national food and cash reserves by vulnerable nations and peoples "to all time lows"; the second in June 2007 "when aggressive price increases exhausted all coping strategies"; and the third when these same nations and peoples "became dependent on external assistance to avoid widespread human suffering and ensure affordable access to adequate food."[26]

The fuel-food crisis of 2007–2008 jarred the international donor community and devastated the global poor. The consequence, as Sheeran pointed out at the time, "is that the bottom billion could become the bottom 2 billion overnight, as those living on US$1 a day see their purchasing power cut in half."[27] Oxfam UK, the British humanitarian NGO, estimated that by 2008 the fuel-food clash had pulled the incomes of 119 million people below the UN's poverty line. By 2010, although the demands on food production by biofuels appeared to have lessened, the alarms and debates about how this crisis of hunger had happened, who it harmed, and whether or not it might return, continued. There was agreement, however, that a global "nutritional crisis" was under way and that it was affecting more than 1 billion of the world's poorest people.

In addition to the increase in global poverty during the first decade of the twenty-first century there was a continuing and parallel trend toward "donor fatigue" among the grain-surplus states. This is a significant theme that runs throughout this book. All of the conditions causing poverty remain: drought and flooding, the AIDS/HIV epidemic, armed conflict, climate change, government mismanagement and political turmoil, the global economic collapse, and declining food production. The urgent need for emergency food relief and long-term development aid also continues. Yet donors with surplus food supplies are sometimes overwhelmed, slow to respond, and often manifest what has been termed "donor fatigue" or "compassion fatigue." "We have the economic and technical means to make hunger disappear," said Jacques Diouf, FAO's Director-General, in 2010. "What is missing is a stronger political will to eradicate hunger forever."[28]

The Millennium Goals

This compassion fatigue has spilled over into two areas: reducing childhood mortality worldwide and meeting the Millennium Goals. To be sure during the first decade of the twenty-first century some significant gains were made. Before the global recession began in 2008, among the most encouraging improvements was the decline in global childhood mortality. In 1960, for example, the number of children dying each year before their fifth birthday was an estimated 20 million.[29] By the late 1980s that number had declined to about 14 million children annually.[30] In 2006 it fell below 10 million (to 9.7 million children) for the first time in its recorded history and to about 8.8 million by 2008. Why? A principal factor was the long-term commitment by agencies and individuals to inexpensive preventative interventions: a fourfold increase in the number of children getting vitamin A; a tripling in the use of insecticide-treated mosquito nets, a basic tool in preventing malaria; more than a 10 percent increase since 1990 in measles immunization; and the expansion of breast-feeding.[31]

But in contrast to these gains unacceptably high levels of child mortality remain and persist. Sub-Saharan Africa and South Asia, two regions at the bottom of most statistical charts, have made little progress. For example sub-Saharan Africa still has the highest child mortality rates; South Asia is home to the most undernourished children.[32] Countries in these regions are intractably poor, unable (or unwilling) to protect their citizens from preventable diseases, chronic hunger, and the horror and dislocation of armed conflict. Measles, malaria, pneumonia, diarrhea, and the ravages of AIDS are common among the ranks of the regions' children and their parents.

Despite these gains and the dedication and hard work of thousands of bright and capable people, progress toward alleviating chronic hunger, disease, and poverty in specific regions is moving very slowly, or in reverse. Take the Millennium Declaration and the Millennium Development Goals, for example. Here is one of the most exciting ideas to emerge in the last sixty years in the struggle to end global hunger and disease. In 2000 members of the United Nations agreed on a universal framework for development in the impoverished world. They courageously took on not only the plight of the bottom billion, but also the next billion—the 2 billion human beings who are the world's poorest and most vulnerable. They created eight Goals and Targets[33] and sought to achieve these by 2015. (Chapter 8 discusses the UN Goals and Targets in more detail.)

But at the halfway point to the Millennium Declaration's target date, the reports were mixed. Millennium Goal 1, which directly concerns us in this book, seeks to eradicate "extreme hunger and poverty" and to cut by half the number of poor living on less than US$1 per day, by 2015. By 2008 fifty-eight countries were on track to reach that goal, but thirty-three countries had made "insufficient" progress, and another eighteen no progress at all. Some "143 million [children] under five in the developing world continue to suffer from under-nutrition."[34] Goal 4, to reduce childhood mortality by two-thirds, showed promise (as detailed above), but in sub-Saharan Africa and South Asia the UN reported, "global progress is insufficient to achieve MDG 4."[35] Goal 6, which also informs sections of this book, pledges to "combat HIV/AIDS, malaria and other diseases." But at the halfway mark malaria remained a killer of more than a million people annually, and "80 percent of these deaths occur in

Sub-Saharan Africa among children under five." In fact, the UN stated, "most countries are falling short of global malaria goals."[36]

There are several reasons for this failure to achieve the Millennium Goals by the midway point. Some of the most important are these:

Inequitable and poorly funded health care systems. This includes access to nutritional information and to safe and plentiful food and water. Also, part of the problem in developing states is retaining trained doctors and nurses, who are drawn to employment elsewhere in their region or to the developed world.

Continuing high levels of violence, civil conflict, and community dislocation in many developing states (discussed in chapter 9). This results in large numbers of dislocated people and in continuing and increasing violence against women. Because women are the principal farmers in many developing regions, this violence also disrupts or halts the planning, planting and harvesting of crops.[37] The consequences include food shortages and entrenched poverty.

The continuing international economic crisis. UN research estimates that this may increase the number of "working poor" globally by 100 million and the number of chronically hungry poor by 104 million. This is being exacerbated by "stagnating remittances, drying-up of capital flows and investment, falling revenues in relation with the contraction in world trade and commodities crisis." The World Bank estimated that by 2010 the developing world had incurred a financial shortage of $700 billion.[38]

The issue, therefore, is not only the international donors' "political will to act," but also their financial ability to continue their global assistance. "Donor fatigue" remains, but it has taken on a new, economically driven meaning.

The "Wealth Paradox"

As indicated above, the core of our analysis, with the exception of the Great Irish Famine, draws its examples and case studies from Africa. Why? Largely because of what we call Africa's "wealth paradox." Ironically, Africa[39] south of the Sahara is rich. The continent is blessed with prodigious natural resources: gold, diamonds, oil, minerals, a vast agriculture potential, and resourceful and well-educated "human capital," including an entrepreneurial market labor force. Multinational corporations and superpowers such as the United States and emerging superpower China[40] compete on the continent for Africa's natural resources; they pump its oil, dig up its ores and diamonds and gold, and farm its limited arable lands.

Yet we encounter a contradiction: juxtaposed with this wealth, Africa's countries and their people rank highest on almost every index of human suffering. The African people are among the poorest in the world; they suffer disproportionately from chronic hunger and such "ordinary" afflictions as dehydration, diarrhea, and measles that leave them too weak to resist common infections. The "nutritional crisis" of the very poor is most evident among Africa's people, the "nutritional transition" of the wealthy less so.

Some 800 million Africans live in fifty-three countries—about one out of every eight people on earth inhabiting 27 percent of the total number of countries worldwide. And because Africa is geographically enormous—three United States would squeeze into its external continental boundaries—we need to bear in mind its broad economic, social, political, and environmental differences. There is no single "Africa" but rather a vast and complex continent and people. Therefore, our perceptions and generalizations about its problems, and our statistics, will be *indicative* rather than *definitive*.

Nonetheless, those statistics help us to define, identify, and articulate our core paradox: the great wealth of Africa matched against the poverty and suffering of the African people. We see this paradox in the following:

  ○ Africa south of the Sahara is the poorest of the world's megaregions. Of the continent's fifty-three countries, only six have per capita GNPs above US$1000 per year; of the fifty-nine countries worldwide whose people live on less than US$1 a day, thirty-five are located in sub-Saharan Africa.[41]

  ○ Of the forty-four countries at the bottom of the Human Development Index, which measures life expectancy, education, and per capita income, twenty-seven are located in sub-Saharan Africa.[42]

  ○ Some thirty-three African countries continue to experience declining per capita food production; their people are food insecure. One in three Africans suffers chronic hunger; in some regions, such as Central Africa, more than half the people are undernourished.[43] In 2009, some 265 million Africans—one in four—were continuously malnourished, an increase of 12 percent over the previous year.[44]

  ○ Africans suffer disproportionately from treatable diseases such as dysentery, malaria, and measles.[45]

  ○ AIDS is the sixth-ranked cause of death globally, but it is the number-one cause of death in sub-Saharan Africa according to the UN World Health Organization's statistics. About 70 percent of the world's HIV-positive people live in Africa. In southern Africa the number may be as high as one adult in every five.[46]

  ○ One African in every five lives in a country severely disrupted by armed, largely internal, conflict.[47] This has caused some 5.1 million displaced Africans to be homeless within their own countries; another 2.3 million wander beyond state borders as international refugees.[48]

It is this paradox of wealth and suffering that places Africa and its people at the center of our investigation into the biology and politics of hunger and disease. If Article 25 of the *Universal Declaration on Human Rights* is to be fulfilled, it will be Africa where that effort starts, and Africa that benefits first and most. As Barack Obama told the people of Ghana in 2009 on his first visit to Africa as President of the United States, "I do not see the countries and peoples of Africa as a world apart; I see Africa as a fundamental part of our interconnected world."

We do the people of Africa a disservice, however, if we discuss only the challenges critical to their future. Those who study the continent and its people in depth—and Shepherd has been working in Africa since 1968—soon discover "the other Africa" removed from that of the statistics of suffering. Disaggregate those fifty-three nations, and one finds complex cultures, diverse and skilled workers, high levels of literacy (for example, more than 90 percent in Zimbabwe at the beginning of this century), and a kindness and respect for strangers and elders that is humbling.

Nor is the news out of Africa all negative: for example, between 2000 and 2005 deaths among children under the age of five had declined by more than 20 percent in Ethiopia, Mozambique, Namibia, Niger, Rwanda, and Tanzania. In Malawi, childhood deaths were down 29 percent.[49] There are more democratic countries than ever before (thirty as opposed to five in 1990) and less violence (three civil wars as of this writing against thirteen at the beginning of the 1990s). One excellent example is Rwanda, the scene of horrific ethnic conflict in the 1990s, where a truth-and-reconciliation system of some 12,000 *gacac* or community courts has now heard more than 1 million cases of genocide. It is, as one observer reported in 2009, "the only nation where hundreds of thousands of people who took part in mass murder live intermingled at every level of society with the families of their victims." The death penalty has been abolished. It is now "one of the safest and the most orderly countries in Africa." The country's GDP tripled between 1994 and 2009. The population of 10 million enjoys national health insurance. Broadband internet service is available in the cities and many parts of the rural areas. The majority of the parliamentarians (56 percent) are women, the highest percentage in the world. The country has even outlawed plastic bags to cut down on litter.[50]

At the political and economic level across Africa, successful and peaceful national elections and presidential successions are occurring more frequently. In Botswana and Ghana, Mozambique and Angola, stability is increasingly the norm, and economic growth the standard. Women are also playing a more central role in African politics. In addition to Rwanda's 56 percent, they make up 30 percent of the parliaments of Angola, Mozambique, South Africa,

Tanzania, and Burundi. And the first woman elected president in Africa, Ellen Johnson-Sirleaf, took office in Liberia on January 16, 2006.

There are promising alliances forming around regional entities such as the Southern Africa Development Community, modeled after the European Union, the Economic Community of West African States, and the East African Federation. Regional cooperation includes water, customs and labor protocols, the removal of trade barriers and even the opening of international boundaries (drawn up by the former colonial powers). Most of these open borders are linking national game parks. The Trans-Frontier Conservation Areas (TFCA) uniting fifteen southern African states offer an outstanding model for environmental conservation, open international boundaries, and economic cooperation. The TFCAS were originally designed to link the national parks across international borders, "from Cape Town to Kilimanjaro." By sharing natural resources (water, land, wildlife) and tourism, and by cooperating on economic opportunities, Africans are attempting to reduce unemployment and encourage transborder economic cooperation. The TFCA model is now being applied to countries in the Carpathian region of central Europe and is being considered in the Middle East.

The key issues that remain for Africa, and the entire developing world, are to address food insecurity, health, and disease; to continue the spread of democracy and the peaceful resolution of conflicts; and to address in meaningful ways the issues that cause poverty. As U.S. President Obama also told the people of Ghana, "Despite the progress that has been made—and there has been considerable progress in many parts of Africa—we also know that much of that promise has yet to be fulfilled."[51]

The Silent Emergency

To the themes of the *diluted promise* of Article 25 of the *Universal Declaration of Human Rights* and the *wealth paradox* of Africa's riches and its poverty, we add a third: the *silent emergency*. These three themes form the heart of our book.

In 1987 UNICEF published a watershed report,[52] "The State of the World's Children." In it James P. Grant, then UNICEF's executive director, warned of the "loud emergency" that drowns out "the silent emergency" that kills millions of people, many of them children, "almost without notice" each year. At that time the "loud emergencies" were often the result of Cold War confrontations in Afghanistan, Sudan, Ethiopia, the Middle East, Cuba, the Koreas, and Central and South America. More recently, we could add the tsunami that swept the Indian Ocean littoral in 2004, the unrelieved starvation and brutal conflict that has settled into the Darfur region of Sudan, the repetitive food shortages and hunger in North Korea, the 2010 earthquake in Haiti, among others. These "loud emergencies" gain our attention and that of the media, and attract large amounts of donations and emergency relief aid. "Loud emergencies" overwhelm the underlying "silent emergencies" that occur globally, every day.

James Grant identified and understood the importance of "the massive world-wide public and political response" to loud emergencies. Two years after the global responses to Ethiopia's second famine, he wrote: "Today, our world no longer allows millions of its children to die in the sudden emergencies of drought or famine anywhere on the planet." But, he continued, "In the early 1940s, for example, an estimated 3 million men, women and children starved to death in Calcutta and Bengal while the world knew little and did less. Such a change is a significant step towards a more truly civilized world."[53]

Yet, the "silent emergencies" continue. We ignore them at enormous human and moral peril. Throughout the last half of the twentieth century and well into the twenty-first, "silent emergencies" killed—and continue killing— hundreds of thousands of people *every week*, without publicity, in forgotten corners of the world. As we write, more than 49,000 people are dying *every day* from the preventable afflictions of diarrhea, malnutrition, tuberculosis, meningitis, hepatitis, malaria, respiratory infections such as pneumonia, and childhood diseases such as measles. These include more than 26,000 children under the age of five who die *every day*, more than half of them from deaths associated with undernutrition and poor sanitation.[54]

Grant called for a "revolution in child survival and child health." He wanted to "defeat infection and undernutrition," childhood killers. He abhorred the fact that the world then, as now, "accepted as *normal*" the deaths of large numbers of young children every year and the fact that other children and their parents continued to live "in malnutrition and ill health."[55] He demanded a change in our global moral awareness—"a change which will make the silent emergency equally unacceptable to the majority of the world's people."[56] We share James Grant's concern. "The silent emergency," he concluded, "is also an invisible emergency."

Our third goal, therefore, is to identify the scientific, medical, and human characteristics of the silent emergency and to make its components and victims known. It is thus to give voice to a moral awakening, and to moral obligation and response.

Today, Grant's warning has taken on a new urgency. As the developed world struggles with the global War on Terrorism, we suggest that among its root causes lie the statistics and anecdotes—the afflictions—detailed here. That is, the basic catalysts to terrorist behavior are found within the silent emergency. Those who are fighting a civilian war in the streets and mountains of Iraq, Afghanistan, and Pakistan, are those without potable water, sanitation, vaccinations, clinics, reliable food sources, education, hope. A microexample from the war in Iraq illustrates this point: during combat operations in Baghdad in neighborhoods with the most severe fighting, U.S. military officers discovered that the sections that had the greatest violence against American troops matched those areas that had no electricity, functioning sanitation, or drinkable water. "They found a direct correlation between terrorist incidents and a lack of services." [57] By extension, improving living conditions—sanitation, water, access to food and health care—in the developing world would seem to be the better, and even less expensive, path to diminishing the violence of global terrorism. As the WFP's Josette Sheeran reminds us, this is "the emergency issue of our generation."

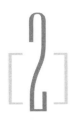

The Framework of Understanding

In this chapter we create a framework for our analysis. Like academics everywhere we start with definitions, which we believe give us a common language and help us to identify and define a problem. Definitions, in turn, enable policy makers to bring institutional responses to address them. If we can say definitively that "starvation" is sweeping across the mountains of Ethiopia, for example, we can then demand that action be taken to feed and aid those who are afflicted. Along with the definitions we suggest further diagnostic "tools" to help us understand the principal or *predisposing causes* of starvation or famine, the *catalytic events* that trigger them, and the actual *medical reasons* people die from hunger or proximate causes of death (poverty being the ultimate cause).

From that base, we discuss the two defining theories—from Malthus and Sen—concerning hunger, starvation, and famine. They, in turn, inform our definitions and principal causes of starvation and famine, and play significant roles in determining our responses. For example, if policy makers in the donor countries believe that rapid population growth impacted by drought has caused a starvation, their response is likely to be short-term emergency food aid and then perhaps longer-term attention to population stabilization and reduction. But if policy makers see the same drought as a triggering event, with poverty as the underlying *principal* cause of the starvation, then short-term emergency food relief will be followed with long-term poverty-alleviation measures such as employment efforts and inputs to farmers. Therefore, definitions, analytical tools, and theories help us to identify the causes of and responses to hunger, starvation, and famine. They create frameworks for policy action. They are instruments to relieve suffering.

None of this is as precise as the sciences of anatomy or physiology. But it is very helpful in determining when, where, how, and especially why people starve.

Definitions: Chronic Hunger, Malnutrition, Starvation, and Famine

A definition is important for diagnostic purposes. Medical definitions tell us about the body's functions and responses. In terms of this book social science definitions tell us of conditions on the ground: who is suffering, how many there are, what their social and economic status might be, what actions they are taking. As mentioned, these definitions also facilitate responses by state, regional, and international actors. How you define something determines how you will act on it.

Here we define chronic hunger, malnutrition, starvation, and famine, and some of their variations. We regard the process leading to famine as a continuum: hunger to malnutrition to starvation to famine. Impoverished people are almost always in one condition or another, and one condition often progresses to the other; sometimes there is a sudden collapse of a community, for example, from chronic hunger into starvation, and even a swing back.

This continuum may shift from being a "silent emergency" to a "loud emergency." A "silent" event, unknown beyond remote communities, may become a "loud" emergency when brought, or forced on, others outside the region and even overseas. When these episodes end, however, the survivors often slip back into their previous condition, usually one of seasonal hunger and chronic malnutrition, in silence.

Here is the spectrum of definitions we use in creating this analytical framework:

Hunger is a recurrent, involuntary lack of access to food. "Hunger occurs when people do not have enough to eat for a healthy, active life."[1] There may be frequent episodes of hunger—such as *seasonal hunger* before a harvest in developing countries, when food stocks from the previous year's harvest have run out, prices are high, and purchasing power among the poor is weak. The UN's World Food Programme (WFP) regularly publishes alarms about seasonal hunger across southern Africa, for example, which it attributes to "the traditional lean season from January to March" when grain supplies are meager just before the harvests.

Food insecurity with hunger occurs when there are limited or uncertain *amounts* of safe (unspoiled) foods, a limited or uncertain *ability* to acquire available food without stealing it, or a lack of access to enough food to meet a person's basic needs *at all times*.

Chronic hunger does not end with a harvest but continues season to season, year to year. It is a condition that occurs daily and over a long period of time (a year or more). It is a significant measure of poverty. It creates physiological, emotional, and social conditions that make people and communities (even regions) vulnerable to events like drought, flood, crop damage by insects, and diseases that stronger people and communities can survive. For example, when the Mississippi River floods large portions of America's breadbasket, there is not widespread starvation. But when a cyclone struck across southern Africa in 2000, more than 7 million people slipped into starvation and required outside emergency responses.

Malnutrition is a deficiency, excess, or imbalance in the diet of specific nutrients essential to good health. Malnutrition can occur in the absence of hunger, starvation, famine, or even weight loss. (Mal-nutrition—that is poor nutrition—in association with obesity is becoming a growing global problem among people in developed countries.)

Chronic malnutrition describes the result of a poorly balanced diet deficient in essential nutrients. It may be a permanent condition of the rural poor in some developing states.

Moving along the continuum, here is where the division between "silent" and "loud" emergencies starts to occur. Our definitions of starvation and then famine link time (duration) to mortality (deaths) and space (geographic locations).

Starvation is the result of long-term suffering from chronic and often extreme hunger in a specific geographic region. As hunger worsens and life is threatened, starvation emerges.

Famine is defined in one analysis as "a shortage of total food so extreme and protracted as to result in widespread persisting hunger, notable emaciation in many of the affected population, and a considerable elevation of community death rates attributable at least in part to deaths from starvation."[2] Several well-known definitions of famine include time, mortality, and geographical space. Carl Mabbs-Zeno suggests that famine "refers to episodes of unusually high mortality in contrast with chronic hunger or malnutrition" with death due to malnutrition and associated diseases over a specific geographical area.[3] John Field writes "Famine is *the endpoint* of a lengthy process in which people in increasing numbers lose their access to food" (italics added).[4] Famine, therefore, may be a crisis of mass starvation—"shortages of *total* food"—and of intensity—"extreme and protracted"—and of *scale*—"widespread"—and *finality* or mortality—"the endpoint." Famine may also be marked by shifting market demand for different foods and by "excess deaths"—deaths that otherwise might not have happened at that time. Most famine-induced mortality tends to occur after the worst of the food crisis is over but while a crisis of infectious diseases still persists.

It is important to note that there may be different definitions of starvation or famine depending on whether one is actually *experiencing* the famine (that is, "inside" it) or *observing* (that is, "outside" it). High mortality may be a distinguishing characteristic of a famine (certainly to those on the outside), but the breakdown and disintegration of a society and its people are the most certain markers and important to those on the inside. We define *famine*—an unusual occurrence—as severe food shortages resulting in *societal breakdown*, followed by *high mortality* as a result of widespread, *persistent starvation and its associated diseases*. Nevin Scrimshaw, the founding director of the Institute of Nutrition of Central America and Panama, ties this together for us:

> The essential element is a relatively sudden collapse in the level of food *consumption* by large numbers of people. Starvation refers to peoples' going without sufficient food, and during famines people do so on such a large scale that mortality is high. . . . [F]amine is not just the result of an extreme and protracted shortage of food, but also an economic and social phenomenon that can occur *when food supplies are adequate to prevent it.*[5]

Generally, starvation and famine as we have defined them here are "loud" emergency conditions that are most frequently characterized by extensive deaths that require fast interventions—or a cold, political calculation of nonintervention. Chronic hunger and its attendant malnutrition are "silent" emergencies found among impoverished people globally that seldom attract urgent intervention. Starvation and famine are generally more confined and concentrated than endemic undernutrition, chronic hunger, and malnutrition. Chronic hunger and malnutrition leave the poor vulnerable to cataclysmic events such as drought, flood, insect infestation, or conflict that may "tip" them over into starvation and famine. Thus, starvation and famine may be the manifestation of long-term, slow-acting systemic conditions.

Some Analytical Tools

We now add some tools to help us determine the fundamental cause(s) of a starvation or famine and other factors that may accelerate it (acting as catalysts, if you will). We break these into what we call the principal or *predisposing causes* and the *catalytic triggers*. Once we determine whether or not starvation or famine is occurring, we can use the following to help understand and perhaps focus the point of our response.

Predisposing Causes of Starvation or Famine

What are the *underlying causes* of a particular starvation or famine? Seeking the answer brings the famine theories discussed below into use. One may argue that the predisposing causes of starvation or famine are Malthusian "acts of God," or the result of accelerating population growth overtaking food production. Or, if one accepts Sen's argument, then perhaps starvation is caused by poverty and vulnerability, or a "loss of entitlements."

In general after consulting the various theories of famine, we sometimes need to merge Malthus and Sen. Both contribute to our understanding. Overall we suggest that poverty is the predisposing cause of starvation and famine, rather than either the clash of overpopulation or collapsing food production. We agree that expanding population is an important element, however, especially in those cases where it is destroying arable land (by requiring it for actual human habitation, for instance) or creating a nutritional crisis (with, for example, increasing food demands). We find that at the household level poverty creates vulnerability that, in turn, makes it possible for catalytic triggers to create sudden catastrophes shifting hunger into a starvation or even a famine. This is, basically, Sen's theory.

Catalytic Causes of Starvation or Famine

These are the immediate agents or triggers that tip vulnerable people over into starvation. They are not always the same, and they sometimes act together. Some examples of these triggers are:

Weak or corrupt governments. Government policies, deliberate or not, such as low prices paid to farmers or delayed payment for farm production, may cause food shortages, malnutrition, and hunger. Governments may also deliberately starve people, as was the case with Stalin in the Ukraine in 1933 and Robert Mugabe in Zimbabwe between 2001 and 2009. National leaders have also shown indifference to feeding people in regions that have opposed them; for example, Haile Selassie and the people of Wollo and Tigre provinces in Ethiopia in 1972–1974. Sometimes national governments ignore starvation in parts of their country for economic (India's Rajasthan state, 2001) or political reasons (China, 1958–1960). From whatever perspective, "bad government" can cause hunger, malnutrition, and even starvation.

War or civil conflict. As we detail in chapter 9, conflict and violence disrupt civil society and are major catalysts to severe food shortages and starvation or famine. Conflict prevents agricultural planning, the planting of crops and their harvest; it disrupts community markets and increases the cost of food. Armies also steal food, plant mines in agricultural areas, deliberately destroy crops and water systems, and kidnap or draft farm laborers as recruits.

Weather: drought or flooding. Prolonged wet or dry weather is a continuing catalyst to food shortages and starvation, especially in rural areas. Ireland in 1816, and again in 1843–1846; the Sahel region of sub-Saharan Africa and the Horn in 1973–1974; Ethiopia in 1984–1986; southern Africa in 2000–2002; India in 2001–2002 offer examples of severe drought or flooding that caused widespread episodes of starvation. The former executive director of the WFP,

James T. Morris, said in 2002 that he identified four "triggers" to the food crisis then spreading across the globe: conflict, AIDS, "collapsing economic systems," and climate. "[Weather is] the largest threat we face," he said. "The scale of WFP's activities has tracked closely with the occurrence of abnormal weather phenomena."[6] Other forces of nature include *Phytophthora infestans*, the fungus that attacked Ireland's potato crop in the 1840s, insect infestations (locusts), rampaging animals such as elephants or hippos, and large flocks of migrating birds. The Red-billed Quelea, for example, travels in flocks of several thousand birds or more and is notorious for destroying food crops in southern Africa.

Single-crop agriculture. Dependency on a single crop creates risks for poor farmers. The destruction of that primary crop—the potato in Ireland, maize in much of sub-Saharan Africa—leaves them without resources to avoid food shortages and prolonged hunger. In Malawi, as we will discuss in chapter 6, the government assured donors that peasant farmers could (and would) switch from dependence on one crop, maize, to another, cassava. This delayed emergency food responses and, because the shift to cassava did not occur, accelerated the country's starvation.

HIV/AIDS. The AIDS pandemic has caused severe disruption of rural farming practices. It is also generating a quiet "nutritional crisis" among farming families in developing states. Of the number of people globally who are HIV positive, 95 percent live in developing countries, and almost two-thirds of that number live in sub-Saharan Africa. About 80 percent of Africans are employed in some form of agriculture,[7] and AIDS and its attendant diseases are decimating rural agricultural workers. Many farms in sub-Saharan Africa and elsewhere are faced with a decreasing (or ill and dying) labor force and are being run by the old and the very young. To survive, these farmers are shifting from staple crops like maize, which is labor-intensive, to root tubers like cassava, which take little labor. There is a parallel loss of nutritional value between the two crops. This, in turn, creates a cycle of diminishing nutrition weakening already undernourished farm workers. As we shall see in chapter 4, diets high in carbohydrates but low in protein (such as one would see with a diet principally made up of cassava) carry a high risk of kwashiorkor—the form of malnutrition caused by primary protein deficiency.

Crowding. Many deaths during the Great Irish Famine occurred in the workhouses or on the "coffin ships" carrying Irish emigrants to North America. We therefore could add "crowding" as a catalytic factor and "cause" of death. People trying to escape starvation crowd into relief camps or other confined areas like makeshift clinics or shelters, where disease spreads rapidly. They are already severely malnourished and may be further weakened from walking long distances. In Ethiopia during 1974–1975 deaths occurred in the relief camps from cholera, typhoid, and dysentery. In addition, the nutrient composition of food in emergency settings has been questioned,[8] with some deaths resulting, although most recently emergency relief nutritionists have concentrated efforts on improving relief food composition and quality.[9]

Lack of Political Will. Over the centuries, private and state donors have been exceedingly generous in their food aid and financial backing to alleviate hunger, malnutrition, starvation, and famine. But the need continues to rise, and the recent global financial recession has made donors unable or unwilling to meet increasing demands for assistance. This has created what some observers call "donor fatigue." The WFP has been especially harsh about this. In 2002, the WFP noted an "unprecedented" crisis across Africa, with more than 38 million people facing starvation, and its executive director at that time said that the only obstacle to ending hunger tomorrow was "the lack of political will" by donors, agencies, and governments. Instead of earmarking funds to eliminate world hunger, he continued, "UN member states have unwittingly adopted policies that make the idea of ending hunger little more than fantasy." With donations to WFP falling, relief operations were also being reduced. Lack of donations for food aid in 2002 caused WFP to cut food for 10 to 14 million people in Ethiopia.[10] In 2003 North Korea needed 1.1 million metric tons (MT), but WFP could distribute less than 430,000 MTS—under 40 percent—because of "an unprecedented slump in donations."[11] (A metric ton, sometimes used as an international unit of weight, is 2204 pounds.) WFP's Morris said: "Hunger today is a creation of politics. And it demands political solutions. . . . Political decisions by some African governments—and by the governments of the developed world—have made it hard for the continent to feed itself."[12]

Proximate Causes of Death

People seldom die from "starvation." Chronic hunger, malnutrition, starvation, and famine weaken the human body, as we will detail, and make it susceptible to disease. This, coupled with unsafe drinking water and poor sanitation common among people suffering from inadequate nutrition, increases the likelihood and severity of opportunistic diseases, such as dysentery, measles, and cholera. In the Great Irish Famine, for example, "prevalent famine fevers" or "relapsing fever" (typhus and typhoid fever, among others) were frequently listed as the cause of a death precipitated by starvation. We review this fully in chapter 10.

Theories of Starvation and Famine

There are many theories about the basic causes and reasons for starvation and famine. These theories may be inexact, not well tested, or require explanation, but like the other tools presented here, they remain essential to policy formation. As the old saying goes: "Where you sit is where you stand," and if your agency or NGO (where you "sit") is formed around a Malthusian (or more likely, a neo-Malthusian) interpretation of starvation's causes, it (and you) will create and implement food relief policies based on Malthus's theory.

Events in the 1970s, as we discussed earlier, stimulated a new set of theories about starvation and famine. Jean Drèze, Amartya Sen, Stephen Devereux, Alexander de Waal, and others challenged the old Malthus-based theories and sought to identify the underlying causes as the result of impoverishment and vulnerability—what we call here *acts of man* rather than acts of nature or God.

For this book we have placed the leading theories about the causes of starvation and famine into two simple clusters. The first cluster, the *acts of God*, discusses Malthus's theory and food supply economics (supply side), also called *food availability decline* (FAD). The second cluster, the *acts of man*, details Sen's theory and food demand economics (demand side), or *food entitlement decline* (FED). Sen won the Nobel Prize in Economic Sciences in 1998 for his work on famine, human development, welfare economics, and poverty. His revolutionary analysis links starvation and famine not to outside forces but to poverty. "Starvation," he writes, "is the characteristic of some people not *having* enough food to eat. It is not the characteristic of there not *being* enough food to eat. While the latter can be a cause of the former, it is but one of many *possible* causes."[13] We ask: Are starvation or famine caused by acts of God—that is, acts of nature such as drought, floods, and so forth—or acts of humans—that is, leaders and governments deliberately or through incompetence starving some people, blocking the movement of food, having their armies lay siege to cities. (We are especially indebted here to the work of Stephen Devereux and his classic, *Theories of Famine.*[14])

The immediate causes of starvation and famine are, in fact, often nuanced. As we analyze the spectrum of suffering, from hunger through malnutrition to famine, we find ourselves incorporating parts of theories rather than choosing sides. We think about these problems inclusively, rather than exclusively. We find poverty and vulnerability (as referenced by Sen) compelling—but not to the complete exclusion of problems caused by excessive population growth (as advanced by Malthus). To do otherwise would, in a medical sense, "miss the diagnosis" and doom our "treatment" to failure.

Acts of God
Is starvation or famine an act of God or an act of human beings? Our investigation into this question starts in Europe as the late Middle Ages drew

to a close; chronic hunger was endemic and starvation and famine common. During the fourteenth and fifteenth centuries, following the Great Famine of 1315–1317, peasants could expect to experience at least one major famine during their lifetimes. Peasants in medieval Britain suffered ninety-five famines; those in France, at least seventy-five. This was seen—usually by those who did not encounter extreme hunger—as God's retribution for their sins ("hunger as punishment"). This was self-defining, of course, because they would not have been peasants if they had not sinned. If one believed that such agony was a form of justifiable punishment, then starvation would end only after prayer, repentance, forgiveness, and redemption. With this interpretation, hunger, starvation, and famine had nothing to do with poverty, corrupt governments, diseases, war, weather, or even greedy landlords. Hunger was simply God's punishment. The astute reader quickly notes the theory's underlying differentiation: those who hold power are blameless because they do not starve; those who are powerless bring starvation on themselves, and they alone must do something about it. Thus we have the creation of an impoverished and voiceless "bottom" for whom chronic hunger and starvation were (and are still) seen as a permanent, even deserved, condition.

As mentioned, and worth reviewing, in 1798 the Rev. Thomas Malthus detailed his theory in *An Essay on the Principle of Population*. The Malthusian theory—and its modern-day neo-Malthusian variations—took for granted that starvation and famine were (and are) natural checks on human overbreeding. Malthus argued that Europe's people were reproducing too quickly and that as a population increases exponentially (that is, 1, 2, 4, 8, 16, etc.), it outgrows (and out-eats) the food supply, which can increase only arithmetically (1, 2, 3, 4, 5, etc.). Therefore, when the size of the population outstrips the capacity of the land to support it, famine inevitably follows.

Europe, Malthus argued, was facing wide-scale starvation and famine as its populations continued to expand rapidly while its agriculture was restricted by limited arable land, simple farming techniques, and poor food distribution. Only when starvation-caused deaths reduced a population to the size that its agriculture could support would famine end. This "positive check" brought a populace back into balance with their food supply. Human suffering, although regrettable, was thus inevitable and natural, caused by careless human overbreeding. The consequences of such overbreeding were part of God's scheme of things. After all, starvation and suffering conveniently struck only those without power or voice, of inferior rank and visage. It was justification of God's will that "peasants always starve."

Malthus, and other proponents, could marshal Scripture in support of their position. Did not God send forth three kinds of punishment for our sins: famine, war, and pestilence? The Bible contains many stories of His hurling "the evil arrows of famine" (Ezekiel 5:16) as a penalty for sin and disobedience. Solomon, at the dedication of the Temple, warned of drought "when heaven is shut up, and there is no rain, because they have sinned against thee." (I Kings 8:35). And was not God's greatest punishment during famine to cause the starving to eat their own children? It was seen as a warning to others: if you disobeyed God's commandments ". . . [T]hen I will walk contrary unto you also in fury; and I, even I, will chastise you seven times for your sins. And ye shall eat the flesh of your sons, and the flesh of your daughters shall ye eat" (Leviticus 26:27–29; see also Deuteronomy 28:53–57). Thus during hungers and starvation devout Christians were admonished by their clergy and governments to repent and pray for forgiveness; in a clever turn, and with astonishing arrogance, those who had plenty even recommended that the starving fast.

Therefore, the "acts of God" position blames starvation and famine on a weakened (and sinful) population outgrowing its food supply and thus becoming vulnerable to natural events such as floods, drought, earthquakes, insect infestations. It does not blame "social, political, and economic issues."[15] Malthusian (and neo-Malthusian) theories have remained central principles of starvation and famine analysis to this date. The basic theory has dominated the responses of food donors and agencies to persistent hunger, starvation, and famine. It has shaped the core of the modern politics of starvation. A Malthusian analysis of the Great Irish Famine, for example, allowed the English (and some wealthy Irish), who were mostly Protestants, to declare that rapid population growth among the Irish peasants, who were Catholics, was outstripping their food supply. When the potato, the peasant staple food, was destroyed by blight, starvation followed. The Irish Famine was therefore viewed as a "positive check" on the excesses of that recklessly breeding population.

In 1936, during the Great Depression, John Maynard Keynes revived Malthus's theory of overproduction (glut) balanced by forces of nature (or God) and moved it into the modern economic theoretical study of supply and demand. Keynes's equation was based on consumer demand (for food, in this instance) and the lack of buying power (poverty). Malthus's work, therefore, became the basis for a "supply side" theory of modern starvation/famine and the policy of emergency food assistance. In general *supply-side theories* concentrate on the precipitating factors ("acts of God") that cause sudden or temporal collapses of food availability. (Therefore, this may also be called *food availability decline* or FAD, discussed below.) That is, starvation occurs when there is a decline in food availability to a level below a population's ability to obtain food and survive.

Food Availability Decline

This neo-Malthusian, supply-side argument is based on the *availability* or *supply* of food. FAD proposes that starvation and famine are caused by sudden collapses in food availability, perhaps the result of drought, floods, insects, war or civil conflicts, or sudden disease outbreaks that disrupt food production and distribution. FAD theory has dominated famine analysis and relief policies since Malthus's time and is closely associated with current food policy and famine management. It has formed the basis of relief aid responses since the early twentieth century. Yet Devereux, de Waal, and Sen among others have identified several weaknesses in this theory.

FAD is focused on supply, but market demand can rise sharply over time creating shortages even when food availability is constant or rising.[16] A more robust theory must explain why food does not come from elsewhere to those who are facing starvation, in the form of trade perhaps or redistribution within a country or region. FAD also does not differentiate an unequal distribution of food—that is, who cannot access food and who can. It does not explain why some groups of people have better access to food than others. "No famine affects all members of a population identically."[17]

Today, as we have discussed, starvation in one region of a country can often be offset by food distributed from another. Indeed, Sen writes, where modern famines have occurred there has been adequate food available elsewhere in the same country. FAD does not distinguish between people who are vulnerable to disruptions of food production and those who are not. "Drought causes crop failure," Devereaux writes, "but *vulnerability* to drought causes famine."[18] Further, as Sen also argues, starvation and famine do not occur in modern, wealthy democracies. Why? There is more government accountability, freer movement of surplus food, wide exchange of information about shortages and supplies, and the resilience to prevent or deflect catalytic causes such as floods, drought, conflict, and others. "It follows that the most damning criticism of FAD theory is that it diverts attention from possibly the most salient fact of all—that famine is first and foremost a problem of poverty and inequality."[19]

Yet the Malthusian theory and FAD still form the basis for much of our policy thinking today. Although few argue that starvation is punishment for sins or a natural check on population growth, policy is formed around the idea of *response* to starvation rather than *treatment* of underlying causes. But are natural disasters, bad luck, corrupt governments, conflict, or population growth the fundamental *causes* of starvation? Can any starvation or famine be blamed on forces outside human influence? In developing states why do peasants experience chronic hunger and starvation, but not government officials, the military, clergy, or landlords (among others)?

Acts of Man

By contrast, the *acts of man* theory (alternatively demand-side theory) argues that starvation and famine are consequences of human activity (or inactivity; nonaction) that can be prevented by modifying economic and political interventions. This may be the result of actions by people for which they are answerable and which they can prevent or alter. Climate, environmental factors, population growth, disease, and so forth do indeed play a catalytic role. But few recorded famines have not been caused by human influence. Three reasons support this view:

1. "There are very few famines in which the rich have starved."[20] If this is the case, we then need to focus on why the poor but not the rich suffer from hunger, starvation, and famine and their attendant diseases.

2. Devereux, Sen, and others argue that almost all twentieth-century famines could have been averted by moving food from somewhere else, often within the same country.

3. There is a close correlation between poverty and starvation (or famine), which have been alleviated in all but the poorest and most unstable countries, "irrespective of their susceptibility" to natural calamities.[21]

For example, the United States, Canada, and Australia all experienced droughts and flooding during the first decade of the twenty-first century, but they endured no ensuing starvations or famines. The Middle East and the Sahel of West Africa receive little rainfall, but widespread starvation and famine are unknown in modern-day Israel and that part of the Arab world. "Famine," writes Devereux, "must be seen as a problem of mal-distribution and disrupted access to food, rather than one of inadequate food production and availability."[22]

Sen created a significant shift in our thinking about starvation and famine. His contribution forces us to look more closely not at the supply side (food availability), but at the demand side (food entitlement) as the fundamental cause of hunger, starvation, and famine. *Demand-side theories* attempt to explain the roles of impoverishment and vulnerability. These theories, discussed below, argue that people do not have enough money to purchase food. That is, poverty is the underlying cause that makes people vulnerable to events that cause chronic hunger, starvation, and famine. This may also be called *food entitlement decline* or FED. Here is another lesson from the Great Irish Famine (that will be discussed more fully later): the Irish peasants starved not merely because of the blight on their staple food, the potato, although that indeed was a factor, but primarily because of their unemployment and poverty; they could not afford to buy food available in their own markets.

Food Entitlement Decline

The famines of the 1970s challenged the idea of a supply-side theory. In some countries, food was being sold in local markets while residents of those villages and regions were destitute and starving. Thus a demand-side theory was put forward to explain the causes of chronic hunger and starvation. This argument is simple: people do not have enough money or *entitlements* (assets such as livestock or household goods) to access food. Poverty and vulnerability combine to cause starvation or famine.

"Famine, a sort-term phenomenon, is inescapably linked to persistent long-term poverty," the Independent Commission on International Humanitarian Issues (ICIHI) concluded in its famine report. "Rich people don't starve. The idea of famines wiping out entire societies, as though the consequence of bad weather were meted out in equal measure to all, is far-fetched. . . . Even in famines there is always some food. Who ever has seen a starving military officer or merchant, let alone an aid worker? It is a question of who has access to that food."[23] Sen, in agreement, writes: "There is, indeed, no such thing as an apolitical food problem."[24] To understand the causes of starvation and famine, he argues, one needs to look at "entitlements."

The core of Sen's argument is simply that people starve because they have insufficient income or accumulated assets (that is, wealth), which leaves them with few choices for acquiring food in times of shortage. Mortality may occur when those "entitlements" collapse (crops fail, livestock die), thus creating starvation, or when "exchange entitlements" shift unfavorably (food prices rise, wages or asset prices fall). Basically, Sen writes, "people starve because (1) they have insufficient real income and wealth *and* (2) because there are no other means to acquire food."[25]

Sen's refocusing of starvation and famine theory offers an analytical framework for more effective famine anticipation, prevention, and relief interventions. For one, it directs policy maker's attention from conventional supply-side analysis of food crises toward an analysis of demand failure. Another strength of the food entitlement decline (FED) or entitlement theory is that while food availability can only define the *regions* affected by famine, food demand analysis helps policy makers identify the affected *classes*. Famine relief measures can then be targeted to those most needing aid. But, Sen warns, "Moving food into famine areas will not in itself do much to cure starvation, since what needs to be created is food entitlement and not just food availability."[26] This might be done by "generating entitlements" through the distribution of free food assistance to those who are starving, or by the setting up of employment or food-for-work programs. This, however, does not always reach highly vulnerable people like the elderly, disabled, or children.

As with FAD theory, there are also flaws in Sen's entitlement theory and FED. For one, FED does not explain "excess deaths that are *not* related to starvation, such as epidemics caused by concentrations of displaced people in unsanitary refugee camps."[27] Further, the disruptive effects of war can upset entitlement responses and policy. So, too, can looting and theft ("extra-entitlement transfers")[28] or a shifting disease environment.[29] The theory also assumes that starving people will consume as much food as they can obtain. But in fact some people facing severe food shortages select basic needs (shelter, clothing, medicine, and fuel) over food; thus, they may see gradual starvation as an acceptable solution. Also, as chapter 6 details, the *rationing* of food supplies is an initial and widespread coping strategy by people facing increasing shortages. The human instinct is toward self-preservation, at whatever other costs.[30] Finally, FED overlooks *extended entitlements* at the intrahousehold level. An infant, for example, has no labor to produce food and no assets to exchange for food. How does it survive? To what relief food does an infant have a "right"?

Sen's defense against these criticisms might be that FED does not offer a broad theory of famine "but aims only to provide a coherent framework for famine analysis."[31] The theory identifies a general cause of famine: "that a famine reflects widespread failure of entitlements on the part of substantial sections of the population." His theory and its subsequent variations have been labeled as insensitive to the historical famine record, apolitical, too economic, too static, and, finally, far too broad for practical application. It is, dissenters say, so limited that it is a tautology, "an elegant, academic way of saying nothing more than 'people starve because they cannot buy enough food.'"[32]

But Sen's theory has turned starvation and famine analysis and response upside down. The simplicity of his argument is challenging. If people starve because they lack real income and wealth and because they have no other means to acquire food, then starvation and famine will never be alleviated by emergency food or even long-term development aid. That can only end with the alleviation of poverty. And that will require a very different set of sacrifices and policy responses from the people of the wealthy nations of the world.

Lessons from the Great Irish Famine [1845–1850]
The Causes of Starvation

The Great Irish Famine, as it is often called, is so deeply imbedded in Irish history—and that of North America—that extensive research into it and the resulting debates and controversies continue today. Entire university departments, centers, and institutes are devoted to its study. The result is a variety of interpretations and analyses. There are the traditional Irish nationalist accounts; the Marxist, Sen, and Malthusian readings; the imperialist, feminist, anti-English, and even the anti-Catholic versions. Not surprisingly, debate about some important and unanswered questions persists: What were the principal predisposing causes of the Famine? Those who study the events in Ireland between 1845 and 1850 (and beyond) disagree about what triggered a nationwide starvation that by 1846 was killing widely across a weakened and impoverished Irish population. Was the Great Famine simply "a tragic ecological accident" or "Ireland's destiny"? Or were the Irish "desperately unlucky"?[1]

Was this indeed a famine? Our definition appears to fit these circumstances: long-term suffering from chronic hunger collapsing into starvation (food shortages and intensity) in a specific geographic area (scale) and resulting in large numbers of dead (the endpoint). Moreover, the Great Irish Famine fits Scrimshaw's additional definition, that famine is "also an economic and social phenomenon that can occur *when food supplies are adequate to prevent it*."[2]

History provides many examples of famines that took more lives than the Great Irish Famine. In the twentieth century alone there was starvation in Ukraine (1932–1933; 9–13 million dead), Bengal, India (1943–1944; 3–10 million), China (1959–1960; perhaps as many as 25 million).[3] Estimates for Ireland from 1845 to 1850, by comparison, range between 500,000 and 2 million Irish dead from starvation-related causes. Yet, "the Great Hunger," as it is also called, has gained a broader and more lasting fame than many other famines, perhaps because millions of Irish fled it to Europe and North America, creating a vibrant diaspora. By 1855, for example, more than one in every four people in New York City was Irish, and the Irish soon made up almost half (44.5 percent) of all immigrants living in that city.[4] "The disaster," two historians write, "which saw the destruction of one Ireland helped to create another Ireland which was not confined within the shores of one small island, for the North American Irish in particular were destined to make a remarkable contribution to the shaping of modern Irish history."[5] The Great Irish Famine became a legendary backdrop for songs, plays, films, and books that even today re-awaken strong feelings among a vast scattering of Irish across Canada and the United States. More than a dozen U.S. states now include the Great Irish Famine in their high school curricula. Montreal's flag still has a shamrock in one corner. On March 17 (St. Patrick's Day) at least seven countries celebrate the Irish among them, including Montserrat, South Korea, and Japan. On this day, many of the people of North America identify themselves as Irish-American: at least twenty-three U.S. and Canadian cities hold St. Patrick's Day parades, Celtic fests, and Irish fiddle contests; some even illuminate buildings with green lights and images of leprechauns.[6]

The Irish Famine also remains a popular case study of Malthusian theory. The Famine is cited as an example of the price paid by the Irish poor for their high rate of reproduction and large families, and, not incidentally, for their Catholicism. (Malthus, after all, was a parish priest in the Church of England.) More recently, however, Amartya Sen (and others) redirected our analysis of the underlying causes of this famine to the poverty of the Irish peasants and their inability to access food available in the markets around them.

The Great Irish Famine further serves as a central support beam in the construction of the nationalist version of Irish history. It is seen, and taught, as "the historical wrong that sealed the fate of the unhappy Union between Britain and Ireland: a partner so uncaring in time of need deserved no loyalty from Irishmen."[7] The Famine continues to shore up the anti-English version of this history: "The Almighty sent the potato blight, but the English created the Famine."[8]

The Irish Famine is also presented as a symbol of the indifference of free-market or *laissez-faire* economics, as then practiced in Europe, to human suffering. It serves as a reminder of the miserly dispersion of benefits from the Industrial Revolution. Since 1801 and through the Famine years, Ireland was a full member of the United Kingdom, with London as its capital. Yet despite daily accounts of starvation under way in nearby Ireland, large sums of money continued being spent in London on the Great Exhibition of 1851, with its elaborate Crystal Palace and its abundance of celebrations.[9]

Analysis of the guiding economic theory of *laissez-faire* as it was applied to Ireland in 1845–1850 gives us a historical reference point in the tension that continues to this day between anti-interventionist and humanitarian responses toward those who starve. Although it is not the goal here to engage in popular debates about the Great Irish Famine, it is nonetheless insightful to hold it up as a distant mirror reflecting on more recent misfortune. The Famine reminds us that even today economic theory drives relief policies with regard to hunger and starvation. Whereas the Irish peasant suffered from the *laissez-faire* economic policy of mid-nineteenth century England, free-market economic theory is thought to have caused hunger and food shortages more recently in sub-Saharan Africa, and particularly the starvation that rose inside Malawi in 2001–2002 and again in Niger and Mali in 2005 (discussed in detail in chapter 7).

Predisposing and Catalytic Causes

Several authors refer to the Irish Famine as "the last famine in Europe." Starvations and famines had essentially disappeared from England by 1600, although during the 1840s starvation visited Ireland and the Scottish Highlands, both as the result of the potato blight.[10] Why did this famine occur? What were the fundamental predisposing causes of the Irish starvation? What catalytic causes may have tipped the Irish poor into the Famine?

Like modern twentieth-century starvations in Africa, India, China, and elsewhere, the Great Irish Famine erupted out of a prolonged, intractable silent emergency. Smaller starvations among segments of the Irish population had been recorded in the late eighteenth and early nineteenth centuries. But chronic hunger, malnutrition, and disease were spreading across an expanding, impoverished Irish peasantry, making them increasingly vulnerable to a catalytic event. There is some agreement about what may have precipitated the Great Famine: the ownership and control of Ireland's arable land, the failing structure of the Irish economy causing extensive poverty among the Irish peasantry, profound shifts in the Irish population from births and emigration, the increased dependency of the Irish peasant diet on the potato, and then its blight. Interpretation of these events, however, quickly divides into two broad and opposing camps: the nationalist, who say that the British government "deliberately used the pretext of the failure of the potato crop to reduce the Celtic population by famine and exile," and those less willing to see conspiracy, but who blame the social and economic systems imposed on Ireland by the British government.[11]

A less nuanced, but equally vociferous, dichotomy occurs over the predisposing causes between those who argue that the Great Irish Famine was the result of a food availability decline (FAD) or a food entitlement decline (FED). The FAD (Malthus or supply-side) advocates point to the rising Irish population and their dependency on the potato for income and sustenance. They see the starvation as the inevitable outcome when the potato blight—the "positive check"—caused a shortfall in this food staple by some 12–15 million tons annually, which in turn triggered starvation. The FED (Sen or demand-side) advocates put forth the poverty of the Irish peasant as the underlying predisposing cause. The Irish economy was heavily dependent on agriculture, which after the Napoleonic Wars increased production of grains for export and grew potatoes for food. With commercialization of farming, the Irish peasantry became increasingly landless. When the economy faltered, farmers and peasant laborers lost work. Incomes fell, the blight destroyed the potato crop, food prices jumped beyond the reach of millions of peasants. Unable to grow other crops and without income, the Irish peasants starved. The FED side argues, therefore, that the dependency of the Irish peasantry on a single crop, "the primitive state of Irish agriculture and the bad relations between landlord and tenant were but different expressions of the same evil, poverty."[12]

Both sides agree that as many as 3 million Irish emigrated out of the country between 1845 and 1860, many to North America, and that perhaps as many as 2 million of those who remained died from the effects of starvation. Ireland did not recover from these economic and social losses until well into the twentieth century.

We examine here three possible predisposing causes of the Great Irish Famine. We believe they are the fundamental and underlying reasons the starvation occurred. Two of them—population and poverty—meet our criteria as principal or predisposing causes. The third, *laissez-faire* economics, falls on the margins of our definition but was such a seminal force that it requires inclusion here. We also argue that all three are similar—and in some instances, identical—to the principal causes of modern starvation in developing states today. We frame the analysis around discussion of the Irish population, economy, and politics before and during the Great Famine.

Population
Population numbers in Ireland (and elsewhere) during the mid-1800s must be considered more descriptive than definitive; nineteenth-century census-taking was a flawed process. Yet the Irish population figures form an important part of FAD analysis. Cormac Ó Gráda tells us that the Irish population quadrupled between 1780 and 1845, from 2 million to 8.2 million on the eve of the Famine. It appears that the pre-Famine population growth rate, in five important locations where starvation was severe, reached about 2.1 percent a year, with a doubling rate of thirty-three years. Just before the Famine struck there were some 700 people per square mile of arable land—the highest density in all of Europe. This rapid population growth and density were not slowed by earlier starvations that occurred in 1800–1801 and again in 1816–1819.[13]

It is thought that expansion of the Irish population came from increasing dependence on the potato, which was easy to grow, nutritious, with a high yield per acre. As Mary Daly, the Irish scholar, writes, "By ensuring good health the potato may have increased the Irish birth rate and reduced mortality levels."[14] In addition the dietary dependency on the potato *alone* may have triggered starvation. This dependence on a single crop, as we shall also see in our discussion of Africa's starvations, made the impoverished Irish peasant vulnerable. When the blight struck, the peasants and laborers had neither the money (entitlements) nor the opportunity to purchase food elsewhere. Would the Irish have starved if the potato had not succumbed to blight? Probably not. But when the potato crop did fail—in three consecutive harvests—millions of Irish were too poor to purchase food, and they did indeed starve.

Population growth, however, is clouded somewhat by the argument that emigration "depressed the Irish population" between 1815 through 1845, when some 1.5 million Irish people left the island. This accelerated in 1845 and 1846 when the Poor Law Extension Act, which made landlords responsible for the maintenance of their own poor, pushed some to clear their estates by paying for the emigration of their tenants. A few landlords did so for humanitarian reasons, but others simply evicted the poor because they could then consolidate their holdings and shift cultivation to cash crops for export.

During the four years of the Famine (1845–1850), 571,704 Irish emigrated to the United States alone. Another 1,174,251 left Ireland and joined them during the next decade (1850–1860).[15] So profound was this flow of refugees that the Irish made up about one-third of all voluntary trans-Atlantic passengers.[16] The voyage was difficult: thousands died on the "coffin ships"—so named because of the way people were packed into them—crossing the Atlantic. In 1847 alone there were 17,465 documented deaths among the Irish at sea. Ranelagh writes "This chaotic, panic-stricken and unregulated exodus was the single largest population movement of the nineteenth century."[17]

Who was left behind? Many of those who could not afford food during the Famine also lacked funds to emigrate. The fare to North America—plus food for three or more months at sea—equaled about a year's wages for a laborer.[18] Those who could emigrate from Ireland, therefore, were the healthier and better off; those who remained were predominately the poor and unemployed, malnourished and weakened by illness and disease. This further deprived Ireland and its agriculture of reliable and healthy human capital and left behind a peasantry caught in a poverty trap inside the country.

Poverty

Poverty made the Irish peasant vulnerable to price fluctuations. As prices for food rose rapidly in 1845 and 1846, and the potato crop again failed across the country, poverty's effect was to separate the Irish peasants into two identifiable groups: those who could purchase food and/or leave the island, and those who could not.

How did the Irish become that poor? First, there was the segregation of the Irish Catholics by English law: the Penal Laws, The Statutes of Kilkenny. These laws of separation were not unlike the twentieth century colonial-era laws in sub-Saharan Africa that separated blacks and whites, reserving the best land for white minority farmers. The Statutes of Kilkenny read like the *apartheid* regulations in pre-1994 South Africa or the Land Apportionment Act of 1930 in Southern Rhodesia (today's Zimbabwe), both of which divided land unequally, with whites getting the more arable acreage and blacks the most marginal, thereby creating an impoverished majority. In pre-Famine Ireland, the result was similar: the entrapment of the Irish peasant worker and family and the restriction of the Irish peasants to less-arable farmland left them with few, if any, reliable economic opportunities. As a result of these and other laws, one-third of Ireland's landholders held two-thirds of all arable land.

On the eve of the Great Famine, therefore, wealth was concentrated among those who not only controlled the most fertile farming areas but also ruled with great power over their tenants. With the "evictions," a large and land-less class of itinerant Irish peasants, perhaps two million, wandered about the country looking for work. These were the "essentially poor."[19] Their profile is not unlike today's bottom billion. They annually struggled through *summer hunger*—the potato gap between the old and new crops that lasted from mid-May through September, a time of hunger and even malnutrition. Anything that caused a poor harvest drew down their resources and created a shortage that carried over into the next year and pushed these Irish peasants into starvation. They formed "a hidden Ireland," not unlike today's global poor or "the other America" of rural and inner-city United States, who suffer from hunger and poverty. "[T]here is no denying the gradual decline in the living standards of the [Irish] poor, the bottom half or so of the population before 1845," writes Ó Gráda.[20] "The poor were wretchedly housed—two-thirds of the entire population huddled into sparsely furnished, tiny mud cottages or their urban equivalents—and [were] poorly clothed, and often hungry for two or three months of every year." Others lived in "fourth-class" dwellings, mud cabins having only one room.[21] When falling wages and rising prices occurred as a result of the potato blight, these Irish were unable to absorb the shock.[22] Those few Irish with income or skills—"entitlements"—could buy food and/or emigrate. Those who lacked money, skills, or other resources were locked into a poverty trap—unable to work, buy food, or leave. Thus, several million Irish fell to the bottom of the economy. They bore the full weight of the Famine.

Malthus's argument of 1798, when applied to the Irish Famine forty-seven years later, played well in London, where anti-Irish sentiment was high. The Irish were often referred to as ignorant, primitive, and sketched in London newspaper cartoons with simian features. To the Malthusians in England, the Great Famine was part of God's plan for humankind, or at least that part of humanity who were Irish. The prevailing view was that there was little or nothing that could (or should) be done to prevent or avert starvation. It was viewed as a "positive check" to bring a sinful population, often depicted as subhuman, back into balance with its food supply. Their suffering, while regrettable, was considered inevitable and natural.

Laissez-faire *Economics*

No famine stands in isolation: the starvation in Ireland rose out of decades of agrarian inequities between tenant and landlord. By 1847, calls for tenant rights were louder than demands for the repeal of the Act of Union with Great Britain. The Great Famine emerged also from the fact that about 66 percent of the Irish population depended entirely on agriculture. Moreover they struggled on small individual plots; almost half of all farms in Ireland at the time of the Famine were less than five acres.[23] "The buoyancy of the British economy" was nowhere to be found in the Irish countryside, and 5.5 million Irish peasants (in a population of 8.2 million) were smallholders, often seasonally unemployed or landless, and trapped by single-crop agriculture. They were "doomed to spend their lives in very great poverty."[24]

The dominant economic theory of mid-nineteenth century Britain was based on the concept of *laissez-faire*. This theory held that it was not the task of government to provide aid for its citizens or to intervene with the free market movement of goods and trade. One might argue that this economic philosophy was a predisposing cause of the Great Irish Famine, but we suggest that this popular economic theory of the time served more as a trigger to Ireland's famine. We test this simply by asking: Did landowners, government officials, or even landed peasants starve under this economic policy? If not, then the fundamental difference was the *poverty* of the Irish peasant, the principal cause of the Great Famine. The *laissez-faire* economic policy of the time was a catalyst that made poverty worse and prevented alleviation of the starvation.

Despite this policy, the initial response in 1845 of the British government under Prime Minister Sir Robert Peel was "prompt, efficient and interventionist."[25] The Prime Minister sent over a Scientific Commission to examine Ireland, which reported that half the Irish potato crop was destroyed, or unfit for use, and correctly identified the cause of the crop's failure as the blight. Against advice from his own treasury ministry, Prime Minister Peel engaged a merchant house in November 1845 to purchase £100,000 of Indian corn and meal from the United States—enough to feed 1 million people for more than a month. "A buffer stock was built without fuss or publicity."[26] At the same time, Peel was convinced that only "the removal of all impediments to the import of all kinds of human food" would disperse the threat of famine in Ireland. One of those impediments was the Corn Laws, which erected a trade barrier around the United Kingdom—of which Ireland was a member—preventing importation of corn even for emergency purposes. Peel's position was difficult: he was head of the Conservative Party, which supported the Protectionist policy and "he was aware that for him to propose repeal [of the Corn Laws] would be considered gross and shameful treachery."[27] Ó Gráda writes "this dramatic reversal of a key Tory policy—the Corn Laws—led to his political downfall eight months later."[28]

Sir Robert Peel was forced to resign in June 1846, and Lord John Russell succeeded him as Prime Minister. Russell took office as more than 90 percent of the potato crop of Ireland failed for the second consecutive year. The winter of 1846–1847 became one of the worst in Irish history and marked "the true beginning of the Great Famine."[29] The second season of failure was unanticipated, despite the previous year's poor harvest, largely because potato acreage was at an all-time high in 1846. The average yield dropped to less than half a ton per acre, compared to 6–7 tons. Supply fell as demand rose, which ignited increases in prices. "Cups," a common type of potato, which sold at less than 2 shillings per hundredweight (or 50 kilos) on the Dublin market in October 1845, more than tripled to 7 shillings within the year. The price of the "lowly Lumper"—the peasant's potato—jumped from 16 pence to 6 shillings. The Irish laborer, already impoverished and hungry, slipped into starvation. "The average agricultural wage per day was now less than the cost of a poor man's food, making no allowance for those dependent on him. Famine loomed."[30]

As the new Prime Minister Lord Russell, like his predecessor, was also in a difficult role: he had pledged himself and his Whig Party to Corn Law repeal. He nevertheless made his approach to the Irish Famine very clear: "It must be thoroughly understood that we cannot feed the people . . . We can at best keep down prices where there is no regular market and prevent established dealers from raising prices much beyond the fair price with ordinary profits."[31] Most members of Parliament put their faith "in the market." Like some modern-day politicians, they also viewed public charity as a sign of weakness that ignored the "inevitability" of the outcome. Such aid would shift the distribution of food "from the more meritorious to the less," as *The Economist* wrote at the time, because "if left to the natural law of distribution, those who deserved more would obtain it."[32] By the winter of 1846–1847 the numbers of Irish dying from starvation "began to mount alarmingly."[33] Press coverage in London was extensive, but most favored the *laissez-faire* position. Matchstick figures of Irish scavengers and fully sketched reports of the dead and dying that appeared in the more liberal press such as the *Illustrated London News* did nothing to shift the British government's course. The Irish were abandoned to the vagaries of a free market and self-correcting pricing mechanism that, if left alone, its proponents promised, would match demand with supply. Ó Gráda writes that even today scholars see this as "Malthusian murder by the invisible hand."[34]

As mentioned earlier, perhaps as many as two-thirds of the Irish peasants[35] were wretchedly clothed and housed during the Great Famine, living in mud huts, malnourished, suffering "summer hunger" from May to September before the autumn potato harvest. There was sufficient food produced throughout the Famine to feed all of them, but it was exported in what Sen calls a "food 'counter-movement'" driven by prices and markets.

As prices for the peasant's staple potatoes started to rise—doubling in less than a year—the Irish grain crop was being exported to England. Cecil Woodham-Smith, the preeminent authority on the Irish Famine, wrote in *The Great Hunger: Ireland 1845–1849* that "no issue has provoked so much anger or so embittered relations between the two countries . . . as the indisputable fact that huge quantities of food were exported from Ireland to England throughout the period when the people of Ireland were dying of starvation."[36] By several accounts, the amounts were staggering:

○ In 1845, some 3,251,907 quarters (1 quarter = 8 bushels) of corn and 257,000 sheep were sold and shipped to Britain. In 1846–1850 another 3 million live animals left Ireland, and in 1847 (or "Black '47," as it was called) 822,609 gallons of butter went to England in the first nine months,[37] which totaled more than 1 million gallons of butter shipped from Ireland during the height of the Famine.

○ Alcohol exported from Ireland to England amounted to 874,170 gallons of porter, 278,658 gallons of Guinness, and 183,392 gallons of whiskey. In Black '47, the total amount was 1,336,220 gallons—almost all derived from food grains.[38]

Thus, despite the collapse of the potato crop, Ireland still produced grain crops in abundance—enough, some experts believe, to feed the entire starving population throughout the entire Famine. But while the potato was considered a "food crop," the grain crops were a "money crop" and therefore part of commerce and the free-market economy. Although there were calls for the exports to be stopped and for grain to be sent back to Ireland, this would have meant repealing the Corn Laws, which protected British grain traders and generated large profits for them. There was strong and powerful political opposition in England to reversing the Corn Laws, as former Prime Minister Peel had experienced. The British government relied instead on a balance of supply and demand controlled by market forces. Thus, grain crops would not be diverted, and throughout the five-year period of the Great Famine, Ireland remained a net exporter of food.[39] Even during the terrible winter of 1846–1847, as hundreds of thousands of Irish poor starved to death in frozen huts or along the roadsides, "Russell and his colleagues never conceived of interfering with the structure of the Irish economy in the ways that would have been necessary to prevent the worst effects of the famine."[40] As Sen points out, the shifting of food from those who were starving and poor to those who were well-fed and had money—the counter-movement—was seen not only in the Great Famine, but also later in Ethiopia 1973–1974 and in the Bangladesh famine of 1974.[41]

Can the Great Irish Famine be blamed on an anti-interventionist economic policy of the day? Some historians propose that the Famine was a problem of scale; for example, an embargo was placed on food exports during the smaller and shorter 1741 famine in Ireland, thus keeping grains inside the country, which alleviated the hunger. But 1845–1850 marked the first time that a British government had attempted to deal with such a huge and prolonged catastrophe as the Irish Famine. Thus encumbered by its own "hands-off" economic policy, it was ill-equipped to intervene had it wanted to do so.

Other historians propose that even had exports been halted, and food retained inside Ireland, perhaps as many as 3 million Irish poor would still not have been able to locate and purchase food. They were the poorest of the poor, at the bottom of Ireland's economy. *Laissez-faire* had been in place for decades before the Great Famine, and "free-trade policies gradually eroded the profitability" of rural-based agriculture in Ireland. Poverty and shortages of food were therefore already in place; "the removal of protective tariffs doomed kelping, fishing and textile production to failure" and thus denied the Irish laborer nonagricultural income. During the Famine, blind adherence to the *laissez-faire* economic policy merely continued an entrenched economic system that allowed exports of food, as well as "the failure of successful public intervention to relieve the starvation."[42] That said, it is an inescapable fact that "Nevertheless, the lack of generosity displayed by the Irish landlords and farmers, together with the rest of the United Kingdom, guaranteed the disastrous outcome."[43] Thus, the economics of *laissez-faire* and the free market can be said to have *assured* Irish poverty and starvation, but perhaps not to have been its principal "cause."

Finally, there was a *core-periphery disparity*. The Irish were poor, rural, far from London, and Catholic. They, like their counterparts today in developing countries, were also generally silent in their suffering. During earlier economic difficulties in the 1830s and 1840s, for example, "the poor in the industrial areas of England impressed themselves more vividly in the political consciousness than the rural poor, just as they did in China in the 1950s . . . and in Ethiopia in the 1970s," writes Liz Young, a geography professor at Staffordshire University, England.[44] It was easier to supply the urban centers of England, and they had a longer history of demand, which they "punctuated by riot" ignited by increasing bread prices, turnpike fees, "and a score of other grievances." Rioting mobs from Lancashire to Glascow and Dunfermline in Scotland quickly got London's attention and aid. The silent starving in Sligo and Skibbereen did not. "Industrial unrest in England," Young argues, "was potentially more revolutionary and more disturbing than dispersed unrest in Ireland."

What have we learned to this point from the Great Irish Famine? We argue that poverty, the result of population growth, land and tenancy restrictions, and dependency on a single staple food, characterized a "silent emergency" that spread among the mid-nineteenth-century Irish peasantry. We suggest here, and will discuss more fully later, that the imposition of *laissez-faire* and free market economic policies prevented substantial relief food aid from entering Ireland and continued drawing out grains and other foods for export. With successive failures of the potato crop, evictions, and loss of employment, those Irish who could not buy food or emigrate, starved.

How many died? In 1841 the population of Ireland was thought to be 8,175,124. This rather precise figure may nonetheless have been smaller than the actual number, given the general suspicion of government census takers by those being counted and the remoteness of parts of the Irish countryside. By 1851, after the worst of the Famine, the population was said to have fallen to 6,552,385. The Irish census commissioners calculated that given normal growth rates there should have been 9,018,799 people had the Famine not occurred. What happened to them?

We know that during the Famine years, 1845–1850, some 571,704 Irish arrived in the United States and another 257,354 landed in Canada, for a total of 829,058.[45] The number of Irish making the 120-mile trip across the Irish Sea to Liverpool, England, with the cheaper fare, shorter voyage, and possibility of easier return, might have matched that sailing to North America. Thus, perhaps 1.5 to 1.7 million Irish emigrated during those five years. Putting the census and emigration together, we estimate that another 800,000 to 1.5 million Irish men, women, and children may have died from starvation-related causes in the Great Irish Famine. Thus, the total losses from death and emigration may be estimated at about 2.5 million (2,466,414) people—a staggering drain on Ireland. Emigration out of Ireland continued for more than a century and produced an unanticipated benefit: it planted and nurtured a vast international dispersion of Irish culture and nationalism.

PART II

The Crisis
of Nutrition

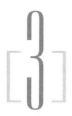

The Basics of Nutrition

Famine: Historical Background

In the preceding chapters we learned about some important statistics regarding the avoidable suffering and millions of preventable deaths associated with chronic malnutrition. Sister Brigid Corrigan, medical director of Pastoral Activities and Services for people with AIDS, Dar es Salaam Archdiocese (PASADA), has said that statistics are people with the tears washed away. One of the goals of this book is to continuously connect the politics, historical record, and current situation of chronic malnutrition and food insecurity directly back to the human conditions to which they relate. To do this one of the requirements is a basic understanding of ourselves as biological organisms, inextricably linked to our need for access to adequate nutrition to fuel our energy needs and provide the building blocks for our own bodies. In this chapter we review the basics of the source of the elements and energy of life and the basic biochemical principles of life. This will be the foundation we will need on which to build our understanding of the mechanisms of nutrition and the consequences of inadequate nutrition.

The history of humans has been marked by the constant pursuit for and attainment of reliable, adequate sources of nutrition. The prehistoric record shows ample evidence of the struggle for food, whether it is evidence in the fossil record of chronic inadequate nutrition,[1] competition between man and animals for the same food sources,[2] or indications of cannibalism.[3] The failure to find food also has its historic record: the first documentable written record we have of famine is found as a hieroglyphic inscription, perhaps from the Ptolemaic Dynasty (300–30 BCE) but felt to describe events at the time of the pharaoh Djoser circa 2600 BCE. This inscription was found on a black granite boulder—named the Stele of Famine—on the island of Sehel, north of the First Cataract of the Nile (and now just north of the Aswan Dam). It is remarkable not only in that it documents the presence of famine in our earliest history but also in the notable precision with which it describes the general picture and the very kind of human suffering we see with famine to this day.

I am mourning on my high throne for the vast misfortune, because the Nile flood in my time has not come for seven years! Light is the grain; there is a lack of crops and all kinds of food. Each man has become a thief to his neighbor. They desire to hasten and cannot walk. The child cries, the youth creeps along, and the old man despairs; their souls are lowered down, their legs are bent together and drag along the ground, and their hands rest in their bosoms. The council of the great ones in the court is but emptiness. Torn open are the chests of provision, but instead of contents there is air. Everything is exhausted.

The Bible is replete with references to famine including chapters of Genesis, Exodus, Ruth, 2 Samuel, 1 Kings, 2 Kings, 1 Chronicles, 2 Chronicles, Nehemiah, Job, Psalms, Isaiah, Jeremiah, Lamentations, Ezekiel, Amos, Matthew, Mark, Luke, Acts, Romans, and the Book of Revelation.[4] Ansel Keys, in his classic text, *The Biology of Human Starvation*,[5] lists 500 early famines but limits those to the British Isles, Northwestern Europe, and the Mediterranean Basin, as well as India—the famines of Africa and Asia are notably absent. There is no lack of evidence for frequent episodes of famine, either in the prehistoric archeological record or the record of recorded history, and the centrality of the pursuit (and control) of adequate and reliable sources of nutrition in human commerce is as true today as it ever was. In fact, we shall make the case in this book that this pursuit is first and foremost the driving force of human behavior—both for individuals as well as for political groups.

Famine: Scientific Study

Although we have the historical records of human famine, there is remarkably little scientific study of the biological processes involved in the progressive, relentless wasting away of the human body during prolonged chronic malnutrition and starvation. This is partially because most famines are observed externally and at a distance and partially because controlled experiments—that is, the purposeful starvation of one or more experimental subjects—would be considered unethical for obvious reasons. Much of the data we have available to us comes from observational studies conducted in the field and at the end of observed famines, many of which date from the period of World War II. They include chronic undernutrition and isolated starvation in Belgium between 1940 and 1944, the Warsaw Ghetto in 1942, the Siege of Leningrad in 1941–1942, Western Holland (the Dutch Winter Famine) from September 1944 through May 1945, and studies of the victims of Nazi concentration camps during 1945.[6]

Textbooks in biochemistry, physiology, and medicine have also used the results of individual trials of fasting (total starvation) in discussing the measurable results, but as Keys points out, there are fundamental differences between total starvation and prolonged semistarvation, the latter of which is the actual reality in essentially all famines. Among the many differences, Keys identifies those he considered elemental: in total fasting the sensation of hunger is essentially abolished after a few days, whereas that same sensation increases progressively in prolonged semistarvation; ketosis (to be discussed in chapter 4) results predictably in the fasting state but not in semistarvation; critical metabolic changes (in the example given by Keys, the edema associated with famine) are never reported in total starvation but are cardinal findings in semistarvation.

Some of the earliest studies of severe food shortages were carried out on the *hunger artists* or *starvation artists* popular in the late nineteenth and early twentieth centuries. These were people, almost all of them men, who isolated themselves and fasted for weeks, charging money for the public to view them. Perhaps the most famous of these was one Professor Agostino Levanzin, a gentleman who volunteered to fast under scientific observation at the Carnegie nutrition laboratory in Roxbury (Boston) and who ultimately claimed he had been "squeezed like a lemon and put out weak and starving" (and not paid).[7]

The most definitive, scientifically accurate studies available to date come from the Carnegie Nutrition Laboratory and the Minnesota Starvation Experiment. The Carnegie study, reported by the Director of the Carnegie Nutrition Laboratory in 1919,[8] was a prospective post–World War I examination of two groups of twelve healthy, normal male volunteers, all students at the International Young Men's Christian Association College in Springfield, Massachusetts. The study was limited in that the intent of it was more to demonstrate the adaptability of the normal human body to a restricted diet (and the safety of a low-protein diet during wartime for the purposes of rationing) as opposed to demonstrating the physiological and psychological effects of prolonged, severe semistarvation. As such, the experimental goal was to reduce the intake of calories in these normal subjects to achieve a 10-percent loss of baseline body weight—a level considered to be completely safe not only in terms of health but also the maintenance of full mental and physical functionality. A second limitation of the Carnegie experiment was that it did not include any study of the effects of dietary rehabilitation or safe refeeding—a critical part of any study on chronic undernutrition from the perspective of the medical community.

The Minnesota Starvation Experiment, directed by Dr. Ansel Keys and colleagues, took advantage of two important facts that coincided in 1944, the year the experiment was conducted. The first was that it became known that there was widespread severe, chronic undernutrition throughout all of occupied Europe, and that the subsequent liberation of these large populations would require knowledgeable dietary rehabilitation on a massive scale in order to mitigate mass famine-related deaths. Second, there was also a large cohort of potential volunteers for a prospective study of true semistarvation. These were the conscientious objectors who, although they were morally or religiously opposed to armed conflict during World War II, were nonetheless willing to subject themselves to substantial discomfort and risk of injury to contribute to scholarly and medical knowledge of starvation. The Minnesota experiment, by far the most definitive prospective study in human semistarvation, addressed the deficiencies of the Carnegie experiment in that the goal was aimed at analyzing the physiological and psychological effects of true semistarvation and included a critical evaluation of dietary rehabilitation methods. Although it included only thirty-six subjects, all healthy male volunteers (only thirty-two were included in the final report), it rigorously evaluated all metabolic, anthropometric, psychological, and behavioral aspects of a true semistarvation diet. This diet was constituted mainly of whole wheat bread, cereals, potatoes, turnips, and cabbage and was meant to reflect the diet of semistarvation experienced in Europe during the war. The Minnesota study diet averaged 1570 calories a day, only 50 grams of protein, and 30 grams of fat with little meat or dairy products. The goal for weight loss averaged 24 percent of the baseline body weight (19–28 percent depending on initial body weight and fat composition).

We discuss the specific details of the clinical manifestations of chronic undernutrition, both from a perspective of macronutrients as well as micronutrients, starting here and continuing in later chapters. There are, however, a few basic introductory points to be learned from these studies.

The reality of the process of starvation is that rarely does a food supply completely and abruptly disappear. There is almost always a prolonged period of caloric deficit resulting in semistarvation. Prolonged semistarvation has permanent, irreversible effects, especially in children, which include intellectual, psychological, and social handicaps that are just as devastating as the more obvious physical deficits, such as stunting of growth or physical deformity. In addition:

- Most individuals can tolerate a weight loss of 5 percent to 10 percent of body weight with little to no loss of functional ability.
- Severe famines are usually attended by loss of 15 percent to 35 percent of total body weight in the general population.
- Weight losses of 35 percent to 40 percent of body weight are invariably fatal.

With this history and the two studies for context, in this chapter we begin our scientific analysis of starvation with a brief review of the biochemistry of life in order to further our understanding of some of the consequences of inadequate nutrition that we consider in subsequent chapters. We ask: How does nutrition "work" in the human body? How does this help us to understand inadequate nutrition, or starvation? In order to answer these questions, first let us discuss the basics of life sciences in order that we can have a foundation to work through the more complex subjects relating to nutrition in biology in general, in normal human biology specifically, and in situations in which adequate nutrition becomes scarce or unavailable.

I believe a leaf of grass is no less than the journey-work of the stars . . .
—Walt Whitman[9]

We are star-stuff.
—Carl Sagan

Thus it is possible to say that you and your neighbor and I, each one of us and all of us, are truly and literally a little bit of stardust.
—William A. Fowler[10]

The above quotes can be inspirational when taken metaphorically (as Whitman undoubtedly intended), but they are no less inspirational when taken literally, as Sagan and Fowler intended. The vast majority of the "substance" of the universe is made up of elemental hydrogen and helium, and as Sagan has pointed out, the other elements can be considered impurities swimming about in these seas of hydrogen and helium. Compared to the stars, the planets have extremely low gravitational fields, so they rapidly lose their atmospheres of the lighter elements hydrogen and helium. What is left, the concentrated "impurities" that are generated by the stellar nuclear reactions, are the heavier elements that make up the bodies of the planets—and our bodies as well. Of these heavier elements, those that are most abundant include carbon, oxygen, nitrogen, and phosphorus. These, in addition to hydrogen, are the atomic building blocks of what we call life. We are, in every literal sense, the stuff of stars.

In addition to these elemental building blocks of life, the energy of life comes directly from the stars—in our case the sun. The current system of biological classification divides that life into three domains. The *Archea* or archaebacteria are in general primitive bacteria (from the Greek *archaea*: ancient or original ones). *Prokaryotes*, which are the majority of the more highly evolved bacteria, are still relatively simple, unicellular organisms without complex, intracellular structure. The *eukaryotes* have more complex cellular structure, including defined nuclei and organelles such as mitochondria, and include more advanced unicellular organisms as well as the multicellular plants and animals. There are some extremely interesting Archaea that can capture energy from geothermal sources and inorganic minerals. These *chemoautotrophs*, felt by some to have been the first life forms to have developed, can then introduce this energy into food chains otherwise isolated from other energy sources. Examples of isolated colonies of organisms dependent on such energy sources can be seen in the deep-sea geothermal vents discovered in 1977 by scientists from the Scripps Institute of Oceanography. Except for these rare and exotic exceptions, however, essentially all of the Earth's life energy is generated directly from the sun's energy by the biochemical process of photosynthesis. The organisms that can capture the sun's energy and transform it into the chemical energy of life are called *autotrophs*. All other organisms that depend on the autotrophs for their access to organic compounds and energy are called *heterotrophs*. Although bacteria, which have only about 1000–8000 genes,[11] are far less complex than humans (we have about 20,000–25,000 genes),[12] it bears mention here that the basic machinery used for running a cell is fundamentally the same! In fact, rates of conservancy of the protein sequences and functionality encoded by the genomes of such disparate organisms as Archea, prokaryotic bacteria, and eukaryotic organisms have been reported to be as high as 70 percent[13] (the point here being that, even if we compare ourselves to bacteria, at a very basic level we are more the same than we are different).

Taking these two broad concepts into account—that the physical matter and the energy of life come from the stars—we can go on to a more detailed understanding of how this all works.

The Energy of Life

We obtain energy from the sun through the process of photosynthesis (from the Greek *photo*: light; *synthesis*: to build or put together). Photosynthesis is the process by which plants capture and convert light energy or photons into the energy of chemical bonds, while at the same time they convert inorganic carbon dioxide and water into more complex "organic" compounds (and oxygen). These compounds can then be broken down at a later time (using the oxygen), and the energy thereby released can be used for the processes of life. The basic formula for the photosynthetic reaction is:

$$CO_2 + H_2O \rightarrow (CH_2O) + O_2$$

where CO_2 is carbon dioxide, H_2O is water, O_2 is molecular oxygen, (CH_2O) is hydrated carbon, that is, carbohydrate, and the energy that drives the reaction comes from sunlight. If we were to perform this reaction with six molecules of carbon dioxide and six molecules of water (and light energy), we would end up with six molecules of oxygen and a six-carbon carbohydrate called glucose:

$$6CO_2 + 6H_2O \rightarrow C_6H_{12}O_6 + 6O_2$$

The biochemical process of photosynthesis takes place in specialized microscopic intracellular organs or *organelles* in the plant tissue called *chloroplasts* and is actually two reactions: the light reaction, which uses the familiar green pigment chlorophyll and converts light energy into chemical energy, and the so-called dark reaction (also called the Calvin cycle, after Melvin Calvin, who received the Nobel Prize in chemistry in 1961), which then uses the chemical energy formed during the light reaction to join molecules of carbon dioxide to form the sugar glucose. As Professor K. Myrbaumick, a member of the Swedish Academy of Sciences, said in his presentation of the Nobel award to Dr. Calvin, "photosynthesis is the absolute prerequisite for all life on Earth and the most fundamental of all biochemical reactions." Although there may be those who would challenge this statement, it has some basis in fact, and one cannot blame the professor for a bit of hyperbole under the circumstances.

One of the convenient things about energy is that it is conserved. This concept is nicely explained by the First Law of Thermodynamics, or the universal law of the conservation of energy, which states that "the increase in the internal energy of a system is equal to the amount of energy added to the system minus the work done by the system and the heat created." Put more simply, the total energy of a system equals the energy put in minus the energy expended (as work) plus heat. Since energy is conserved, if the energy put in is more than the energy expended, the system will store that excess energy, a concept that is very important in biological systems. This will become evident when we discuss the physiology of nutrition and malnutrition, but for now this simple statement will suffice. If you eat more calories than you burn, you will store energy (and gain weight). If you eat fewer calories than you burn, you will lose weight. The energy that is expended as physical work or heat is called kinetic energy (from the Greek *kinesis*: motion). Energy that is stored is called potential energy.

With this basic knowledge of the source of matter and energy, we can now turn to how it applies to nutrition; that is, how do we take matter and energy from the environment and incorporate them into our bodies?

Metabolism

The processes by which living organisms extract energy and the building blocks of life from the complex molecules produced by photosynthesis, or store energy and organic molecules for later use are encompassed by the term *metabolism*. Metabolism can be divided into two types of processes: *catabolism*, which is the breakdown of nutrients to obtain energy; and *anabolism*, which is the synthesis of the components of the living organism such as proteins and nucleic acids. Some of the processes of catabolism are also called *respiration* (different from the process of breathing, which is how most of us understand the term). Anabolism is also called *biosynthesis*.

Respiration

Respiration is the array of biochemical processes by which living organisms break down nutrients in order to convert the potential energy stored in the chemical bonds into a biologically usable source of energy. This drives the biosynthetic processes as well as producing the kinetic energy associated with all but the most sedentary of organisms (even most plants have some form of active motion). To illustrate this concept, let us look at the reverse of the basic photosynthetic reaction, or the respiration of the simple sugar glucose.

THE METABOLISM OF CARBOHYDRATES. Glucose is a six-carbon sugar with the chemical formula $C_6H_{12}O_6$. The process by which the six-carbon glucose molecule is metabolized into two, three-carbon pyruvate molecules is known as *glycolysis* (from the Greek *glycos*: sweet; *lysis*: rupture or dissolution). It is also known as the Embden-Meyerhof pathway (Otto Meyerhof was awarded the Nobel Prize in Physiology in Medicine, along with Archibald Hill, for his work on muscle metabolism and lactic acid. Apparently Gustav Embden had to be content with having his name come first on one of the most important, fundamental biochemical processes known).

Glycolysis takes place in the biochemical soup inside of cells called the cytoplasm and is a nearly universal pathway in biological systems. Even as one of the simplest of biochemical reactions, glycolysis is actually quite complex, but it can be chemically summarized as:

$$C_6H_{12}O_6 + 2ADP + 2Pi \rightarrow 2CH_3(C=O)COO + 2ATP$$

where the six-carbon glucose has been split into two three-carbon pyruvates, and the potential energy in the chemical bond that was holding the two three-carbon fragments together has been converted to potential energy in a high-energy phosphate bond. This reaction is part of the glycolytic pathway in which adenosine diphosphate has an additional inorganic phosphate added to form adenosine triphosphate or ATP. *It is ATP that is ultimately the biologically usable form of energy that drives all of life's processes.*

Glycolysis is one basic metabolic pathway, but of course it is not the whole story. The process of glycolysis can (and does) occur without the need for oxygen, and it is therefore an anaerobic process. The product of glycolysis—pyruvate—can then follow three potential pathways of endpoint metabolism. Some organisms, such as yeast, anaerobically metabolize the pyruvate further into ethyl alcohol and carbon dioxide in the process we know as fermentation (first described by Louis Pasteur in 1857). If anaerobic metabolism occurs in animal tissue, the pyruvate is metabolized into lactic acid (which is indirectly involved in the acute muscular discomfort associated with extreme exercise). These two pathways are not particularly desirable endpoints both because the end products are toxic and because they are not efficient—only one of the five carbon-to-carbon bonds in the glucose has been used to make the biological energy source ATP. Luckily, as the environment in which life evolved, so did the biochemical pathways of living organisms. Remember, the primal atmosphere of the Earth was not an oxygen-rich environment. As the Earth cooled and lost its hydrogen and helium, an early atmosphere was most likely formed by gases emitted through volcanic activity. If we assume these gases were similar to volcanic gases today (after all, it is only 4.5 billion years later) the early atmosphere would have been mostly composed of water vapor (95 percent), carbon dioxide (1–2 percent), various sulfur-containing compounds, nitrogen (in both the elemental form and as ammonia), and methane.

The earliest organisms were chemotrophs, but as plants evolved the mechanisms of autotrophism (the conversion of light energy into chemical bonds via photosynthesis), they also were able to use the carbon dioxide, "fix" the carbon into organic compounds, and in the process change the composition of Earth's atmosphere to an oxygen-rich (21 percent), carbon dioxide–poor (0.038 percent) mixture. As the oxygen content of the atmosphere increased, biochemical pathways evolved to take advantage of oxygen's unique chemical ability to accept electrons (and therefore oxidize other elements with substantial transfer of energy). The pathway by which living organisms accomplish this is called the Krebs citric acid cycle or tricarboxylic cycle (after Hans Adolph Krebs, who shared the Nobel Prize in Physiology in 1953 with Fritz Albert Lipmann for his discovery of coenzyme A).

The citric acid cycle is also a highly complex process involving many intermediates, enzymes, and cofactors. The important points to remember are these:

The early products of metabolism, in this case pyruvate, are further altered to form the "activated" two-carbon product called acetyl coenzyme A or acetyl CoA. It is this active molecule that enters the citric acid cycle to join with oxaloacetic acid to form the six-carbon compound citric acid. The pathway then goes through a number of enzyme- and cofactor-mediated reactions during which the two added carbons are sequentially "stripped off" of the substrate molecule as carbon dioxide, producing energy for the cell to use or store and regenerating the oxaloacetic acid (hence the term *cycle*). The bottom line of this is that all metabolic breakdown of nutrients occurs as two-carbon fragments, constrained by the laws of physics and chemistry.

The Krebs citric acid cycle is the final common pathway for oxidation of all fuel molecules. Proteins and fats are themselves broken down into small carbon fragments (by processes other than glycolysis), which are then activated to form acetyl CoA so they can be further metabolized by the citric acid cycle.

The citric acid cycle does not occur in the cytoplasm in more evolved cells (eukaryotes), but in organelles called *mitochondria*. It is of more than passing interest that mitochondria structurally and functionally resemble chloroplasts. This is not surprising, considering that the citric acid cycle can be considered to be essentially the reverse reaction of photosynthesis. Photosynthesis captures energy from the sun; inorganic carbon, hydrogen, and oxygen (as carbon dioxide and water) from the environment and produces organic compounds. Mitochondrial respiration extracts that energy for immediate use or storage as ATP, and in so doing breaks the organic nutrient down into its inorganic components, carbon dioxide (CO_2) and water (H_2O): a very elegant system indeed. It should be noted here that the citric acid cycle is only one of many cycles of intermediary metabolism. There are many more, involved in either the breakdown of nutrients to produce energy or the synthesis of new, complex biomolecules. The products of the citric acid cycle are used by the organism not only for energy but also as precursors for this biosynthesis.

As luck would have it, this is not the end of the story. Each turn of the cycle produces one GTP (guanosine triphosphate), which is then converted into ATP. The bulk of the energy of the chemical bonds is transferred to the two coenzymes nicotinamide adenine dinucleotide (NAD^+) and flavin adenine dinucleotide (FAD). These are respectively easier to remember as a form of vitamin B$_3$ (niacin) and a form of vitamin B$_2$ (riboflavin). It is these coenzymes that then utilize oxygen in the process known as *oxidative phosphorylation* and transfer the energy stored in their activated bonds by transferring the electrons to molecular oxygen, in the process forming the high-energy phosphoanhydride bond in ATP.

There are two obvious benefits to this aerobic process. The first is that, as the process is regenerating, no toxic products build up. The second is that it is highly efficient—all of the carbon-to-carbon bonds in glucose (or any other nutrient) are converted to energy. If we again do the math, each six-carbon glucose molecule will yield two ATPs from glycolysis and then an additional total of thirty-six ATPs from the two turns of the citric acid cycle that result from each molecule of glucose (we get two pyruvate molecules from each glucose molecule). This is a nineteenfold increase in available energy when we compare the anaerobic process of glycolysis to the aerobic process of the citric acid cycle coupled to oxidative phosphorylation.

Although the details of the above process are fascinating, they are outside of the parameters of this discussion. There are two specific points we wish to call attention to, however, that are particularly relevant. The first is that the biochemical processes that drive these reactions are dependent on biological catalysts called enzymes, a term coined by Friedrich Wilhelm Kühne in 1878 from the Greek *en*: in and *zyme*: leaven (as in to ferment). Enzymes are for the most part proteins. This is important because, as we shall see, if you do not have the building blocks to make your own proteins, such as enzymes, you cannot carry out life's processes (starvation at the cellular level). As we shall see in chapter 8, this is one of the reasons that protein malnutrition is particularly insidious. The second point is that these biochemical reactions, in addition to requiring the action of enzymes, also require micronutrients that are the catalytic cofactors we have discussed. Without these the process cannot be complete. These catalytic cofactors are needed in only very small amounts (hence the term *micronutrient*), but without them, life stops.

In addition to the niacin and riboflavin discussed above, another excellent example is found in the catalytic cofactor (or enzyme prosthetic group) thiamine, which we know as vitamin B_1. It is an essential cofactor for three important enzymes in the further metabolism of glucose: pyruvate dehydrogenase, α-ketoglutarate dehydrogenase, and *trans*-ketolase. If you do not have a significant background in science, do not let the long chemical names bother you. The important point here is, as complex and elegant as these enzymatic reactions might be, without vitamin B_1 they grind to a halt, and the organism dies. We discuss some other examples of the importance of micronutrient deficiency in chapter 8.

THE METABOLISM OF FATS. Fatty acids, the biological molecules that make up fats in our diet, differ from carbohydrates structurally in that they are long chains of carbon atoms that are bound with single bonds to one another, and otherwise bound only to hydrogen (saturated fats) or bound to one another with a variable number of strategically placed double bonds, and therefore bound to less hydrogen (monounsaturated or polyunsaturated fats). Fats do not contain the hydroxyl group (OH) that carbohydrates contain and hence are not hydrated. We discuss this further in the next chapter.

The metabolism of fats follows a different pathway, known as β-oxidation, so called because the biochemical reaction involves the second, or β carbon in the chain. This process involves activating the long carbon chain with coenzyme A to form an acyl CoA, which is then shortened in each step by two-carbon fragments to form acetyl CoA which can then be cycled through the citric acid cycle (note the repetition of the two-carbon fragment here). Since fatty acids have many more than six carbons, metabolism of fats can generate more energy than carbohydrates. For example, the fatty acid palmitic acid (as the name would suggest, a major component of palm oil) has the chemical structure $C_{16}H_{32}O_2$. Fully metabolized, one molecule of palmitic acid would yield 129 ATP, compared to the thirty-eight derived from the complete metabolism from one molecule of glucose. Although this is not a completely fair comparison, since glucose has only six carbons with their attendant bonds and palmitate has sixteen, the carbon atoms in the glucose have already been partially oxidized (they are each bonded to an oxygen), and these partially oxidized carbons carry less energy than the unoxidized carbons in fat do. As we will see later, this is one of the characteristics of fats that differentiate them as a nutrient, that is, there are more calories in a gram of fat than there are in a gram of carbohydrates or protein.

THE METABOLISM OF PROTEINS: THE SPECIAL CASE OF NITROGEN. The four most important elements in life, in terms of amount at any rate, are carbon, oxygen, hydrogen, and nitrogen. We have learned in the preceding sections that the carbon, oxygen, and hydrogen in our bodies come originally from carbon dioxide and water. Organic nitrogen, however, follows a different path. Molecular nitrogen, or N_2, makes up the majority of our atmosphere at 78 percent. It is a relatively inert gas, and for the purposes of most life forms it is inaccessible for biological functions. The majority of organically accessible nitrogen is created by the process of nitrogen fixation by a group of specialized prokaryotes known as *diazotrophs*. These bacteria, either as free-living forms or living symbiotically in the roots of certain plants (most of which are legumes) are able to convert molecular nitrogen into ammonia (NH_3), which can then be further converted to more complex organic molecules (either by the bacteria or associated plants) such as the amino acids, which are the basic building blocks of proteins. The amino acids are each metabolized by very specific enzymes. Amino acids can be broken down and converted into glucose (and then used as energy) by the process of *gluconeogenesis* (literally, "new glucose formation"), and we discuss this process in more detail in chapter 4. More frequently, as we discuss in chapter 8, they are conserved, recycled, and used in the process of biosynthesis.

The Macronutrients: Carbohydrates, Fats, and Proteins

We have laid the groundwork for understanding the basic biochemistry of how we convert the energy in our food into energy and biosynthetic precursors for our own use. Now we discuss the nutrients themselves: their energy value as well as special biochemical characteristics that might add to their nutritional value over and above their caloric content. The importance of this is that in understanding why we need these nutrients we can then understand what happens when we do not have them.

In regard to energy value, we measure our nutritional intake in the form of calories (from the Latin *calor*: heat). What we mean by calories in terms of nutrition is actually, in terms of scientific measurement, kilocalories or a thousand calories—a calorie being the amount of energy required to raise the temperature of 1 gram of water 1 degree Celsius. Although in scientific terminology a nutritional calorie is capitalized as Calorie (or called a kilocalorie or kcal), for the purposes of this book when we use the term *calorie*, we are referring to the nutritional value of food in kilocalories. For purposes of this discussion, let us consider a daily caloric requirement for an average adult to be 2500 calories a day and build a macronutrient diet based on historical intakes.

Carbohydrates

Carbohydrates are the most plentiful of biological molecules and can be defined chemically as organic molecules containing carbon, hydrogen, and oxygen with the latter two components present in a ratio of 2:1 (the same as in water—hence the name, *hydrated carbon* or carbohydrate). Carbohydrates can serve both as a source of nutrition as well as a source of structure and support, such as the cellulose in plants or the chitin found in the exoskeletons of insects. With regard to the former, although cellulose is by far the most abundant carbohydrate in the Earth's biomass, it is nutritionally inaccessible to all but the most simple of prokaryotic organisms—even termites and cud-chewing ungulates such as cows depend on the bacteria in their guts to digest the cellulose in their diets.

The nutritional forms of carbohydrates are found either as simple sugars (mono- and disaccharides) or more complex molecules called starches (polysaccharides). The simple sugars include the monosaccharides glucose, fructose, and galactose. The two major dietary disaccharides are sucrose (table sugar, which is made up of one molecule of glucose joined to one molecule of fructose) and lactose (milk sugar, made up of one molecule of glucose joined to one molecule of galactose). The main polysaccharides are amylose (plant starch), glycogen (animal starch), and of course cellulose, which as we mentioned cannot be considered a direct source of nutrients for us.

Carbohydrates provide 4 calories per gram of nutrient. An average diet in a developed country would contain about 300 grams of carbohydrate—about three-fourths of a pound—mostly in the form of the plant starch amylose (65 percent by weight) but with a significant contribution from the disaccharide sucrose (25 percent). The remainder is made up of glycogen and lactose, and the total caloric value would be 1200 calories.

Fats

Dietary fats are for the most part triglycerides. (Although cholesterol and a group of compounds called phospholipids are also dietary fats and are nutritionally important, we can limit our discussion to triglycerides for the purposes of caloric needs.) Triglycerides are complex molecules made up of three fatty acids bound to a three-carbon molecule called glycerol (hence *tri*-glyceride).

Although both the fatty acid molecules and the glycerol molecules are important metabolically, the caloric value of triglycerides is primarily found in the fatty acid chains. As we discussed earlier, complete metabolism of a given weight of fatty acid produces substantially more ATP than does metabolism of the same weight of sugar. For this reason fat provides 9 calories per gram and is the most energy dense of the macronutrients.

There are two other characteristics of fats that make them important as a macronutrient. The first is that, although humans can synthesize most of the fatty acids from ingested carbohydrates, there are two fatty acids, α-linolenic acid and linoleic acid, that we cannot synthesize. These are called essential fatty acids; since we cannot synthesize them they must be present in our diets. The other characteristic is that fat, unlike starches, which are the storage form of carbohydrates, can be stored without the need for water of hydration. Because the storage of carbohydrate energy (in the form of glycogen in the case of animals) requires the additional storage of water, the caloric density of the stored carbohydrate is reduced effectively from 4 kcal/gram to 1–2 kcal/gram. If we look at the average amount of stored energy in a 70-kilogram (150-pound) man, it works out to approximately 110,000 kcal, the vast majority of which is stored as 12,000 grams (26 pounds) of triglycerides. If we wanted to store that energy as carbohydrates, given the above reduction in caloric value and the attendant hydration, we would have to store between 55,000 and 110,000 grams of carbohydrate, or 120–240 additional pounds. Our 150-pound man would have to weigh between 270 and 390 pounds in order to store an adequate amount of energy. So it is easy to understand why the characteristics of the high caloric density of fat and the ability to store it without an additional water burden make triglycerides an essential nutritional source both for kinetic as well as potential (stored) energy.

If we turn our attention back to dietary requirements, given the caloric requirements of a 70-kilogram man in a developed country as 2500 calories a day, and given the caloric value of fat at 9 calories per gram, an intake of 100 grams of dietary fat (with 95 percent of that coming from triglycerides) will add 900 calories to the 1200 we obtained from our carbohydrates, giving us a total of 2100 calories.

Proteins

Proteins are highly complex, specialized biomolecules. Their distinctive place in biology, over and above the fact that the word itself is one of the rare instances in the English language when the "*i* before *e*" rule does not apply, was recognized early on: the term was first used by the Swedish chemist Jöns Jacob Berzelius in 1838 from the Greek *proteios*: of the first rank. He was referring to his impression (in some respects quite accurate) that protein seemed to be the principal substance for animal nutrition that plants produce for herbivores (and that are then passed on to carnivores).[14] We discuss their fundamental importance in the diet (and in malnutrition) in chapter 8, but for now let us consider the basics of their chemistry and structure.

Proteins are made up of chains of smaller molecules called amino acids. Amino acids are made up of carbon, hydrogen, oxygen, and unlike the fats and carbohydrates, they contain nitrogen as well (two of the amino acids also contain sulfur). Their basic structure is a molecule with an amino group (NH_2) and carboxyl (acid) group (COO) bound to a carbon atom called the α carbon. Each amino acid then has a different side chain that determines its chemical behavior in terms of reactivity and how it affects the ultimate structure and function of the protein. There are twenty naturally occurring amino acids, and all organisms utilize the same twenty amino acids in constructing their proteins. Human beings can synthesize eleven of these amino acids from dietary carbohydrates, but just as in the case of the two fatty acids we cannot synthesize, there are nine other amino acids we cannot synthesize, and these are called essential amino acids. These must be present in our diets. The presence and quantity of the essential amino acids in any dietary protein are used in defining whether that protein is a high-quality dietary protein or a low-quality dietary protein.

Amino acids form the structure of the protein molecule by linking together in what is called a peptide bond, formed by the removal of a water molecule (an OH^- from the carboxyl terminal of one amino acid and an H^+ from the amino terminal of another). We will discuss this chemical reaction, called condensation, in chapter 4.

The protein molecule itself has a complex three-dimensional structure, and this final structure is called its conformation. That conformation is determined by a protein's primary, secondary, tertiary, and quaternary structures. The primary structure is determined by the linear sequence of amino acids in the chain, called a polypeptide chain, which is itself determined by genetic sequence. A secondary structure develops due to attractive forces called hydrogen bonds between the different amino acids in the chain, causing the chain to twist or fold in a particular manner, for example as a helix or pleated sheet. The tertiary structure is then formed by additional folding of the polypeptide chain into a more compact, globular structure (you have heard of *globins*, such as in hemoglobin, immunoglobulins, etc.). Finally, some proteins are made up of more than one polypeptide chain, and it is this association of multiple chains (which may have identical or differing primary, secondary, and tertiary structures) that determines the quaternary structure of these proteins.

As noted, we discuss the special case of proteins as they relate to how they are utilized nutritionally and why proteins play such an important part in chronic malnutrition in chapter 8. For the current discussion, let us limit our attention to the fact that proteins, like carbohydrates, have a caloric value of 4 calories per gram. Assuming that all ingested protein is used as an energy source (which we will see is not the case), in order for us to reach our stated goal of a daily intake of 2500 calories for our imaginary 150-pound man living in a developed country, he would have to eat 100 grams of protein a day. To recap his diet:

300 grams of carbohydrate at 4 calories a gram = 1200 calories
100 grams of fat (triglyceride) at 9 calories a gram = 900 calories
100 grams of protein at 4 calories a gram = 400 calories
Total = 2500 calories

The Micronutrients: Vitamins and Minerals

The macronutrients we consume supply the energy and building blocks we need in order to grow, function, and replenish our tissues and energy stores. We need other nutrients, however, that do not have intrinsic caloric value but are otherwise critical for the biological processes we call life. Although these nutrients are generally needed in relatively small or even trace amounts, they are no less critical to our health, well-being, and ultimately our survival. We learned in the section on metabolism that there are essential cofactors required for certain enzymatic reactions to occur. Three of the cofactors we discussed are the vitamins B_1, B_2, and B_3. Other cofactors necessary for biochemical reactions would be considered minerals, such as magnesium, and there are other types of vitamins that function in biochemical processes other than the metabolism of nutrients.

Vitamins as a group are biomolecules that function as cofactors or coenzymes in a number of critical bodily processes. The name comes from the early recognition that there were vital factors, necessary in trace amounts, for certain biological processes to proceed, and that the factors first recognized were in a chemical group called amines—hence *vital amines* or *vitamines* (specifically the term was used to describe the discovery in 1912 that an amine extracted from the residual of rice polishings could be used to prevent beri-beri). The *e* was dropped when it became known that there were vitamins, such as vitamin C, that are not amines. Vitamins can be separated into two groups—fat-soluble and water-soluble. The fat-soluble vitamins include A, D, E, and K. The water-soluble vitamins include the B-complex of vitamins—thiamin (B_1), riboflavin (B_2), niacin (B_3), pantothenic acid (B_5), pyridoxine (B_6), biotin (B_7), folic acid (B_9), and cyanocobalamin (B_{12})—and vitamin C. In the case of human beings, these are all essential dietary elements. The only one we can make ourselves is some amount of vitamin D in our skin—and that only when we are exposed to enough direct sunlight.

The term *dietary minerals* is something of a misnomer, as most of these elements are actually in the ionized state when biologically active. A good example of this is sodium chloride, which when ingested becomes sodium ions and chloride ions, present in our blood, cells, and all other bodily fluids. For the purpose of this discussion, however, the term *minerals* will serve, and it refers to chemical elements other than carbon, hydrogen, oxygen, and nitrogen that are necessary for the structure and function of living organisms. The major minerals, in order of amount, are: calcium and phosphorus, present in large amounts in our skeletons and cells; potassium, present in our cells and blood; sulfur, an important element in many of our proteins; sodium and chloride, present in our blood and cells; and magnesium, an important mineral cofactor in many biochemical processes. The trace minerals (needed in much smaller amounts) include iron, a necessary central element of the oxygen-carrying protein hemoglobin; manganese; copper; and iodine (which we shall see is a critical element in normal hormonal control of growth, development, and normal metabolism).

We discuss the specific disease states associated with isolated deficiencies of some of these micronutrients in chapter 8. The important point to remember now is that all of these micronutrients, be they vitamins or minerals, are essential for a human being to maintain a healthy existence. Therefore, the absence of any one of them will kill or disable a person as readily as insufficient calories; sometimes in medically interesting but quite unpleasant ways.

Water

As poet W. H. Auden (1907–1973) wrote, "Thousands have lived without love, not one without water." Life originated in the seas, and terrestrial organisms are able to live on land only because they (and we) carry their own internal seas with them. There is no known life form that does not depend on the presence of water. As an example, both basic processes of photosynthesis and cellular respiration either use water as a raw material or produce water as an end product. Water is considered the "universal solvent," and most if not all biochemical reactions take place in an aqueous environment, even if water is not consumed or produced by the reaction.

Our bodies are 70 percent water by weight, and our basal metabolic requirement for water—that is, the amount of water we need just to exist without doing anything—is about 700 milliliters a day, or approximately 1.5 pints. Our bodily processes require (and recycle) 8 liters of water a day. A generally accepted minimum daily requirement for an average, active adult, needed to replace the losses associated with breathing, sweating, and transporting wastes in our urine and feces is 2.5–3 liters a day (about 2.36–2.8 quarts).

Although 70 percent of the Earth's surface is comprised of water, 97 percent of that water is salt water, and only 3 percent is fresh water. Of that 3 percent fresh water, 69 percent is locked away as ice in the polar ice caps and in glaciers (90 percent of this is in Antarctica, accounting for over 60 percent of the world's fresh water). Thirty percent of the fresh water is "ground water," that is, water either in the subsurface soil or in deeper collections called aquifers. An aquifer is defined as an underground stratum of water-saturated rock (or unconsolidated material such as sand or gravel) from which water can be extracted by a well or that naturally supplies water to a spring or other surface source. Some aquifers are huge, such as the Ogallala Aquifer in our Midwest, formed from alluvial deposits during the late Miocene and early Pliocene epochs (about 5 million years ago). The Ogallala Aquifer extends from South Dakota in the north to Texas in the south, and the water from this aquifer is used to irrigate much of our most productive farmland (up to 30 percent of all irrigated farmland in the United States is irrigated from this aquifer). As is true of many of the largest aquifers, the water in the Ogallala Aquifer is considered to be *paleowater* or fossil water— deposited there at the end of the last ice age. As such, this water source is not renewable at the rate it is being used—according to the U.S. Geological Survey, 21 million acre-feet of water were removed from the aquifer for irrigation in the year 2000,[15] about equal to the annual discharge of the Colorado River. Stated in another way, the removal of water from this major resource is four times the estimated recharge rate. Only 1 percent of the Earth's fresh water is what we would recognize as surface water, that is, lakes, streams, and rivers (of some interest, 20 percent of the world's liquid, fresh surface water is found in Lake Baikal in the Russian Federation, and 20 percent is found in the Great Lakes of North America). In total, only about 0.3 percent of the water on our planet is available or suitable for human use. As the figures presented above for the Ogallala Aquifer suggest, this resource is neither unlimited nor renewable.

These worrisome statistics aside, there remain huge quantities of fresh, potable water on the planet. The problem is more one of access than it is of scarcity, very much in the same way that Amartya Sen's theory of loss of access and entitlement to existing food sources (discussed in chapter 2) conflicts with the Malthusian concept of population growth outstripping the Earth's ability to produce adequate nutrition. The fact is that 20 percent of the world's population—that is 1.3 billion people—do not have access to a reliable source of safe drinking water, and 40 percent—2.6 billion people—do not have access to adequate sanitation. The consequences of this are devastating in regard to human suffering and death. The contrasts between the "loud" emergencies and the "silent" emergencies are a thread throughout this book. This is one of the silent emergencies, described in an article in *The Lancet*, one of the world's most prominent medical journals, as a silent humanitarian crisis. This lack of access to safe drinking water and adequate sanitation, which are fundamental requirements for survival, is responsible for the preventable deaths of 3900 children *every day* (1.4 million preventable deaths a year). The article goes on to point out that this "robs the poor, especially women and children, of their time, health, and dignity."[16] In addition to this insidious waste of human capital, diseases transmitted through water or human excrement are the second leading cause of death among children worldwide, after respiratory disease, as we discuss in some detail in chapter 10.[17] To reiterate this contrast between the loud and silent emergencies, far more people suffer the ill effects of poor water supply and sanitation than are affected by the most prominently covered events in the media today, war and terrorism.[18] One cannot help but to ask the question: Is there a link between so many people's lack of access to the basic human needs and the proliferation of war and terrorism?

The Millennium Declaration

We introduced the *Millennium Declaration Project* in chapter 1.[19] Of the many goals and targets, goal 7—ensuring environmental sustainability—has as one of its targets (target 10) to "halve, by 2015, the proportion of people without sustainable access to safe drinking water and basic sanitation." Although this may seem to relegate improving the access to safe water and basic sanitation to a relatively small role in the larger project, it should be noted that the full report recognizes that sound water resources management is necessary to achieving all of the *Millennium Development* goals and that the current situation "thwarts progress towards all of the *Millennium Development* Goals." As so strongly stated in chapter 1 of the report of the *UN Millennium Project Task Force on Water and Sanitation*: Water is life.

Water is life for people and for the planet. It is essential to the well-being of humankind, a vital input to economic development, and a basic requirement for the healthy functioning of all the world's ecosystems. Clean water for domestic purposes is essential for human health and survival; indeed, the combination of safe drinking water, adequate sanitation, and such hygienic practices as hand washing is recognized as a precondition for reductions in morbidity and mortality rates, especially among children.

Water is also critical to other facets of sustainable development—from environmental protection and food security to increased tourism and investment, from the empowerment of women and the education of girls to reductions in productivity losses due to illness and malnutrition.

The Meaning of Life (as Seen by a Biochemist)

As Darwin stated, "We must, however, acknowledge, as it seems to me, that man with all his noble qualities . . . still bears in his bodily frame the indelible stamp of his lowly origin."[20]

In this chapter we have reviewed the basics of the chemistry and biochemistry of life in order to enable us to understand some of the consequences of inadequate nutrition that we encounter in subsequent chapters. Although it would be neither feasible nor desirable to discuss the myriad other processes occurring at a molecular level in essentially every living organism, it is useful to consider what we are actually talking about when we discuss the concept of life from a scientific viewpoint.

The Earth was formed 4.5 billion years ago. Life formed on this planet 4 billion years ago, so for the vast majority of its history Earth has been inhabited. How did life arise so quickly (in geologic terms) in such a sterile, inhospitable environment as the primordial planet must have offered?

As we noted earlier, the primitive atmosphere of the Earth was quite different from what it is today, composed mainly of gases released by volcanic activity such as methane, ammonia, and water vapor, and lacking in oxygen. In 1922 the Soviet (Russian) biochemist Alexsander Oparin theorized that organic compounds would have been created in this atmosphere by constant exposure to electrical storms. This was considered purely hypothetical until thirty years later when Stanley Miller, at the time a graduate student working in the laboratory of Harold Urey at the University of Chicago, did a relatively simple experiment. He put ammonia (NH_3), methane (CH_4), water (H_2O), and hydrogen (H_2) into a glass flask and exposed this laboratory equivalent of Earth's primitive atmosphere to electrical activity to reproduce the effects of lightning. When the contents of the flask were analyzed after a week of this exposure, they were found to contain a number of organic compounds (including amino acids, the building blocks of proteins), confirming the real possibility that Oparin was correct in his theory that life, or at least the biomolecules associated with life, had initially been created by a nonbiologic, or *abiotic*, process.

These biomolecules, when examined in isolation, exhibit all of the physical and chemical characteristics of inorganic molecules. Yet, as pointed out in Lehninger's textbook *Principles of Biochemistry*, "Organisms possess extraordinary attributes, properties that distinguish them from other collections of matter." What are these distinguishing characteristics, according to Lehninger?[21]

1. A high degree of chemical complexity and microscopic organization—manifest in each biomolecule having a specific sequence of its subunits, a specific three-dimensional structure, and highly specific spatial relationships to all of the other interactive molecules in its environment.

2. Systems for extracting, transforming, and using energy from the environment, enabling organisms to obtain and extract nutrients, to process and internalize them in order to build and maintain their own internal structures, and to perform mechanical, chemical, osmotic, and electrical work. (According to the laws of the universe, inanimate matter tends toward entropy or disorder, as we shall shortly discuss.)

3. A capacity for precise self-replication and self-assembly, from bacteria to human, able to replicate each structure from the smallest subunit to the organism as a whole with remarkable fidelity and remarkably few errors.

4. Mechanisms for sensing and responding to alterations in their surroundings.

5. Defined functions for each of their components and regulated interactions among them.

6. A history of evolutionary change.

It is characteristic number 2 that most concerns us in this book. This is the crux of how we relate biologically to our environment—taking energy and matter from the environment and using it or storing it to build and maintain our own bodies. We have discussed the First Law of Thermodynamics—the conservation of energy—earlier in this chapter. As one might expect, there is a Second Law of Thermodynamics, and it is this—the total entropy or disorder of the universe is continuously increasing, that is, everything tends to go from a more complex form to a less complex form. Everything, that is, except life forms. Living organisms collect and use matter and energy to maintain their complexity at the expense of the complexity of the environment. For example, when we eat a complex molecule such as a starch, we process it into the simple molecules of water and carbon dioxide, and use its energy to build and maintain our own bodies, or to perform our own tasks. So not only do we internalize environmental energy for our own use, but we also defend the order of our internal universe by increasing the disorder of the external universe.

This characteristic of extracting energy and order at the expense of the

environment and the specific metabolic pathways used, both catabolic and anabolic, is essentially identical in all living organisms—indirect but compelling
biochemical evidence for a common origin for all life. It is this fundamental
trait shared by all life forms, the pursuit of nutritional energy in a constant
struggle against the Second Law of Thermodynamics, that is a central theme
of this book—life is the one counterpoint to this otherwise "absolute" law of
the Universe.

The Anatomy and Physiology of Nutrition

Form follows function.
—Louis Henri Sullivan (1856–1924)

God is in the details.
—Ludwig Mies van der Rohe (1886–1969)

The above quotes, although not meant to refer to biological systems, illustrate the following important points about biological processes: on a macroscopic, microscopic, and molecular level we are built exactly to perform the functions of life. The details of how this all evolved, how it all works, and how it all fits together are where the real beauty is.

The first point is stated in Mr. Sullivan's astute observation. (Louis Henri Sullivan was an architect at the turn of the twentieth century, is considered by some to be the creator of the modern skyscraper, and was mentor to one of the great architects of the twentieth century, Frank Lloyd Wright.) What Sullivan meant by his statement, of course, is that buildings (and everything else) should be designed according to the purpose for which they are meant. This is a good idea. And as one studies life's processes in finer and finer detail, the exquisite truth of this observation as it applies to biological systems becomes clear—the function that an object, animate or inanimate, is meant to perform by definition determines its ideal form, and vice versa. This brings us to the second quote. Although there is some controversy as to its origin, majority opinion generally attributes it to Ludwig Mies van der Rohe. Van der Rohe was also an architect, also a colleague of Frank Lloyd Wright, and while his observation was also meant to be interpreted in terms of artistic expression, it is equally applicable to the ultimately simple complexity of life. The fundamental point of the information in this chapter is this: everything about the structure and function of living organisms, down to the smallest detail, is perfectly adapted (engineered?) to do exactly what it is meant to do. So whether you believe in the Darwinian concepts of mutation and natural selection as the engineers of these forms and functions or adhere to the belief of intelligent design (and an intelligent designer), it is hard to deny the beauty and perfection of life.

We have reviewed the basic biochemistry of life—how elements and energy are incorporated into organically accessible forms to be used by living organisms and how they can be internally transformed into usable energy and raw material for energy and biosynthesis. But those are only the basic steps at a cellular level. How do macroorganisms, such as ourselves, internalize, process, and assimilate the macronutrients and deliver them to the internal environment in utilizable forms? What are the physical and functional strategies that living organisms have evolved in order to do this effectively and efficiently?

Anatomy and Physiology of Nutrition

The anatomy of nutrition is the physical structure of the gastrointestinal tract, and the physiology of nutrition is the functional means by which we transform our food into usable form. For purposes of clarity we divide this discussion into two segments: the anatomy of the gastrointestinal tract followed by the physiology, which we then discuss in terms of the two separate processes of digestion and absorption.

Why do we have to know this? Do we need to understand the basic facts about how we obtain and process our nutrients in order to understand or remedy the consequences of malnutrition? The answer, of course, is yes. To give just one example, substantial percentages of certain adult populations are deficient in the enzyme lactase. Lactase is an essential enzyme needed to digest lactose, the sugar found in milk products. People with this deficiency experience severe abdominal pain and diarrhea when they ingest any substantial amounts of milk products. How foolish it would be then, with all the best of intentions, to provide a malnourished population with this lactase deficiency large amounts of nutrient-rich powdered milk and cheese to supplement their diets (yet this has indeed happened, or we would not be using it as an example).

Anatomy

Although the gastrointestinal tract is fundamentally one long tube, each of the segments is perfectly adapted to perform its particular function.[1] The human gastrointestinal (hereafter GI) tract can also be viewed as the means by which we most intimately interact with our external environment, by internalizing external nutrients and incorporating "them" into "us." As an analogy, our respiratory system is similar in this particular regard, albeit far less intricately incorporative, as it basically just exchanges the inorganic gases oxygen (which is, of course, incorporated into our tissues) and carbon dioxide and water vapor (which are waste products of our metabolism). While we also interact extensively with our environment through the senses of touch, temperature sensitivity, and pain as well as through our other highly developed senses of smell, sight, and hearing, these interactions are much more interrogatory and less incorporative.

THE MOUTH. The mouth is lined with a protective mucosa, called stratified squamous epithelium, which differs from skin only in that it does not develop the protective layer of keratin that is essentially made up of the nonliving skeletons of the living cells in the dermis below. Three sets of major salivary glands, the parotid, submandibular, and sublingual glands, secrete saliva that serves lubricating, antibacterial, and digestive functions. The teeth, of course, have the cutting, tearing, and grinding functions associated with mastication (chewing), the breaking of food into manageable size for swallowing.

THE ESOPHAGUS. The masticated, lubricated food travels through the pharynx and is swallowed as a bolus, or compact mass, to travel through the esophagus. The esophagus (Greek, *oeso*: to bring or transport; *phagus*: eaten) is a muscular tube whose sole function is to transport the bolus of food from the pharynx to the stomach. Its structure is perfect for this task as a muscular tube lined again with the protective stratified squamous epithelium. There are dual muscular layers to the esophagus, as is true for most of the rest of the GI tract. There is an inner circular layer of muscle covered by an outer longitudinal layer of muscle. This configuration has evolved ideally suited to produce the characteristic "milking" motion called *peristalsis* by which food and digested material are moved along the GI tract. This muscular configuration is continued throughout the remainder of the GI tract and will not be reiterated in the following sections.

THE STOMACH. The stomach has three basic functions: the holding of food while it is initially processed for further digestion; the mechanical blending and maceration of food with the early digestive fluids; and the beginning of chemical and enzymatic digestion. As one might predict from these functions, the stomach is a capacious organ capable of holding the contents of a complete meal so that it can be slowly processed and released into the small intestine for further digestion. The mixing and macerating process is accomplished by the stomach's muscular walls, with muscle fibers being distributed in multiple planes in addition to the circular and longitudinal planes needed for peristalsis. Finally, to maximize the stomach's ability to produce digestive chemicals (in the form of acid and enzymes), the surface area of the gastric mucosa is increased by the formation of multiple folds or *rugae*.

THE SMALL INTESTINE. The small intestine is the site where the majority of digestion and absorption occurs. It is made up of three separate segments: the duodenum (so called because it was generally felt to be twelve fingers long), the jejunum (so called because its function was originally not clear, and it was felt to be bland or boring), and the ileum (from the Greek *eilios*: twisted). The delineation between these segments is somewhat arbitrary and based as much on their function as on their anatomy. The duodenum is the site of the majority of digestion, whereas absorption takes place throughout the small bowel. Because the small bowel is the site of the majority of nutrient absorption as well as digestion, it becomes functionally very important that it have the largest surface area possible. It is for this reason that the mucosa of the small intestine has three basic structural forms that markedly increase its surface area. The first, on a macroscopic level, is the formation of folds, analogous to the gastric rugae, called *valvulae connivantes* or the folds of Kerckring. These folds increase the functional surface area of the small intestine threefold. The mucosal area is further increased by near microscopic projections called *villi* (singular *villus*, Latin for "shaggy hair"). Each villus is a small (0.5–1.5 mm) finger-like projection made up of a single layer of epithelial cells covering a central core of capillaries and lymphatics, bringing the products of digestion only one cell layer away from the circulatory system. Think about that: structurally, you are only one cell away from your external environment. Functionally, this is critically important.

The presence of these millions of villi gives the mucosal surface of the small intestine the appearance of fine velvet, and increases the absorptive surface of the mucosa by another tenfold. The epithelial cells lining the villi have a finely divided, microscopic brush-like membrane on the apical surface facing the intestinal lumen, the brush border or microvilli, which increase the absorptive surface an additional twentyfold. Taken together, these physical adaptations give the small intestines a surface area available for absorption of 250 square meters—the size of a tennis court or small parking lot.

THE LARGE INTESTINE. The large intestine, or colon, has the function of peristalsis, storage, and to a lesser degree absorption of whatever water has not been absorbed in the small intestine. As such, it shares the same muscular walls as the rest of the GI tract, is larger in diameter than the small bowel to accommodate its storage function, and has a less well-developed mucosal surface with an absorptive function quantitatively considerably less than that of the small intestine.

Physiology

As we discussed in the previous chapter, there are three macronutrients: carbohydrates, fats, and proteins. In addition to being macronutrients these are also macromolecules, and as such they must be broken down into their basic building blocks—monosaccharides, fatty acids, and amino acids, respectively—before they can be absorbed and assimilated.[2]

As we saw in the preceding chapter on the formation of peptide bonds, the basic reaction of biosynthesis involves the removal of a hydrogen ion (H^+) from one molecule and the removal of a hydroxyl ion (OH^-) from another to form a covalent bond between the two reacting molecules, producing a molecule of water. This is called *condensation*. The chemistry of digestion is basically the reverse of this process; that is, a molecule of water is used to split the covalent bond between two larger molecules, using the energy from this bond to incorporate the H$^+$ and OH$^-$ into the resultant subunits in a process called *hydrolysis*. In the case of carbohydrates, the molecules involved are all monosaccharides or sugars, products of the initial digestion of disaccharides and starch; in the case of fats, the covalent bond is between a fatty acid and glycerol; and in the case of proteins, the covalent bond is the peptide bond between two amino acids. Despite the chemical similarity between these reactions, the enzymes that catalyze them are specific only for their precise substrates and the resulting products. Why is this important? Again, consider the previous example of lactose intolerance—all of the proteases (enzymes that break down proteins) and lipases (enzymes that break down fats) in the world will not help someone with this deficiency to digest or to obtain any nutrition from lactose in her/his diet.

DIGESTION OF CARBOHYDRATES. All carbohydrates are composed of *saccharides* (Greek *sacchar*: sugar). There are only three major carbohydrates in our diets: the disaccharide sucrose, known as cane or table sugar (or saccharose); the disaccharide lactose, known as milk sugar; and the polysaccharide we call starch. Saccharose is made up of two basic sugar molecules—one molecule of glucose and one molecule of the simple sugar fructose (so called because it is a dominant sugar in many fruits, as well as other naturally sweet foods such as honey). Lactose, the sugar found naturally in milk, is made up of a molecule of glucose and a molecule of the simple sugar galactose (from the ancient Greek *galaktos*: milk). Plant and animal starches are long-chain polymers of glucose that vary depending on the amount of branching that is present (more in animal starch), whereas cellulose, the most abundant of all organic polymers, is a large polysaccharide molecule made up entirely of glucose. Although there is a substantial amount of cellulose in human diets, we do not have the enzymes to break it down into its constituent glucose molecules. This is going to become a most important point, which we consider when we discuss access to nutrients and the advent of agriculture.

Carbohydrate digestion begins in the mouth, catalyzed by the salivary enzyme *ptyalin*, which is a type of enzyme called an α-amylase. It is this enzyme that is responsible for the fact that even a pure starch, such as wheat flour, tastes a bit sweet to us when we eat it. Only about 5 percent of ingested starch is broken down in the mouth, mostly into the disaccharide called maltose, which is constructed of two glucose molecules bound together. The salivary amylase continues to be active in the stomach until its activity is destroyed by the low pH of the acid environment, so that a total of 30 percent to 40 percent of dietary starch is eventually digested before the gastric contents enter the small intestine. When the gastric contents pass through a sphincter called the pylorus to enter the first part of the small intestine, or duodenum, they are called *chyme*. At this point pancreatic secretions that are very high in bicarbonate ions neutralize the pH of the chyme, and at the same time the pancreatic α-amylase, which is a much more powerful amylase than ptyalin, converts the rest of the dietary starch into maltose within fifteen to thirty minutes. The dietary carbohydrates are now all in the form of the disaccharides sucrose, lactose, and maltose. As these come into contact with the brush borders of the enterocytes, the cells lining the intestine, the disaccharidases sucrase, lactase, and maltase, embedded in the cell membranes, further break them down into their component monosaccharides glucose and fructose, glucose and galactose, and two glucose molecules, respectively. These monosaccharides can then be absorbed and assimilated.

DIGESTION OF PROTEINS. Proteins are complex, biologically active macromolecules made up of chains of the twenty naturally occurring amino acids. These chains are called peptide chains. As we learned in the previous chapter, proteins have complex structures that include the primary structure of the sequence of amino acids in the peptide chains as well as secondary, tertiary, and quaternary structures. For the purposes of digestion only the primary structure is of importance, for the following reason. Proteins (and nucleic acids for that matter) are extremely sensitive to certain forms of external stress, such as heat, or the extremes of the range of pH such as very acid or alkaline environments. When they are exposed to these stresses, proteins go through a change of structure, generally losing their secondary, tertiary, and quaternary structures, while their primary structure remains unchanged. This change results in a loss of function and can be seen physically in ways such as loss of solubility, aggregation, or change in viscosity. A perfect everyday example of this is the change in an egg white when an egg is dropped into a hot skillet. This process is known as *denaturation*. Any ingested protein that has not already been denatured by cooking or other process of food preparation is immediately denatured when it mixes with the acid environment in the stomach.

Digestion of proteins begins in the stomach. There is no protein digestion to speak of in the mouth. As noted, any protein not already denatured is immediately denatured as it mixes with the acid gastric juices, leaving only the primary structure to be dealt with in the further process of digestion. The acidity of the gastric juice is created by the presence of hydrochloric acid, which is produced and secreted by specialized cells in the gastric mucosa known as *parietal* or *oxyntic* cells. In addition to the hydrochloric acid, the gastric mucosa also produces an enzyme called *pepsin*. Pepsin is a protease (enzyme names always end in the suffix *-ase*, with the prefix relating to the substrate on which it acts—hence protease for proteins, saccharidase for sugars, and lipase for fats or lipids). Pepsin is a highly specialized protease for two reasons. The first is that it is only active in an acid environment with a pH of 2.0–3.0 (the lower the pH, the more acid the environment). The second is that it specifically acts on the connective tissue collagen.

Collagen is a ubiquitous protein (the most abundant in mammals) and is a component of structural connective tissues such as bone, cartilage, and the intercellular matrix that holds our cells together. In fact the word comes from the Greek word *kolla*, which means "glue." Collagen is notoriously impervious to all proteases, except for pepsin in an acid environment. The activity of pepsin in the presence of hydrochloric acid is therefore able to digest the collagen in ingested protein, making the other protein components present in the exposed cellular material accessible to subsequent digestion by the proteases in the small intestine. How the stomach avoids digesting itself in this hostile environment is a fascinating question that is only partially understood. In certain pathological (disease-causing) states this does occur and causes the medical conditions we know as peptic ulcer disease and gastritis.

As the chyme enters the small intestine, its acidity is neutralized by the bicarbonate-rich pancreatic secretions. The pancreas also releases multiple proteases such as trypsin and chymotrypsin. The trypsin and chymotrypsin break the proteins down into smaller peptides, so that other specific enzymes can then begin to sequentially cleave amino acids from the carboxyl terminal of the smaller peptides. The smaller peptides so formed come into contact with the brush border of the enterocyctes, which have specific peptidases embedded in their membranes. These further degrade the peptides, and the amino acids produced are transported into the intracellular environment. Any small peptides that are absorbed intracellularly are further cleaved into their constituent amino acids by intracellular enzymes, so that ultimately 99 percent of the products of protein digestion entering the blood are free amino acids. Rarely, larger peptides can be transported directly into the blood, and in extremely rare circumstances more intact pieces of proteins are absorbed. Those instances would be considered potentially pathological and can be the cause of severe allergic or immunological disorders.

DIGESTION OF FATS. As we mentioned in the previous chapter, the vast majority of our dietary fats are triglycerides, complex macromolecules composed of three fatty acid chains bound covalently to one glycerol molecule. Because of their chemical composition and lack of a hydrated structure, that is, lack of the oxygen present in the hydroxyl ion, fats are not water soluble. The explanation for this lies in the fact that the atoms of different elements have differing abilities to attract the electrons they might share with other atoms. This atomic characteristic is called *electronegativity*, a concept first proposed by Linus Pauling in 1932, which contributed to his being awarded the Nobel Prize in Chemistry in 1954. (Pauling also was awarded the Nobel Peace Prize in 1962, and he remains the only individual to have been awarded two Nobel prizes that were not shared with other individuals.) Molecules in which hydrogen is bonded with another element that strongly attracts the electrons they share in their covalent bonds (such as oxygen, nitrogen, or fluorine) demonstrate the characteristic of electronegativity and therefore are polar; that is, the molecules develop a positive pole (where the hydrogen atom is) and a negative pole (where the electron-attracting heavier element is).

We can think of this as a molecular magnet. Water is a perfect example of this, and it is a highly polar liquid. Water molecules are highly attracted to one another because of this polarity with the positively charged hydrogen atoms being attracted to the negatively charged oxygen atoms of the adjacent water molecule. This attraction results from the formation of *hydrogen bonds*. Hydrogen bonds are not as strong as covalent bonds where electrons are shared between different atoms, but they are stronger than the weak, interatomic forces known as *van der Waals forces*, and they play an important role in the chemical and physical behavior of compounds that develop hydrogen bonding. The physical characteristic that most concerns us here is that substances that develop hydrogen bonds, that is, are polar, will mix with one another, whereas nonpolar substances will not mix with polar substances. As we noted, fats are long carbon chains with multiple hydrogen atoms but few oxygen atoms (only on the glycerol molecule). For this reason they do not have the characteristic of electronegativity; they are not polar, and they do not mix with polar solutions such as water. For an everyday example, we may think of what happens when we try to clean a greasy frying pan without soap—the fat or oil droplets just float around in the water but will not dissolve or disperse.

The above minilesson in physical chemistry is relevant for the following reason. The enzymes responsible for the digestive processes are all proteins and are water soluble. They are therefore only able to act on substrates that are presented to them either in solution or on a water interface. It is easy to see, then, that in a large globule of fat floating separately in an otherwise water environment, only the fat on the surface of the globule (and not the majority of fat on the inside of the globule) would be digestible. Our bodies handle this problem in the following way. Among the many constituents secreted into the duodenum by the pancreas, the liver adds its own secretions of two special organic compounds that make up the liquid we know as bile: the bile salts and the phospholipid called lecithin. Both the bile salts and lecithin share a physical characteristic that makes them *amphipathic* compounds—that is they have both hydrophilic (polar) and hydrophobic (nonpolar) properties.

Because of their polar and nonpolar attributes, lecithin and bile salts are able to act as emulsifiers. An emulsifier is an agent, usually with surface activity (surfactant), that has the ability to dissolve partly in water and partly in fat and cause otherwise immiscible liquids to mix into a stable, blended form called an emulsion. A good example of an unstable emulsion is an oil and vinegar salad dressing, which will quickly separate if not constantly shaken. This is actually an accurate picture of what happens to fats in the stomach; they are mechanically, but not chemically, emulsified. In the duodenum, however, the emulsifying action of lecithin and bile salts acts to chemically emulsify the fats as well, so that the resulting liquid becomes a suspension of microscopic fat droplets suspended in the otherwise water-based chyme. An excellent, everyday example of this is the effect of detergent (another emulsifying surfactant) in allowing the grease on dirty dishes to "mix" with the water in your sink so that the dishes can be cleaned. The physical effect of this in the digestive process is that the surface area of fat now accessible to the water-soluble fat digesting enzymes, or pancreatic lipases, is markedly increased. Just as the anatomy of the digestive tract demonstrates the development of folds on the absorptive surface from a macroscopic level (rugae in the stomach, valvulae connivantes in the small intestine) to the microscopic level (villi and microvilli in the small intestine) in order to increase the internal absorptive area many hundredfold above what would normally be present in such limited space, the process of emulsification does the same in the case of fat digestion on a molecular level.

As the lipases break the triglycerides into smaller components—for the most part fatty acids and monoglycerides—the bile salts play another major role. The enzymatic reaction that the lipases catalyze is highly reversible, so that if the fatty acids and monoglycerides were to remain in continuous contact with each other and the lipase, they would be converted back to triglycerides. The reason this does not occur to any significant extent is that the bile salts form submicroscopic droplets called *micelles*, units that arrange so that their hydrophilic (polar) ends are on the outside of the droplet (in a water environment) and their hydrophobic (nonpolar ends) are internally directed (away from the water environment). The fatty acids and monoglycerides created by the activity of the pancreatic lipase can then sequester themselves in the hydrophobic interior of the micelles, and they are then brought into contact with the brush borders of the enterocytes. Since the cell membrane of the enterocytes is a lipid bilayer, the fatty acids and monoglycerides are highly soluble in the membrane and passively diffuse into the cell, where they can then be transported into the central circulation—in the case of the fats, the lymphatic vessel or *lacteal* in the center of each villus.

Absorption

Once nutrients are broken down into their molecular components by the process of digestion, they still need to be transported from our internalization of the external environment—the bowel lumen—into our bodies' internal milieu. This is the process called *absorption*.

Absorption occurs through four basic mechanisms: active transport, passive diffusion, facilitated diffusion, and endocytosis.

In order to understand the challenges faced by cells in transporting substances across their limiting membranes, a brief review of the concept of osmosis is in order. Life on a microscopic level occurs in solution, and as we have noted previously, the *solvent*, or liquid phase, of biological solutions is water. The *solute*, or dissolved substance, may be something as simple as a sodium ion, as complex as a protein, or even a gas or another liquid. It is a physical trait of solutions that, when two compartments with different solute concentrations are separated by a semipermeable membrane (and a cellular membrane would fall into this category), water will pass from the compartment with a lower solute concentration into the compartment with a higher solute concentration until the solute concentrations equalize. The force generated by the movement of water in a system such as this is called its osmotic pressure. Osmosis is a passive process; that is, it does not require the expenditure of energy.

In order for osmotic pressure to develop, it requires some sort of gradient, be it a gradient of molecular particles, a chemical gradient, or, in the case of ions, an electrical gradient. Generally we refer to this as an electrochemical gradient. Movement in the direction of an electrochemical gradient, or "downhill," may occur passively, whereas movement against an electrochemical gradient, or "uphill," requires the expenditure of some form of energy—in the case of cellular transport, ATP.

THE SODIUM-POTASSIUM PUMP. The sodium-potassium pump is a mechanism fundamental to multiple cellular functions. It is the basic means by which substances, be they ions, nutrient molecules, or cellular messengers, are transported into the intracellular environment against an electrochemical gradient. Although the details of function and the specific substance being transported differ depending on the function being served, the underlying "engine" that drives the function is the sodium-potassium pump (and the underlying fuel for the pump is ATP).

The two ubiquitous *cations* (positively charged atoms or molecules) of life are sodium and potassium. Simplistically, life's processes are driven by a gradient of sodium (Na$^+$) and potassium (K$^+$) ions generated by living cells (the related *anions*, negatively charged ions—in this case chloride [Cl$^-$], follow passively). All living cells expend energy to generate this gradient, increasing the intracellular concentration of potassium compared to the external environment and conversely decreasing the internal sodium concentration relative to the external environment. In addition to the formation of this chemical gradient, a small but significant electrical gradient is established at the same time. As these processes create an electrochemical gradient, they require energy in the form of ATP to maintain. The process involves the enzymatic cleavage of the terminal phosphate bond of a molecule of ATP to form ADP (adenosine diphosphate) and a phosphate ion, so the pump is also called the sodium-potassium ATPase.

This works in the following way. Cellular membranes are basically monotonous lipid bilayers—sheets of molecules of phospholipids, molecules with a polar (water soluble) head group and a long, hydrocarbon (fatty or lipid) tail. The membrane is formed by two layers of these molecules, with the polar heads arrayed on the outside and inside of the membrane, facing the aqueous extracellular and intracellular environments, and the fatty hydrocarbon tails sandwiched in between. This membrane is protective and semipermeable to water, some ions, and some small fat-soluble molecules. For the purposes of this discussion we will assume this structure is otherwise biologically inert. (It isn't, actually, and it plays a major role in cell signaling, cell death, and so on.)

Embedded within the cell membrane are numerous, highly specialized molecules that function in an immense range of biological functions, one of which is the active transport of sodium and potassium. The protein involved in this function is embedded in the membrane as a transmembrane protein; that is, it spans the external and internal environments. In its resting state it has a receptor configuration, open to the interior of the cell that has a high affinity for sodium and the capacity for accepting three sodium ions. Once the sodium ions are bound in this receptor, the protein is phosphorylated by the cleavage of a phosphate from a bound molecule of ATP (hence the term *ATPase*), releasing energy and changing the tertiary conformation of the protein. In this new conformation, the receptor is now opened to the exterior of the cell and has a lower affinity for sodium, which now finds itself released on the other side of the cell membrane into the extracellular environment. Two potassium molecules are then bound to the receptor, which causes dephosphorylation of the protein; the protein molecule reverts to its original conformation, the receptor is now open to the interior of the cell, and the potassium ions are released internally. In this way the intracellular environment is made relatively sodium-poor and potassium-rich. Since we are exchanging three sodiums for two potassiums, an electrical gradient is established as well, making the interior of the cell electrically negative relative to the exterior—hence an electrochemical gradient. When the cell dies, this gradient quickly fades and vice versa; that is, if this gradient is disrupted to any significant degree, the cell dies.

It is through the dynamic tension created by this gradient that many cellular functions are accomplished, and it is via the sodium-potassium pump that the work of establishing this gradient is accomplished. (Jens Christian Skou, a Danish physiologist, discovered this mechanism in 1956 and shared the Nobel Prize in Medicine in 1997 in recognition of this important contribution.)

ACTIVE TRANSPORT. Active transport is the movement of atoms and small molecules across cell membranes mediated by specific membrane-bound proteins against an electrochemical gradient and therefore requiring the expenditure of energy. The basic example of active transport is the sodium-potassium pump, but depending on the structure and function of the specific membrane protein, two or more different types of molecules may be transported together in the same direction (*symporter*) or the opposite direction (*antiporter*). As an example, we can look at the active transport of glucose across the intestinal epithelium by the symporter SGLT-I (coded by a gene on chromosome 22q13.1 for the curious). SGLT-I is a member of a family of sodium-glucose transporting proteins found in the intestines and kidney. It functions by using the energy derived from the creation of a "downhill" sodium gradient to "drag" glucose across the intestinal brush-border epithelial membrane into the intestinal epithelial cell. The glucose is then transported out of the cell and into the circulation with the existing electrochemical gradient, mediated by a second type of membrane-bound transporting protein called a *uniporter*.

FACILITATED DIFFUSION. *Facilitated diffusion* is the process by which molecules that are not fat soluble (and therefore cannot passively diffuse through the cell membrane) can be transported across the membrane down the solute gradient. The process occurs through specific transmembrane proteins or pores that can be opened and closed depending on cellular signaling such as a transmembrane voltage, physical stress such as pressure, or specific *ligands* (substances that bind to the exterior or interior of the cell membrane and act as signals).

The simple sugars and small peptides and amino acids are transported both by active transport and facilitated diffusion. As noted earlier the micelles created by bile salts serve the function of "ferrying" the fatty acids that have been hydrolyzed from the triglycerides in the diet away from the highly reversible digestive process catalyzed by the lipase to bring them into contact with the intestinal epithelial brush border. As the fatty acids are nonpolar, they can easily diffuse across the lipid bilayer of the cell membrane by passive diffusion.

There is one other means by which nutrients can gain access to the circulation. Larger peptides and small proteins can sometimes be absorbed by the process called *endocytosis*, basically the same process we know as phagocytosis as when an amoeba engulfs its food. Although this process serves some necessary biological functions (for example, this is how iron is absorbed), it can be potentially dangerous. As we discuss in chapter 10, our bodies' immune systems function in general by a very sophisticated process of recognizing and remembering specific portions of foreign proteins (called antigens). It is due to the occasional absorption of large peptides or small whole proteins by the process of endocytosis that some food-related proteins can be presented intact to our immune systems and be the cause of food-induced allergies.

We started this chapter with the quote "Form follows function," and as this relates to absorption, we have seen how the small intestinal absorptive area is multiplied by the large folds (valvulae connivantes), villi, and brush border. Its structural form enhances its absorptive function. To fully understand how elegant this structural/functional congruency ultimately can become on a cellular level, we should consider the structure of a single villus.

If we were to look at a cross-section of the villus, we would see that the exterior side—that side presented to the intestinal lumen, which is essentially an extension of the outside environment—is covered by intestinal epithelial cells one layer thick. The luminal or, as it is called, apical portion of that cell is finely divided into the brush border and is bathed in the intestinal fluids and its digested nutrients. The internal, or basal, end of the cell abuts on a microscopic blood vessel called a capillary. Therefore nutrients absorbed by the brush border of that cell only have to travel the distance of one microscopic cell before coming in contact with our internal circulation (the capillary in the case of sugars and amino acids; a lymphatic vessel called a lacteal in the case of fats). That is 10 microns—ten millionths of a meter. For comparison sake, the period at the end of this sentence is more than fifty times larger than that. This same relationship holds in the other organs where our bodies interact vitally with our external environment, such as our lungs and kidneys. It is not an exaggeration therefore to say that we are physically separated from our external environment by the slimmest of boundaries, and therefore we are intimately interactive with it.

The Biochemistry of Nutrition and Starvation

If we think about it, our bodies are constantly being asked to adapt to changing environmental conditions; hot or cold, wet or dry, and relevant to this discussion, fed or fasting. Each of these conditions requires specific and significant physiological responses from our bodies, which exquisitely maintain our internal homeostasis.[3] For example our internal temperatures are maintained within a very tight range at 37 degrees Celsius (98.6 degrees Fahrenheit). Any prolonged shift by the relatively slight amount of 3 degrees—to 34 or 40 degrees Celsius (93 or 104 degrees Fahrenheit)—will quickly incapacitate and eventually kill us. The same can be said for the levels of electrolytes in our bodies (another term for the ions of sodium, potassium, chloride, and bicarbonate), formed elements of our blood such as red and white blood cells, and the nutrient molecules from which our cells derive energy and the building blocks we need to grow and maintain our own bodies. A normal concentration of glucose in our bloodstream between meals is generally considered to be between 70 and 100 milligrams (mg) per 100 milliters (or 1 deciliter [dl]). Any number above this, in the fasting state, is consistent with glucose intolerance or prediabetes, and if greater than 125 mg/dl, diabetes (these numbers are slightly controversial, but they are adequate for the purposes of this discussion). The lower level, however, is more tightly regulated, as symptoms that can significantly affect our bodies' functions may begin to appear at levels lower than 70 mg/dl. While the appearance of symptoms and their severity depend in part on the rapidity with which serum glucose levels drop as well as the absolute number, if they drop low enough the resulting hypoglycemia can rapidly lead to brain injury and death. The latter is due to the fact that, although most of our cells can use either carbohydrates in the form of glucose or fats in the form of fatty acids to derive energy and maintain themselves, our brain cells are exquisitely and entirely dependent on glucose (except for one special circumstance, as we discuss later in this chapter).

It is in large part because of our brain's absolute dependence on a steady supply of glucose that the homeostasis of our blood glucose levels is so critically important, but between our intermittent intake of food and our varying levels of physical activity, our bodies are constantly seeing substantial fluxes in the supply and demand for this basic nutrient. How do we maintain our blood glucose levels within such relatively tight parameters despite these swings in intake and utilization? How do these regulatory functions relate to the two opposing functions of our metabolism mentioned in the preceding chapter: anabolism (or biosynthesis), and catabolism (or respiration)? The science of metabolism is complex, and the detail is beyond the scope of this book, but there are some basic facts and precepts we should understand.

THE FED (ANABOLIC) STATE. As the food we eat is digested and absorbed, blood levels of the ingested nutrients begin to rise. Although this includes the simple sugars (glucose, fructose, and galactose); fatty acids and monoglycerides; and various amino acids, it is only the glucose levels that stimulate the secretion of the major anabolic hormone *insulin*.

Hormones (from the Greek: to set in motion) are chemical messengers that carry signals from one cell or group of cells to another group of cells; chemical messengers can have a local (*paracrine*) effect or distant (*endocrine*) effect in relation to the secreting cells. In the latter case the hormone is secreted into the bloodstream and will therefore affect all cells and organs that have a receptor for it. Insulin is a peptide (small protein) endocrine hormone synthesized and secreted exclusively by specialized cells found in the body of the pancreas, but the receptors for its actions are ubiquitous. As we saw earlier in this chapter, the pancreas plays a major role in the digestive process by secreting enzymes (and bicarbonate ions) into the small intestine. This is an *exocrine* function, defined as secreting substances into ducts or the lumens of other organs. Other exocrine glands include sweat glands, salivary glands, and mammary glands. The endocrine glands function without ducts and secrete their products directly into the bloodstream. Examples of endocrine glands include the adrenal glands, the thyroid gland and, in this case, the endocrine portion of the pancreas. The specialized cells in the pancreas that serve this function are called *β cells*, and they are found in isolated pockets embedded in the tissue of the pancreas called the *islets of Langerhans* (the name insulin itself comes from the Latin for island—*insula*).

As noted, insulin is the major anabolic hormone; that is, it is associated with storage of nutrients and growth. Its secretion is stimulated by rising blood glucose levels associated with a meal and signals the cells of the body to transport the glucose in the blood into their intracellular environments for use as energy and for storage. Insulin is not just the signal for this transport but is in fact necessary for the body's cells to transport glucose internally. It is this fact that causes the apparently paradoxical situation seen in juvenile-onset (or type 1) diabetes mellitus. Despite blood glucose levels much higher than normal (three-, four-, and even up to seven- or eightfold higher than normal), in the absence of insulin the body's cells cannot internalize the glucose, so the body's cells behave as if there is no glucose available: the cells behave catabolically, and the person's body mass melts away. In addition to being necessary for the internalization of glucose molecules into cells, insulin signals the liver and the skeletal muscles to store glucose in the form of the animal starch glycogen and signals the adipose (fat) tissue to internally transport the circulating fatty acids and store them as triglyceride. Excess calories, in the form of carbohydrate, can be stored as synthesized triglycerides or used to synthesize amino acids (in the case of the nonessential amino acids) that become new functional protein.

THE FASTING (CATABOLIC) STATE. During the fasting state the body is faced with the opposite problem. Rather than having to deal with excess glucose in the blood, the level has to be maintained despite continued usage by the cells of the body to keep us alive and functioning. During the fasting state insulin levels fall (although not to zero), and the actions of the major catabolic hormones cortisol, glucagon, and epinephrine dominate the metabolism. (It should be pointed out here that the steroid hormones are broadly grouped into three main types: the glucocorticoids, cortisol being the major one, involved in the metabolism of glucose and other nutrients; the mineralocorticoids, involved in the homeostasis of the electrolytes sodium and potassium; and the sex hormones.) The catabolic hormones stimulate the breakdown of glycogen into its component glucose molecules, the breakdown of stored triglycerides into its component fatty acids and glycerol, and the production of new glucose molecules, mostly in the liver, by the process of *gluconeogenesis*. Gluconeogenesis is the main process by which the body maintains homeostasis of the blood sugar levels that are critical to the continued function of the human brain. *De novo* glucose is derived from products of intermediary metabolism such as pyruvate, lactate, and products of the citric acid cycle. Most of the amino acids are glucogenic; thus, they can be utilized to synthesize new glucose, but most fatty acids cannot be used to make glucose (although the glycerol derived from the triglycerides is glucogenic).

Twice now we have mentioned the reliance of the human brain on glucose for its energy. Why this emphasis? In chapter 11 we explore the biological basis for political behavior, and as part of that discussion we try to understand what characteristics, if any, differentiate us from other animals. One physical characteristic that clearly differentiates us is the relative size and development of our brains, especially the neocortex that is the part of the brain responsible for language and consciousness. The human brain accounts for approximately 2 percent of a 150-pound human's weight—but 20 percent of resting oxygen consumption and energy requirements. (The first experiments on this subject were done by Seymour Kety at the University of Pennsylvania in the 1950s.)[4] Our brains are completely reliant on glucose for energy. Completely starved of oxygen or the energy source of glucose for as little as two minutes, the brain suffers irreversible, and at the present state of medical technology, irreparable injury. And yet, as we shall see in chapter 5, humans evolved as hunter-gatherers, well adapted to circumstances of frequent, at times prolonged, fasting. Considering the evolution of the glucose-hungry human brain at the same time that reliable food sources might have been intermittent at best, and at times unreliable, is there a biochemical adaptation humans might have evolved along with our highly developed brain that allows us to starve and survive the ordeal with our brains intact?

KETOGENESIS. In order to understand this very important adaptation, we turn to the outstanding review of the subject of starvation in man written by George F. Cahill Jr., MD, published in the *New England Journal of Medicine* in 1970 and still relevant and elegantly to the point today.[5] As we discussed in chapter 3, and as Dr. Cahill points out, our bodies store energy in the form of fat, protein (mainly in muscle), and carbohydrate in the form of the animal starch glycogen (in liver and muscle). Let us say that an average 150-pound (70-kilogram) man would store 33 pounds as fat, 13 pounds as protein, and a minimal 0.5 pounds as glycogen. We can see that man has two major forms of energy storage: protein and fat, and, for reasons we go into in more detail in chapter 8, protein is relatively spared as an energy source. Fat, therefore, is our major form of storing potential energy for future needs. But as we have learned above, the brain cannot use fat for energy, and we cannot make adequate amounts of glucose from fat. The latter point is specifically relevant to the size of our brains relative to the rest of our bodies. Large mammals, such as black bears and certain cetaceans (whales), go through very long periods of fasting, but they are able to produce enough glucose throughout these long periods of fasting to keep their brains functioning. There are two basic reasons for this. The first is that their brains use a relatively small percentage of their energy requirements when compared to the rest of their bodies. The second is that they have massive fat stores compared to the size of their brains, so that as they metabolize their stored triglycerides, there is enough glycerol (which is glucogenic) created that can be converted to glucose without cannibalizing skeletal muscle protein for its glucogenic amino acids.[6]

This is not the situation in human beings. From data obtained in early experiments (on hapless medical students) in the first part of the twentieth century, we know that in one day an average, fasting male might burn 1800 calories, derived from 75 grams of skeletal muscle protein and 160 grams of triglyceride from adipose tissue. Daily availability of glucose approximates 180 grams derived from gluconeogenesis. A total of 144 grams of this glucose (80 percent) is consumed by our central nervous system (mostly the brain) and is completely metabolized through the citric acid cycle to carbon dioxide and water. There are other tissues in the body that depend on glucose, and these other glycolytic tissues such as erythrocytes (red blood cells), leukocytes (white blood cells), bone marrow, parts of the kidney, and peripheral nerves also metabolize glucose but convert it primarily to lactate and pyruvate. These intermediate products of glucose metabolism, as noted above, can be reconverted into glucose by a process called the Cori cycle. As you might expect, this requires energy in the form of ATP. The energy required to convert two molecules of lactate into one molecule of glucose comes from the oxidation of fat in the liver. This glucose can then be released into the bloodstream, once again metabolized into lactate, and recycled once again. In this way the body can indirectly convert fat into glucose by this "energy shuttle"; that is, glucose-dependent tissues indirectly obtain their energy from fat. In addition, protein is spared by limiting the need for gluconeogenesis.

As these biochemical processes are initiated, triggered by a complex interplay of hormonal messengers, the rest of the body's cells alter their metabolisms by converting from the primary use of glucose (which now must be conserved for use by the brain) to the use of a fuel created by the metabolism of fat. In the fasting state, the citric acid cycle activity is diminished, so as fat is partially oxidized through the process of β-oxidation, the acetyl CoA produced is converted in the liver to acetate (two carbons) and then to the four-carbon compounds acetoacetate and β-hydroxybutyrate. These two compounds are known as *ketone bodies* and are the important products of ketogenesis and of the state known as ketosis. These small products of fat metabolism are important for the following reasons. First, they can be used by most tissues as sources of energy, replacing the need for glucose. Second, they are water soluble (unlike their parent fat molecules) and can therefore enter the central nervous system and be accessible to the brain. So as the Cori cycle is activated, and the process of gluconeogenesis is diminished by that "energy shuttle," the tissues of the body that are not glucose dependent switch to utilization of the ketone bodies released into the circulation by the liver, sparing the available glucose for the brain and other glucose-dependent tissues.

In summary, the biochemical adaptations that occur in the brief fasting state use two sources of energy: skeletal muscle protein and adipose tissue triglyceride. There are three pathways of metabolism of the resultant fuels: complete glucose metabolism in the brain via glycolysis and the citric acid cycle; metabolism of glucose in peripheral glucose-dependent tissue such as red blood cells by the glycolytic pathway such that the resultant intermediate products can be reconverted to glucose using fat-derived energy; and metabolism of fat and its intermediate ketone bodies by the remainder of the body's tissues. The latter two pathways are specifically aimed at sparing the body's protein and reserving all available glucose for the brain. Think of this as a great ballroom dance; the conductor is the array of hormonal messengers (led by insulin), the orchestra is the liver, and the dancers the rest of the body.

As Dr. Cahill points out, as one transitions from brief to prolonged fasting, certain inconsistencies must be explained. If we do the math, we can see that the 180 grams of glucose that we can measure being produced during brief fasting cannot be accounted for from the sum of 20 grams of glycerol derived from triglyceride metabolism, 36 grams of lactate and pyruvate recycled in the Cori cycle, and the 75 grams of amino acid derived from protein metabolism. This gap is most likely filled by the utilization of stores of liver glycogen, which are rapidly depleted (and not repleted in the fasting state). Of even greater concern is the following. If we continued to break down 75 grams of protein a day to provide adequate glucogenic amino acids for even the diminished gluconeogenesis necessary to provide adequate glucose for the brain, we would have depleted our body's protein by one-third within a few weeks, a state that is not consistent with survival.

And yet man can survive for months in a state of starvation. What other biochemical adaptations allow us to conserve protein and yet maintain the function of our energy-avid central nervous system? As it has been shown that urinary nitrogen excretion, and therefore protein metabolism, markedly diminishes in starving man, either the brain must decrease its energy consumption (which would lead to a state of diminished consciousness and function inconsistent with survival), glucose must be produced from fatty acids (a process not significantly demonstrated in animals), or the brain must be able to adapt to another fuel source. The latter explanation is indeed the case, and as reported by Owen and colleagues in the *Journal of Clinical Investigation* in 1967, on prolonged fasting the brain converts from glucose oxidation to the fuels of ketosis—acetoacetate and β-hydroxybutyrate.[7] As Dr. Cahill points out, it is this simple biochemical adaptation that allows weeks of starvation to be extended to months, while sparing gluconeogenesis and body protein. Cahill further goes on to point out that "in an approximate manner, the phylogenic capacity for fasting ketosis to develop parallels the development of the central nervous system, and man, with his large brain, may show the greatest degree of adaptation to keto acid utilization by this organ."[8] In this particular case biochemical form (the physiology of the fasting state) beautifully follows anatomical function (the high energy needs of our highly evolved brain). We should also learn from this that as we evolved physically, there was a parallel evolution of our biochemical function.

Summary

In summary, our bodies are anatomically and functionally perfectly engineered from the macroscopic level through the microscopic level and down to the molecular function of our biochemistry. We are able to take in complex nutrients from our external environment, process them physically and chemically into their basic constituents, and internalize them for our own use to producing the energy and building blocks needed for our own growth and survival. In addition, we are able to direct the storage and use of these nutrients in specific and discriminating ways to maximize the function of vital organs and minimize the survival disadvantage that might be imposed by periods of inadequate nutrition. We will see in chapters 8 and 9 why this is so critically important and how prolonged periods of inadequate nutrition, from either a total caloric or specific nutrient deficiency, can have disastrous results.

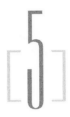

Agriculture The Birth of Civilization . . . and Famine

Man's life in the natural state would be "solitary, poor, nasty,
brutish, and short."
—Thomas Hobbes, *Leviathan*, 1651

Let us not forget that the cultivation of the earth is the most
important labor of man. When tillage begins, other arts follow.
The farmers, therefore, are the founders of human civilization.
—Daniel Webster (1782–1852)

Why did agriculture develop? The sentiments of the seventeenth-century English philosopher Thomas Hobbes stated above suggest that humans' lives in our ancestral environment would be incentive enough to find a better way. The archeological record, however, suggests that members of early agrarian societies were potentially worse off than contemporaneous hunter-gatherers. Evidence suggests that, at least in some cases, they were less well-nourished, had more serious diseases, and died at younger ages. Furthermore the above quote from the great American statesman Daniel Webster seems like a rather simplistic, overreaching claim for a very complex process. Yet Webster was known as an intelligent, eloquent, and ethical political leader of the nineteenth century; in 1957 the U.S. Senate named him one of five of the most outstanding members of the Senate in history. So what did Webster mean when he made the bold comment above? If we agree he was correct, why and how did agriculture evolve as our dominant strategy for access to nutrition after millennia of success as hunter-gatherers, and why, as the chapter title states, is it a prerequisite for famine?

Jared Diamond, in *Guns, Germs, and Steel*,[1] outlines the present thinking on why and how agriculture developed when it did.

According to Diamond, there are five factors that explain why agriculture became the predominant lifestyle for early man.

- Decreased availability of certain wild foods, perhaps in part due to man's increasing proficiency as a hunter.
- Increased availability of other wild foods suitable for domestication, due to the end of the Pleistocene glaciation about 10,000 years ago.

- The development of technologies that had originally been developed for collecting and storing wild foods, but were then applicable to processing the larger quantities that could be produced by agriculture.
- An autocatalytic process during which an increasing population caused an increased demand for food, which in turn led to pressures to produce reliable supplies of foods on a predictable basis.

Agrarian societies have substantial competitive advantages over hunter-gatherer societies as the former's sedentary lifestyle is conducive to producing more children, and only a proportion of an agrarian population is needed to produce enough food for all, allowing others to develop additional skills (like making tools and weapons).

Although Diamond presents a coherent and useful explanation for the development of agriculture 10,000 to 13,000 years ago, there are, in fact, a number of competing hypotheses as to why and how agriculture developed. Raphael Pumpelly, a professor of geology at Harvard University in the early 1900s,[2] first suggested an oasis theory, suggesting that an increasingly drier climate forced humans and animals into close proximity, which drove the process of domestication, a theory later expanded and popularized by the archeologist Vere Gordon Childe[3] (about whom we say more later in this chapter). There is a *feasting hypothesis* suggesting that man's natural tendency to exert dominance led to the development of agriculture in order to enable would-be rulers to host feasts (and control the food supply).[4] Saur and Binford have proposed and expanded a *demographic theory* of increasingly large sedentary populations requiring more abundant and predictable food supplies (one arm of Diamond's autocatalytic process).[5] There is an *evolutionary/intentionality theory* proposed by David Rindos suggesting a coevolution of plants and humans[6] (which to our minds is basically an explanation of the process of domestication). Since agriculture developed and evolved de novo in a number of independent sites and spread throughout areas of human habitation at varying speeds, it is most probable that all the factors addressed by these theories, as well as others not mentioned here, played a significant role in man's discovery and expansion of the basic concepts and further development of agricultural science. Diamond's fifth point, however, is directly pertinent to the title of this chapter and speaks to Webster's important observation. The development of agriculture enabled increasingly large percentages of agrarian populations to engage in other pursuits, developing surpluses of food and other goods but, more importantly, developing their uniquely human capital. For this reason the development of agriculture was the enabling factor for the birth and evolution of what we call civilization.

Agriculture began at a time well before recorded history, in fact, at least 4000 years before the first written language. For this reason our knowledge of events leading up to and driving the early evolution of agriculture is fragmentary, incomplete, and still the subject of debate. What is not in question is the fact that agriculture did evolve to the point that it is unarguably the dominant means by which the vast majority of Earth's population produces and procures its food supply. Clearly, there are social and cultural benefits to having only a relatively small percentage of a population engaged in producing our food supply, allowing the population to grow, and leaving others free to engage in other forms of commerce and recreation. Should that food supply fail, however, a situation will develop that would not occur in a population dependent on hunting and gathering for its sustenance.

In the hunter-gatherer society, the population is limited necessarily by two basic facts. The first is that the nomadic lifestyle of the hunter-gatherer imposes the need to limit the birthrate so that only one babe-in-arms is present in a family at any one time. This practice is seen today in the few remaining hunter-gatherer societies, where fecundity may be limited biologically by lactational amenorrhea (continued lactation and breast-feeding tends to suppress ovulation and menstruation), culturally by sexual abstinence, or even by the more brutal methods of abortion or infanticide. The second fact is that the population will be naturally limited to the number that can be reasonably (and reliably) sustained by the nutritional output of uncultivated land (a somewhat Malthusian concept, as we discussed in chapters 1 and 2). For this reason, hunter-gatherers live in units of moderately sized extended families or, at the most, tribal societies, as opposed to the more "advanced" groupings of towns and cities found in agrarian cultures. Although members of a hunter-gatherer tribe may go hungry, or one or more of their food sources might occasionally fail, it is highly unlikely that all of their food sources would fail over such a wide region that large-scale famine would develop. The same cannot be said for agrarian societies. Only 0.1 percent of the biomass of an uncultivated acre might be available as nutrient to a human (mostly because most natural biomass is in the form of cellulose, which we cannot digest), whereas up to 90 percent of the biomass of a cultivated acre may be edible. Therefore, a far greater number of people can be supported on much less land, and when larger numbers of people than can be sustained by the natural production of the land are dependent on the production of food by a small percentage of that population and food production fails, the result is famine: malnutrition, starvation, and ultimately death on a large scale. This is especially easy to understand if the population is dependent on a relatively undiversified crop, such as the potato, as we shall see when we discuss the Great Irish Famine of the mid-nineteenth century. It is for this reason that the title of this chapter credits the development of agriculture with the birth of civilization—but also the birth of the possibility for widespread famine.

So it seems that Webster was right in his assessment, and over the long term possibly Hobbes as well, albeit for the wrong reasons.

Development of Agriculture
as a Model for Human Divergence

We may develop the line of thinking a bit further in order to understand that the development of agriculture led to a divergence of our biological, social, and technological evolutions. There are a number of attributes that seem to differentiate us from the other animals with which we share this planet, although actually defining these differences can be quite difficult (and frequently controversial). One of these differences is that human beings have embarked on a degree of social and technological evolution that has outstripped our biological evolution in regard to our relationships with ourselves and our environment. All life forms modify their immediate environment to a greater or lesser degree and in some cases make modifications that may have more far-reaching environmental effects. For example many microorganisms produce biologically active substances that make their immediate environments more "user friendly" for themselves or more "user unfriendly" for organisms that might compete with them for nutrients. An example of the latter is the mold *Penicillium chrysogenum*, which produces and secretes a substance in its immediate vicinity that inhibits local growth of bacteria that might otherwise compete with the mold for nutrients. This was incidentally noted by the bacteriologist Alexander Fleming in 1928 and led to the subsequent isolation and purification of the antibiotic penicillin, for which Fleming (and Florey and Chain) shared the Nobel Prize for Medicine in 1945. Larger animals, such as elephants, have substantial effects on their local environments that end up having far-reaching effects on the greater environment, such as maintenance of savannah grasslands. The most extreme example of this in nature is the effect that early plant life had on the earth's atmosphere and the eventual evolution of other, oxygen-requiring life forms. Most of the interactions of living organisms with their environments, however, are, as Charles Darwin pointed out, very much in the other direction; that is, environments dictate the form and function of the organisms living in them by the dual processes of mutation and natural selection, the two drivers of evolution.

According to the fossil and archeological record, *Homo sapiens* differentiated from earlier hominids about 250,000 years ago, although there is genetic evidence based on analysis of mitochondrial and Y-chromosome DNA that the ancestor of modern humanity appeared on the African continent only about 60,000 years ago[7] (the actual timeline is controversial, and discussion of this is well beyond the scope of this book). Two traits of early *H. sapiens* were the use of language (which markedly changed and accelerated our social evolution) and our ability to conceive of and use tools (which markedly changed and accelerated our technological evolution). Despite the significant effects of these traits on the lives of our early ancestors, those developments had relatively little effect on our ancestral environment. The far-reaching effects they might have had on early humans were limited in extent and scope to their immediate local environment.

Biologically, we evolved to live in that ancestral environment as hunter-gatherers. What that means, in essence, is that early man took advantage of the nutrition available in his environment in an opportunistic fashion, gathering plant material such as seeds, fruits, and grains, and easily accessible animals such as insects, grubs, and the occasional unlucky reptile, amphibian, and small mammal. Larger mammals and birds were hunted. Language certainly aided our hunting ability in terms of group cooperation, and the development of increasingly sophisticated weapons of individual destruction made us more successful in killing the large mammalian prey available at the time. Nonetheless, as a species we did little to actively alter our environment on a large scale, although, as we noted above, there is an argument that one of the drivers of the development of agriculture was the disappearance from the environment of large prey due to the success of Paleolithic hunters at the end of the Pleistocene epoch.

As agriculture evolved and became the dominant way in which humans lived and provided for their nutritional needs, cultures developed that led to the growth and evolution of increasingly complex and sophisticated civilizations, allowing people to develop skills beyond those needed for subsistence, as well as surpluses in food and other goods. A more advanced understanding of this is in the concept of capital—especially human capital. Adam Smith (1723–1790), the Scottish philosopher and economist who is considered the father of modern economics (and the father of the concept of "the invisible hand of the market"), described four forms of fixed capital (that is, areas of investment that lead to revenue without themselves being consumed): machines, buildings, improvement of land, and human capital.[8] The last is defined as any trait or skill that enhances an individual's ability to be productive within his specific environment. Such traits include innate abilities such as intelligence and physical prowess, although education, training, and experience played an increasingly important role as societies (and their related technologies) evolved. There is an excellent description of human capital and its value, as well as the suggestion that a proximate if not ultimate cause of poverty is the lack of investment in human capital, in Charles Wheelan's book *Naked Economics*.[9] Many executives and managers ascribe to the concept that their workforce, their human capital, is the most important asset of their enterprise. The most successful of these managers actually believe it.

An unfortunate consequence of this expansion of societies, however, is that civilized populations became dependent on a mode of food production that is inherently risky due to either unanticipated acts of God or unanticipated (or flagrantly purposeful) acts of man, as discussed in chapters 1 and 2. A more subtle outcome is that abundant food sources have given us the freedom to invest time and resource into our growth as intellectual organisms as opposed to physical organisms, allowing our social and technological evolution to move apace exponentially, while our biological evolution continues, at least visibly, at the Darwinian pace it has always followed.

There is a major consequence of this almost instantaneous (in terms of geologic timeframes) explosive growth of our intensely agricultural society. As agriculture has become more technologically industrialized, it has become dependent on the unfettered, unsustainable use of energy derived from fossil fuel (an unrenewable source of ancient solar energy) as pointed out by Michael Pollan in his book *The Omnivore's Dilemma*.[10] This, along with other forms of pollution associated with our social and technological evolution, has markedly altered the earth's atmosphere, biosphere, and climate. By those yardsticks we have unquestionably changed our planet's environment far more than the environment has changed us, to some extent reversing the direction of cause and effect as generally accepted in the Darwinian view of our natural world. Of some interest in this regard, the explosive growth of agriculture as a catalytic influence on our social and technological growth did not occur so much as a process of evolution as it did by a process of revolution.

The Agricultural Revolutions

Natural scientists view geologic change relative to timeframes that are, in part, determined by whether we are referring to abiotic processes (nonliving chemical or physical aspects of the environment) or biological processes. For example the growth of mountain chains due to the shifting of tectonic plates would be an abiotic process, whereas the change in the Earth's atmosphere, from a relatively carbon dioxide–rich atmosphere to an oxygen-rich atmosphere due to the action of photosynthesizing plants, is a biological process. On a geologic scale, time is measured by eons, eras, periods, epochs, and stages, with the definition of each epoch being identifiable events within definable eras. Thus, an era contains multiple epochs. We are now in the Cenozoic era which began 65.5 million years ago with the Paleocene epoch measured geologically by the Cretaceous-Tertiary extinction event of the dinosaurs. Furthermore, we are in the Neogene period, which began with the Miocene epoch 23 million years ago measured by the appearance in the fossil record of modern birds, mammals, and the first apes. Finally, we are in the Holocene epoch (which began 11,430 years ago, measured by the end of the most recent glaciation and the rise of human civilization). To summarize this confusing time scale, we are in the Holocene epoch of the Neogene period, of the Cenozoic era. Note that, although we are measuring these relatively recent epochal events in terms of the biological fossil record, the causes of these changes were in fact abiotic: for example, a catastrophic event such as a possible giant meteorite causing a "nuclear winter" or multiple factors leading to generalized global warming or cooling leading to shifts in glaciation.

Unlike these geologic timeframes, substantive changes that are brought about by active human behavior occur in much shorter time periods and are usually termed revolutions (as opposed to epochs). Revolution (from the Latin, *revolutio*: turnaround) can be defined as a fundamental change occurring in a relatively sudden timeframe. The word may be used to refer to social/political upheaval, as in the American Revolution; a sudden shift in our view of the universe (and our place in it) as in the Copernican Revolution; or in our present use of the term to describe relatively abrupt changes in how we interact with our environment.

For the purposes of this discussion, we can broadly choose four recognized revolutionary periods in human history that are related to agriculture: the Neolithic Revolution, which led to the shift to agriculturally based subsistence and the birth of civilization as we know it; the Muslim Agricultural Revolution, which led to major advances in agriculture and increased urbanization; the British Agricultural Revolution, which is felt to have spurred (or at least to have been autocatalytic with) the Industrial Revolution; and the Green Revolution, which is the agricultural component of the Postindustrial Revolution (increasingly apparent as an ill-advised triumph of technology over biology).

The Neolithic Revolution[11] (also called the First Agricultural Revolution), a term coined in the 1920s by the Australian archaeologist Vere Gordon Childe, refers to the period between 12,000 and 8000 years ago, when the transition occurred from a nomadic hunter-gatherer lifestyle to agriculture and a more settled, sedentary lifestyle. This transition is considered to be the birth of human civilization. In addition to the ensuing effects on human sociological and technological evolution, this change in focus for the acquisition of his food caused a major shift in man's relationship to, and attitude toward, his environment that was markedly disparate from the worldview of the hunter-gatherer.

As pointed out by Lewin and Leakey in their book *Origins*,[12] the hunter-gatherer considered himself part of nature, whereas the farmer's goal is to control nature and bend it to his will. As the farmer works to create fields, plant, cultivate, and harvest crops and accumulate the excess food and additional "wealth" associated with the freeing up of people and time to devote to other enterprises, he must also expend time and effort to protect and defend the fruits of his labor against others who might take them by force. This behavior has been postulated to explain why our cultures evolved not as cooperative, communal societies but as more insular, inwardly directed societies aimed at protecting the rights of personal ownership and defending "us" against "them." An additional outcome of this shift to ownership and differentiation between "insiders" and "outsiders" is felt to be the advent of slavery—the belief that one man can own the work effort or the actual person of another human being. Although it may well be true that the fossil record and early written history supports this observation, we believe there is substantial evidence in the sciences of ethology (animal behavior) in general and human behavior in specific to suggest that we are, to some extent, biologically hardwired to be quite comfortable with an "us-them" paradigm and therefore willing to allow others to suffer indignities, suffering, and deaths that we would fight to our last breath were anyone to attempt to impose them on us. (This theory will be further explicated in chapter 11.) We can recognize as well that Western social, philosophical, and religious frameworks tend to be conceptually binary in nature—good versus evil, right versus wrong, heaven versus hell—and therefore antithetical to integrative models. Whether this is a cultural trait that enhances a hardwired tendency or is in fact a direct result of genetically hardwired behavior is an intriguing question beyond the scope of the current discussion. We present evidence in chapter 11 that it is both.

The Neolithic Revolution was the point of transition from a hunter-gatherer lifestyle to an agrarian lifestyle resulting in the birth and growth of civilizations. As we have said, this was almost certainly triggered and sustained by a multiplicity of events, including the abiotic geologic and climatic transitions as well as the biotic interactions between man and his environment—the plants and animals with which he interacted. Agricultural practices evolved over the ensuing millennia, with a possible "secondary products revolution" involving the increased utilization of domesticated animals for more than just meat but also milk, wool, leather, burden, and transport, which occurred during the third and fourth millennia BCE.[13]

The next quantum change enabling substantial increases in food production did not occur until what has been termed the Muslim or Arab Agricultural Revolution during the eighth to thirteenth centuries. Rather than being associated with transforming geologic shifts, these changes were a product of the advances in culture, science, and technology associated with the expansion of Islamic influence throughout the Old World. In addition to the creation of a global economy of the time, which led to the dispersion of previously isolated agricultural crops (sugar and cotton being among the most important), this era also saw the introduction of new concepts of crop rotation and, most importantly, mechanized irrigation.[14]

Agriculture did not change substantially in Europe throughout the Middle Ages, but a number of practices coalesced in England during the eighteenth century to bring about yet more improvement in agricultural productivity, a development termed the British Agricultural Revolution. There are four developments that are commonly cited as driving this process: enclosure, mechanization, four-field crop rotation, and selective breeding. *Enclosure* was the process by which the open-field, postfeudal practice of subsistence farming converted the use of common land to the more efficient, albeit exclusive, husbandry of the land by selected individuals. Although this led to more efficient use and increased productivity of the land, it forced large segments of the population to move to less rural areas to find work and in effect caused them the loss of entitlement to the food produced on the land to which they formerly had access. As we noted when we discussed Amartya Sen's theory on famine, this was a critical development. *Mechanization* was the technological development of machines capable of taking advantage of these large plots of land, the most famous inventor of which was Jethro Tull, who is said to have invented the seed-driller.

Perhaps more important to the actual advancement of crop productivity were the modern plow, which markedly improved the farmer's ability to rapidly prepare land for planting, and the horse-collar, which allowed the use of the faster, more nimble horse as compared to oxen (the yoke used to hitch oxen to a plow would choke a horse if used to pull any significant weight). Farmers in earlier times had used three-crop rotations, requiring significant areas of land to remain fallow in order to regain their fertility; but in the eighteenth century a four-field crop rotation was developed, adding clover (a legume that fixes nitrogen and adds it back to the soil) and turnips (that could be used to feed livestock) and allowing the farmer to leave less land fallow. Finally, major advances in the understanding of selective breeding of livestock resulted in larger, more productive animals.

The importance of the increase in agricultural productivity at this time is not limited only to the improved productivity of available food but also to the fact that the concurrent substantial growth of the population could be supported and was therefore available as a workforce (and as a ready-made market) for the Industrial Revolution.

The final agricultural revolution for us to consider is the *Green Revolution*, a term first used in 1968 by William Gaud, the former director of the U.S. Agency for International Development. Norman Borlaug, considered to be the father of the Green Revolution, in 1943 introduced to Mexico the proven agricultural techniques (use of pesticides, petroleum-derived nitrogen fertilizers, advanced irrigation techniques, and genetically modified crops) that had been fruitful in industrialized nations, with a level of performance that attracted the attention and support of the Rockefeller Foundation. Subsequent gains followed in India in the 1960s, fending off predicted famines both in the short and long term. Borlaug was awarded the Nobel Peace Prize in 1970 for his work in increasing the world food supply. He has attracted substantial criticism, however, both from adherents to Thomas Malthus's original theory that growth in the food supply can never keep up with the growth of human populations, as well as from environmentalists who point to the substantial negative environmental effects of industrialized agriculture from the perspectives of overuse of petrochemicals (both as fuel for the industry and as fertilizer for the crops), pesticides, introduction of genetically modified organisms, and decreased biodiversity caused by intensive monoculture. In addition, the ultimate failure of this strategy in Asia was evidence that it was not the panacea for our species' need for increasing amounts of food.

Two points are illustrated by the preceding outline of the development and subsequent evolution of agriculture over the past 10,000 years. The first point is that the growth of agriculture, since the original "revolution" in the Neolithic period, has been fueled more by social and technological advancement than by biological evolution, and so it has potentially reached an inevitable Malthusian endpoint, outstripping the Earth's biological capacity to contain it and possibly our biological capacity to manage it. The image that this possibility brings to mind is that of a social-technological "tiger-by-the-tail" scenario wherein we are all okay—as long as we can hold on to the tiger's tail. The other image brought to mind is that of an inadvertent, global Ponzi scheme—the eventual denouement of which one does not care to imagine. Although a disastrous outcome may not be inevitable, the loud call for consideration of a second Green Revolution, with an eye toward healing and maintaining a healthy environment while producing a sustainable, accessible food supply for the world's population, is a call we must heed.[15] Unanswered questions remain, however. Is a second Green Revolution necessary? Is a second Green Revolution even feasible? Our answer: perhaps, but a functional, sustainable solution will not be produced by technology alone, unless it is accompanied by substantial changes in the way we approach the problem morally. This is a critical point we explore further in the next section.

The second point implicit in the foregoing discussion has to do with the fact that producing more food does not necessarily achieve the goal of ending world hunger. In fact, as discussed in chapters 1 and 2, hunger, chronic malnutrition, and famine frequently occur in the presence of adequate food for all. The problem lies not in the presence or absence of food but in people's access to it. Consider the story in Genesis of Joseph.

When Joseph had been sold by his brothers and brought down into Egypt, he gained the favor of the Pharaoh and prospered.[16] He had gained the reputation for being able to interpret dreams by correctly interpreting the dreams, and the fates, of the Pharaoh's cupbearer and chief baker, so that when the Pharaoh had a dream that no one could interpret, he called for Joseph.[17] The Pharaoh had dreamt that he had seen seven healthy, fat cattle come out of the river, followed by seven sick, thin cattle, which proceeded to eat the healthy ones. He then dreamt that he saw seven healthy, full heads of grain on one stalk, followed by seven sickly, withered heads of grain (blasted by the east wind) that proceeded to consume the healthy ones. Joseph interpreted the dreams as God's future intent. The seven healthy, fat cattle and seven full heads of grain represented seven years of plentiful harvest and the seven sickly cattle and seven withered heads of grain represented a subsequent seven years of crop failure and famine. Joseph counseled Pharaoh to choose a wise man to administer the crop production during the years of plenty and to put by one-fifth of all produced to feed the population during the time of famine. Pharaoh chose Joseph, who efficiently did as he had counseled. During the ensuing seven years of famine that appeared as Joseph had predicted, the stores of grain that Joseph had amassed were able to avert famine in Egypt while people in other lands starved.[18]

Although there is clearly a lesson to be learned in this fact alone (and many other lessons in the full story of Joseph and his brothers), there is another, more insidious warning in this biblical allegory. As the people of Egypt became progressively dependent on Joseph's stored grain, they were forced to buy it from him until they ran out of money. They next were forced to trade their livestock for food, and finally had to relinquish the ownership of their land to Pharaoh in exchange for the grain that Joseph had stored (but they had produced).[19]

These are the classic "coping strategies" we see in modern famines, and at the end of it all, the people had lost their entitlement to the food produced on their own land. This was a critically important transition between the Neolithic hunter-gatherer conceptualization of being an intrinsic inseparable part of the land and the agrarian-based cultures' concept of land (and chattel) ownership (or disenfranchisement). As we have seen, this concept of loss of entitlement is a fundamental element of the contemporary theory of famine expounded by Amartya Sen.

In considering these two points—the fact that our attempts to constantly increase our agricultural outputs technologically, at substantial harm to our environment, in order to stave off a Malthusian outcome on the one hand, and the fact that just producing more food will not answer the loss of entitlement factors elucidated by Sen on the other hand—it becomes evident that there is an unfortunate synergy between the Malthusian and Senian factors of famine.

The Tragedy of the Commons

In 1832, during the Michaelmas term, the Reverend W. F. Lloyd, MA, delivered two lectures at the University of Oxford, based on the Malthusian concepts of population growth and agricultural sustainability.[20] He made an interesting observation in regard to preventive checks (or moral restraint), which was that "systems of equality, with a community of labour and goods, are highly unfavorable to it [moral restraint]." As explanation he noted that in cases in which two men agree to labor jointly, the effort of one man results in his enjoying only half of the benefit of that work, as the other man also receives benefit. In a situation in which a "multitude" shares the benefit, but he makes the total investment, there is essentially no incentive at all for the individual to either invest in the shared resource or demonstrate prudence in its consumption. In 1968, Garrett Hardin, a professor of biology at the University of California, Santa Barbara, elaborated on this concept in an article in *Science* that he titled "The Tragedy of the Commons."[21] Hardin uses the example of men pasturing their cattle on common land. Each man is given incentive to increase the size of his herd, as the benefit of each animal accrues only to him, while the cost of supporting each additional animal is borne by everyone. Of course, the end result is overgrazing and loss of the commonly held resource as the pressure on its use causes that resource to become unsustainable. In an article in *The Encyclopedia of Environmental Sciences*, DeYoung notes that this is actually not a new concept, quoting Aristotle's observation that "what is common to the greatest number has the least care bestowed on it."[22] The crux of Hardin's (and Aristotle's and Lloyd's) point, however, was that there is not a technological solution for this problem and that the solution will depend on our ability to alter "human values or ideas of morality." As the world's economies and societies become increasingly globalized, this concept becomes central in our understanding that the inequities in access to resources, be they food, health care, or other benefits of a healthy economy, are manifestations of this drive to utilize available resources viewed as "common assets," with no attention paid to the fact that they are limited, frequently unrenewable, and unprotected. As Hardin himself recognized on considering his essay, it should have been called "The Tragedy of the Unregulated Commons."

How is this relevant to our discussion about agriculture? We have seen global resources as "up for grabs" (see section on "land-grabbing" in chapter 13), common resources that no one has the responsibility for conserving, and as Hardin and others predicted, we have behaved with the philosophy of "every man for himself, and the devil take the hindmost." We started this chapter discussing the advent and growth of agriculture as humankind's dominant strategy for producing and ensuring adequate nutrition, and the interaction of that revolutionary development, in some respects the ultimate disruptive technology if you will, with our innate characteristic as social animals that led to the birth and growth of civilization. How did we arrive at the present point in our discussion? Why is there such a gap between what the physical sciences tell us "what is" and what the social sciences tell us "what should be?"

A good deal of the answer may lie in the fact that we are biological entities, constrained physically and to some degree mentally (as discussed in chapter 11) by that very biology. We are also social and technological beings, at least in our orientation. Why do we appear to be stymied by what appears to be a simple moral problem well within our economic and technological means to solve? Why do we appear to be doomed to continuously repeat a history from which we never seem to learn? Is it that we are looking for technological solutions to moral problems? There is an imbalance between our biological capacity to functionally solve the problems we have created with our social systems and our technology; that is, we can produce enough food for all but cannot create the systems of personal responsibility that would ensure access to that food for all. We are driven to develop the technology, but perhaps a biological predisposition to make the fruits of that technology universally available is what is lacking. We have the biological predisposition to solve our problems technically, but this is a problem that requires a moral solution.

The questions with which we are now faced appear to have neither obvious nor straightforward answers. Our social evolution has outpaced our biological evolution, and our technological evolution has outstripped both. In terms of our food supply, we appear to be at a possible technological dead end. Perhaps we have indeed reached a Malthusian endpoint that we have merely postponed by progressively increasing our ability to improve agricultural yields, albeit with the use of technologies that will ultimately prove these yields to be unsupportable by our environment and unsustainable in regard to restricted and unrenewable resources. On the other hand, hundreds of millions of people today suffer from chronic malnutrition, despite adequate resources to provide them with food or the means to produce it. We are avidly consuming limited (and irreplaceable) resources trying to feed ourselves by using the technologies, policies, and cultural values of yesterday to deal with the problems of tomorrow. This is not an original observation; it is a point that has been made before, perhaps most notably by Wangari Muta Maathai, who in 2004 became the first African woman (and the first environmentalist) to be awarded the Nobel Peace Prize "for her contribution to sustainable development, democracy and peace."[23]

Might it be that we have not socially evolved as much as we would like to believe? Will further understanding of the biological and political realities lead us to insights for a sustainable future?

Lessons from the Great Irish Famine [1845–1850]
Nutrition

Along with the politics of starvation, we have in the last three chapters examined the biology of nutrition and malnutrition. Here, with nutrition as our theme, we transpose that analysis to the Great Irish Famine, which offers several lessons about the central role that poor nutrition and food shortages play as "catalysts" to starvation and famine. As mentioned, a large peasant and laboring class in mid-nineteenth-century Ireland became increasingly dependent on a single food staple, the potato. The potato was a cheap and nutritious crop, easily grown on small plots, which allowed increasing acreage to be converted to production of grains for export out of Ireland. For the Irish, this was a prescription for disaster.

As our first Lesson detailed, the "predisposing cause" of that disaster was the poverty and vulnerability of the Irish peasant worker and peasant families. The agents of Irish poverty were "changes in entitlements," reduced wages, and reduced access to food that in turn eroded the peasants' ability to withstand the loss of their basic potato diet. We do not, however, simply dismiss the Malthusian argument that Irish population growth and its impact on the food supply played a significant role in the Famine, although recent research indicates that the Irish population was emigrating at a steady enough pace since 1800 to offset a Malthusian "positive check" (starvation) of the Irish people.[1] And, as discussed in chapter 1, Malthus's later work seems to shift his focus from population and the "positive check" of starvation to a lack of employment opportunities and thus to poverty.

Here we explore the Great Irish Famine as an early example of the more current nutritional crisis that is occurring among the world's very poor. We discuss the "catalytic causes" or "triggers" of the Famine. We examine the potato's nutritional value and central place in the Irish diet. When that single crop failed not once but for three successive harvests, starvation increased, and Irish peasants succumbed by the hundreds of thousands to diseases "that thrived in its wake."[2] We next detail the Great Famine relief efforts, one of the first examples of international food aid and one that mirrors responses today. By 1846–1847, in the absence of concerted government response, private relief groups from Europe and the United States stepped in to provide aid to the

Irish poor in the form of donations of money and food and in the operation of soup kitchens and food-for-work schemes.[3] There were questions about the nutritional value of relief food and accusations of contaminated shelters; some religious groups tried to take advantage of the plight of the starving Irish and demanded their conversion to Protestantism before feeding them. All of these are important concerns, and they continue to occur even today among relief agencies, donors, and some religious-based aid groups.

"Catalytic Causes"

What were the *catalytic causes*—the triggers—of the Great Irish Famine? Whereas *predisposing causes* of starvation and famine are often long-term, slow-acting, and connected, the catalytic causes are more likely to be short-term, sudden incidents such as a flood, a cyclone, or an insect infestation. But they may also be repetitive events, such as a prolonged drought or the failure of a staple crop over the course of several harvests. The single important factor is that catalytic causes strike vulnerable populations, with catastrophic effect.

In the Great Famine the possible list of causes is long and debatable. We believe, however, that Ireland in 1845–1850 closely follows Scrimshaw's definition of famine discussed in chapter 2: that large numbers of the impoverished Irish peasantry went "without sufficient food" for long periods and suffered from chronic hunger and malnutrition; that their economic and nutritional poverty made them vulnerable to "a relatively sudden collapse in food consumption" that affected "large numbers" of them, resulting in high mortality. We argue that the failure of the Irish diet—the result of the potato blight—is a principal catalytic cause of this famine. We look closely at three characteristics of this catalytic cause: the dependency of the Irish peasant on the potato, its nutritional content, and its sudden collapse.

Dependency on the Potato

The potato, first domesticated in the Andes and carried to Europe in the sixteenth century, reached Ireland by way of Spain about 1590. The potato soon became a staple crop in Europe, where it underpinned the Industrial Revolution as a cheap source of calories that liberated workers from the land; by doing so, it took on a major role in free-market trade and economic development. In Ireland the potato also played a central part in the evolution of the island's agriculture and history. It proved to be both a blessing and a curse. The potato was cheap to grow, but it spoiled easily and could not be stored for more than a year. The only way to use the potato as a buffer stock against future shortages was to convert it to another food, most often by feeding it to pigs. "For those [Irish] on the lower rungs of the economic ladder the only cash transaction of the year was the sale of the pig, which together with working as an agricultural labourer for his landlord, helped to pay the rent on the plot of land."[4]

The potato grew almost everywhere it was planted. Observers in Ireland and nutritionists[5] elsewhere calculated that an acre of Irish farmland could feed 2.08 people on wheat but 4.18 people on potatoes. Irish farmers developed several varieties of potato, and most favored the "notorious 'lumper,'" which was productive even in poor soil.[6] By 1845, Ireland's peasant farmers were planting potatoes on as many as 2 million acres—about two-thirds of Ireland's tilled land. The poverty of the island was compensated for by heavy manual labor. These laborers worked the ground with great care: spade cultivation, ridging, generous doses of lime, manure, and sea-sand—carried great distances in many cases—to enrich and lighten the soil. Yields were high, and before the blight potatoes fed more than 4 million of the Irish people, for whom it was the basic food, and most the island's pigs and fowl. Before the Famine, about 1 million tons of surplus potatoes and some 450,000 tons of grain were also annually exported to England, further integrating the Irish economy into that of Europe.[7]

On the eve of the Great Famine, the potato had become a crucial element in the Irish agricultural system that had evolved since the mid-eighteenth century. While the potato was Ireland's staple *food* crop, grains became the *money* or export crops. By raising potatoes for consumption at home, and because of the fact that potatoes took half the acreage of corn, oats, or wheat for the same nutritional value, more Irish farmland could be converted to grains and pasture for sheep and cattle, all for export. In effect the potato and the land-holding class structure allowed Ireland's agriculture to gradually evolve into a kind of granary for the rest of the United Kingdom. That the agricultural system was, in turn, driven by a free market economy outside Ireland was of little or no benefit to the Irish poor. Land confiscation caused the abandonment of smallholder farming. Smaller plots, usually less than 10 acres, prevented the Irish laborers from switching crops after the blight in 1845 because they could not produce sufficient quantities of other foods on the same amount of land.

Dr. Liz Young of Staffordshire University has proposed that the Great Irish Famine was marked by an uneven economic and social polarization. Irish peasants were a marginalized people. Landlords dominated political and economic life. This differentiation is clearly seen in their diet. Those with 50 acres or more "ate well, and the famine passed them by unscathed while 'family farmers' with about 20 acres were less vulnerable than the 1,300,000 labourers and poor peasants." They made up the bulk of the 3 million or so at the bottom, whose annual income was about £15 to £20. They suffered unevenly, depending on where they lived and their access to relief aid; for example, 75 percent of the male population on the Donegal estates was "economically vulnerable,"[8] well below the number in, say, Antrim.

Most historians agree that the fragile Irish economy, more than anything else, made the country vulnerable to a catalytic event. Food collapse, a withering labor market, and evictions ("clearances") all crushed the already impoverished Irish peasant laborer, and when potato production dropped from about 14.8 million tons in 1844 to less than 4 million tons annually between 1846 and 1849, starvation was inevitable.[9]

The Potato Diet and Undernutrition

The potato was considered "a nutritional miracle."[10] An easily grown, high-yielding crop, it is rich in proteins and carbohydrates, in micronutrients including thiamin, niacin, folate, and—perhaps most historically and nutritionally important—vitamin C. Although deficient in vitamins A and D, the potato shielded the Irish poor from scurvy, rare in Ireland, and pellagra, both of which were endemic elsewhere in Europe. In the United States, for example, where corn was the staple food at this time, pellagra was widespread, especially in the South.

Just before the Famine, most of the people in Ireland ate potatoes in some form as part of their diet.[11] The Irish laborer's consumption was impressive. An adult male would eat between 5 and 7 kilograms of potatoes a day (12–14 pounds), the equivalent of today's supermarket bag. Modern dietary analysis suggests that "the Irishman's gargantuan meals of potatoes and buttermilk provided all the proteins, calories and minerals he needed."[12] There were, however, some dietary cautions. As noted, the potato did not store well; it was easily damaged when shipped. Potatoes prepared in advance, perhaps for field laborers, were prone to contamination, especially when mixed with buttermilk. "The result would have been diarrhoea, and children aged less than 6 months would have been especially vulnerable." The potato is also "a bulky and coarse food" with digestive risk "for the ailing or weaning child."[13]

The Potato Blight

Other countries in Europe grew potatoes and experienced crop diseases. But these countries had developed faster during the Industrial Revolution and benefited more. They could withstand the shock of the potato blight.[14] The arrival of *Phytophthora infestans* in Ireland was first noted in the press on September 6, 1845. It is thought that the spores of the blight were carried by wind, rain, and insects, and perhaps came to Ireland from Britain and the European continent, and that a fungus affected the potato plants, producing black spots and a white mold on the leaves. This rotted the potato into a pulp. The fungal hypothesis was scoffed at by most experts. After all, hadn't Europe also suffered a rainy season? Yet there was no "potato famine" there. The disease was diagnosed as a kind of wet rot. Ó Gráda calls it "a tragic ecological accident."[15]

The failure of successive potato harvests from 1845 through 1848 caused not only starvation, but also the withdrawal of the population's main source of vitamin C. Along with famine large numbers of the Irish poor now faced scurvy, a vitamin-deficiency disease, which appeared among them for the first time in decades.[16] This outbreak prompted medical doctors to connect the potato with scurvy prevention, which enabled them to add the potato as a possible prophylactic mechanism in addition to lemons and limes.

The importance of the common potato as a source of nutrition continues to this day. By 2010, the potato was the world's fourth most important food crop, after maize (corn), wheat, and rice. The United Nations (UN) declared 2008 The Year of the Potato and noted that it provides a high number of calories, grows quickly and widely, and uses less land than its three principal competitors. This gave the potato the same clout that it had enjoyed in Europe and Ireland in the mid-nineteenth century: The UN stated that the potato "will contribute to the achievement of the Millennium Development Goals, by helping to alleviate poverty, improve food security and promote economic development."[17] To do this, UN agencies and other experts were by 2009 encouraging smallholder farmers in the developing world to increase their potato crops. Despite the Great Irish Famine, as *The Economist* noted, in the twenty-first century potatoes "are now the icon of globalization."[18]

Early Famine Relief Operations

The Great Irish Famine is also an example—ironically—of concern by others for those in peril. It offers early examples of humanitarian relief efforts, feeding operations, and food-for-work schemes. These are common responses today, as we discuss in chapters 6, 7, and 9, but in 1845–1850 such efforts were considered a unique, even risky undertaking. As described earlier, in 1845 British Prime Minister Robert Peel directed his government to purchase corn from the United States for Ireland. He also established a Relief Commission to accelerate and oversee that grain importation and the distribution to the Irish poor. The amount of relief food, mostly corn, was too small to replace the lost potato, although it held down food prices for about a year. A public works relief scheme was also initiated. After Lord John Russell replaced Peel as prime minister, however, he abolished the Relief Commission, placed relief work in the hands of civil servants, and ordered that the Irish pay for all Irish work relief. Food riots soon broke out.[19] Tens of thousands died from hunger-related causes during the winter of 1846–1847, but "Russell and his colleagues never conceived of interfering with the structure of the Irish economy in the ways that would have been necessary to prevent the worst effects of the famine."[20]

Food-for-Work Schemes

During the Irish Famine, proposed *food-for-work schemes* included "reproductive" work like land reclamation, drainage projects, and estate improvement. The goal was to increase farm output using the starving as labor, but official preference for roadwork and quay construction won out. None of this mattered, however, since there were too few public works projects for the demand.

By October 1846 as the Great Famine worsened, hundreds of projects employed more than 100,000 people. But they were unevenly distributed—20,000 were helped in one county, Clare, while the whole province of Ulster accounted for only 1200. An evaluation of public works jobs put the number of people needing employment at 2,385,000 in 1846–1847, and the number of desperately poor at 80,000. Public works projects had been set up to handle 100,000; at its peak in March 1847, the number had expanded to 750,000.[21]

Although the British spent some £10.5 million on relief efforts, much in the form of loans, most of that came after the winter of 1846 and was too little, too late. Moreover, Lord Russell's efforts were "in stark contrast" to what his government spent on other projects at the time, "including £20 million to compensate slave plantation owners in the West Indies following emancipation and £70 million to fund an ill-advised adventure in the Crimea."[22]

The public works were disbanded in the spring of 1847, partly because of complaints in London about the high cost and the concern that food-for-work was absorbing farm labor.[23] Yet they were called "a tremendous achievement." About 90 percent of the outlays were indeed spent on wages, and the large bureaucracy took only 7 percent. But too often the work had no purpose. It also benefited only those still healthy enough to undertake the labor. The scheme further widened the gap between the younger, healthier Irish and those at the bottom, yet failed to provide enough funds to fight starvation. On average these workers earned about 12 pence a day, "enough for a family of four to subsist on in normal times, but now literally a starvation wage . . . What was lacking was the *purchasing power* to command subsistence at prevailing prices."[24] There is reason to believe that had those on public work received a better wage during the pivotal winter of 1846–1847, it is possible that they might have created enough of a consumer market to attract food supplies *into* Ireland.

Humanitarian Aid

In 1846–1847 an "alarming increase in mortality" from starvation and fever caused the British government to establish soup kitchens in what was one of the first instances of international humanitarian relief aid, now also a common response. The Soup Kitchen Act of January 25, 1847, called for relief kitchens to be set up in each of Ireland's election districts. The kitchens were seen as less likely to "crowd out" other employment. By March 1847, The Destitute Poor (Ireland) Act had directed that Famine Soup, or "gruel," be defined as "any food cooked in a boiler, and distributed in a liquid state," and that it be served directly to the starving. The Soup Kitchen Act made available the Famine Pot or Work House Pot, a cast-iron soup container of varying size supplied by the government. By the summer of 1847, some 1,850 soup kitchens run by local relief committees supported by the government were serving perhaps as many as 3 million people daily. In most kitchens those who were destitute received their soup free; those with wages paid.[25]

Soups were created by a variety of well-intended people: Alexis Soyer (Soyer's Soup), the French chef of the Reform Club of London; a Mrs. Neale of Castleconnell, County Limerick (Mrs. Neale's Soup Recipe); and Grattan's Soup concocted by the Right Hon. James Grattan of Vicastown, County Laois. Most called for large vats of water in which some beef, onions, and other vegetables were stirred along with barley and salt. The proper mixture of minerals and vitamins seems to have been unknown, and the Famine Soup's food value was considered low. Over time visitors to the soup kitchens suffered diarrhea or scurvy, which of course the potato had helped them avoid.

Famine Soup was ladled out to those who lined up before the Famine Pot, pans and bowls in hand. Many Irish considered this debasing and humiliating, with reason: Some were called "soupers" even for generations after the Famine. Others waited for their handouts while enduring pleas from donors to convert from Catholicism.[26] Yet the soup kitchens were seen as "by far the most effective of all the methods adopted by government to deal with starvation and disease."[27]

Private relief committees formed in Ireland and Great Britain. Some had helped with food shortages in 1822 and 1831. Most prominent were the Irish Relief Association and the British Association for the Relief of Distress in Ireland and the Highlands of Scotland, which was first organized in London in 1847 by Lionel de Rothschild, the banker and philanthropist. The Society of Friends (Quakers), both Irish and British, and other Protestant churches ran many of the soup kitchens. The Quakers operated a large program county by county and also provided grants and unguaranteed loans for Irish agriculture and fisheries. But perhaps most important, they almost alone among the church-based relief groups did not attempt to convert the Irish Catholics.

The relief assistance was unusual for the time but familiar today. It was also global and generous. Donations to purchase food came from India, the Ottoman Sultan, Pope Pius IX, and even Queen Victoria herself. Canada shipped food and money. A New York City newspaper reported in March 1847 that some $1,250,000 in supplies was leaving that port each week for Ireland, matched by some $5 million from across the United States.[28] The French, Dutch, Germans, and Swiss also contributed. Even the Native American Choctaws gathered $710 in donations and sent it to Ireland—just sixteen years after their own "Trail of Tears" marked by forced evictions and starvation.[29]

The government soup kitchens ended prematurely, amid protest, at the end of September 1847. The Soup Kitchen Act had been passed as a temporary measure to sustain the starving until the autumn 1847 harvest. Immediately after that, Sir Charles Trevelyan, assistant secretary to the treasury, announced that the Great Irish Famine had ended. According to one historian, "In Trevelyan's opinion the famine was the 'direct stroke of an all-wise and all-merciful Providence,' apparently operating on Malthusian lines, to civilize the Irish."[30] He withdrew almost all British financial contributions to the relief effort.[31] Although the harvest of 1847 was notable for the absence of widespread blight, it brought in only 25 percent of what was expected. The 3 million Irish who had been sustained through the spring and summer of 1847 by Famine Soup, however meager, were now on their own. The Central Relief Committee of the Society of Friends (Quakers) continued their soup kitchens on a diminished scale through 1847 and into 1848, for which the Irish remember them with fondness to this day. The "callous act" of ending the kitchens, however, "prolonged the crisis," and "roadside deaths were still commonplace in the winter of 1848–49."[32]

Proximal Causes of Death

Mortality is an important analytical and policy tool, as we noted in chapter 2 and discuss in greater depth in chapters 6 and 7. It is especially helpful to know both what causes excess deaths among the starving and what other factors might indicate the vulnerability of those suffering prolonged chronic hunger. This knowledge assists in targeting responses and policies. The Irish Famine is, unfortunately, an excellent example of this analysis. So, too, is the 1973–1974 famine in Ethiopia, where starvation-related deaths spiked and then continued at a lower level before spiking again almost 10 years later, in both cases triggered by drought. Accounts of the Irish deaths also humanize the Great Famine's statistics and create a place in the larger Irish Famine narrative for their voices.

By 1847, the number of deaths directly from starvation in Ireland was starting to fall, while deaths from starvation-related diseases were rising. Opportunistic infectious diseases took those weakened by malnutrition and severe hunger. The young and the old died "disproportionately." Death was an equal opportunity reaper, unencumbered by geography. Many of the Irish died alone "by the countless thousands" along the roads, in woods, fields, and bogs. Some died when exposed to other famine victims. Hospitals and clinics or dispensaries, set up in 1845–1846, became dangerous places even to work: 36 of 473 medical officers appointed by the Board of Health "died of the occupational hazard of famine fever."[33]

Death was also seasonal, with peaks during wintertime, especially in 1846–1847 and again in 1848–1849, perhaps the result that year of a cholera outbreak, for example, or the shutting of the soup kitchens. Death was everywhere: Dysentery, smallpox, typhus, "famine fever," cholera, and even eating killed the Irish. "So many had been starving for so long that when they were given food . . . the danger of death actually increased." The death of one man who died suddenly at Skibbereen was noted: "'Carthy swallowed a little warm milk and died."[34] Others, weakened, were chased by packs of dogs and died from the exhaustion. One woman spoke of seeing famine victims who "fell dead out of their standing and the dogs eating at them. They mustered up . . . in bunches like, them that felt getting weak, and then they went away to some place out, and one done what they could for the other till they died."[35]

As autumn passed into winter, "the nettles and blackberries, the edible roots and cabbage leaves on which hundreds of people had been eking out an existence disappeared; flocks of wretched beings, resembling human scarecrows,"[36] combed the empty potato fields. Half the children in Skibbereen's workhouse died in October, most from diarrhea. In County Mayo, one observer saw "a strange and fearful sight . . . the streets crowded with gaunt wanderers" and later in Galway, "walking skeletons."[37] A dispensary doctor found seven "wretches" seeking warmth under a single cloak: "One of them had been dead many hours, but the others were unable to move either themselves or the corpse."[38]

Even those who could emigrate did not escape: it is estimated that 40 percent of the Irish fleeing the Great Famine died from disease before or immediately after their arrival in North America.[39] Typhus, "recurring fever," and dysentery were the principal killers, but voyagers also encountered ice, snow, and gales that delayed them at sea for up to three months with little rations and increasing malnutrition. Some fell overboard or suffered injury on the ship. Thousands of others died at medical facilities in Canada; the U.S. ports at Boston and New York were frequently overwhelmed. The *Mary*, carrying forty-six people from the Famine in Cork, Ireland, was refused landing by port authorities in Boston "owing to [the] destitute condition" of its passengers. They were fortunate. On May 28, 1847, the *Virginius* appeared off Nova Scotia, Canada. She had left Liverpool with 476 passengers fleeing the Great Famine, the medical superintendent at Grosse Isle reported, but by the time she arrived ". . . 106 were ill of fever, including nine of the crew, and the large number of 158 had died on the passage, including the first and second officers and seven of the crew, and the master and the steward dying, the few that were able to come on deck were ghastly yellow looking spectres, unshaven and hollow checked, and without exception, the worst looking passengers I have ever seen." The "fever" he spoke of was typhus rapidly spread by lice on the crowded ships. At the time, it killed as many as 70 percent of those infected.

Right behind the *Virginius* came the *Jas. H. Shepherd* also out of Liverpool, with 228 on board, 26 of whom had died during the voyage, and 105 who were ill including all but 6 members of the crew. Arrivals in Canada overwhelmed immigration and medical officials. The agent at Quebec reported that on May 11, 1846, for example, that there were thirty-one ships approaching his station with 10,636 passengers on board. In 1847 alone, Grosse Isle reported 9,572 deaths; New York had another 703. That year there were 17,465 *documented* deaths at sea,[40] and at least 197 children lost both parents during the sea voyage and arrived as orphans in North America.[41]

Children suffered and died disproportionately. The Great Irish Famine set a marker unfortunately still seen today in the developing world: high mortality among young children. In many ways the marginal economy of Ireland before, during, and after the Great Famine matched those of sub-Saharan Africa and South Asia now. Malnutrition, infection, diseases, the food-energy requirements of subsistence farming families all have similar characteristics and similar outcomes. The hunger of the "potato gap" matches the seasonal hunger found among today's rural poor in their developing country communities.

During the Great Famine children under age 10 and men and women over age 60 made up less than one-third of the Irish population at the time, but they were three-fifths of the Irish dead.[42] And long after the Famine ended, the deaths continued: "The death rates in 1850 and 1851 were equal to that of 1847–1848, indicating the protracted nature of the Famine."[43] Between the deaths and the emigration, Ireland today remains the only European country where population is less than it was in the mid-nineteenth century.[44]

The Great Irish Famine created a narrative of remembered wrongs and the belief that a humane government would have done much more to alleviate such suffering. Within twenty years, the Great Famine also became the basis of political demands for Irish sovereignty. Famine memories, in Ireland and North America, transformed into Irish nationalism.

To be sure, there were direct and measurable benefits from the Irish emigration, and at least one significant lesson learned. Those who took in the Irish— Great Britain, Canada, Australia, and the United States—gained immediately from Irish adult immigrant labor. In one exquisite twist of history, the influx of large numbers of Irish men in the 1840s and 1850s into Boston and New York provided, starting in 1861, five regiments of Irish infantry (the Irish Brigade)[45] that fought in the Civil War against the Confederates, who were supported by the British. The bravery and service of the Irish troops helped preserve the Union of the United States, assure its sovereignty as a nation and its progress toward becoming the world's leading democracy. By 1870, just 20 years after the starvation and upheaval of the Great Famine, more than 1 million Irish lived in the United States and another 300,000 in Canada. They and other new immigrants gave voice and substance to the American democracy, which in turn inspired and stirred other peoples in the colonial world, as well as in Ireland, and foreshadowed the end of almost 300 years of the British Empire.[46]

PART III

The Genesis of Response

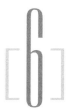 **Responses on the Ground**

Our next two chapters are about "knowing," and "responding" to what is known. How do we learn that chronic hunger, malnutrition, starvation, or famine is occurring? What are the response choices? How does relief food actually reach those in need? Are these responses influenced or distorted by whether or not one is "inside" (experiencing) or "outside" (observing) the event? The answers to these questions create the framework for this section. They help us determine whether or not starvation or famine is taking place, what the scale of that famine might be, what the possible causes are, and when, where, and how donors might intervene. They also assist our efforts to answer two of our fundamental questions: Who starves? And why?

Two new case studies assist us in addressing these questions: Malawi in southern Africa, and Niger and its neighbor Mali, in West Africa. Malawi interests us because in 2001–2002 well-meaning international financial institutions, the World Bank, and the International Monetary Fund (IMF), required that the Malawi government incorporate free-market economics—a twenty-first-century version of *laissez-faire*—into its economic system. This may have heightened Malawi's chronic hunger and inadvertently caused its starvation. In Niger four years later, hundreds of thousands of impoverished Africans also suffered prolonged and "extreme hunger" in part because of the imposition by the same international financial institutions of almost identical economic structures. Although *laissez-faire* is not identical to "free-market economics," what concerns us here is that, in both the Irish Famine and the more recent African cases, there was advocacy and imposition of an unquestioned economic theory without consideration of its human costs. The Niger-Mali case study also offers an interesting turn: Mali, among the five poorest countries on earth, with "precarious health and sanitation conditions," experienced severe food insecurity, drought, and locust invasions, as did its neighbor. But while Niger's people starved, those living in Mali "escaped" famine.[1] We explain why below.

The Pathways of Response

Almost all starvations and famines—except those that are "artificial"[2]—begin as "silent" emergencies. People who suffer chronic hunger, malnutrition, and "the hungry months" just before the harvests are especially vulnerable.

How do we, outside these events, know *when* starvation occurs and how far along it might be? How do those "inside" the event know, and how do they define a time of starvation?

Nevin Scrimshaw's definition, discussed in chapter 2, is again helpful here much as it was in analyzing the Great Irish Famine. Scrimshaw emphasizes the *range* of a starvation, its "high" mortality, and, most important to this chapter, the *occurrence of social and economic changes*.[3] We use Scrimshaw's definition as an insightful tool. He argues that one of the early characteristics of starvation is social disintegration, which begins in the household and ripples outward through the community and region. There are ways to see this taking place and to measure it.

How Do We Know? The "Outsider" Observation

Those who are not starving will see and define starvation and famine differently from those who are. To the "outsider" the one signal of a rising starvation is that people alter the patterns of their lives. These are often called *survival strategies* or *coping strategies*. These strategies identify behaviors that people adopt to get them through a short-term shock. As chart 6.1 illustrates, coping strategies can be diagrammed. They often follow a progression that moves from easily reversed actions (such as eating food reserves) along a downward curve toward increasing irreversibility (such as outward migration). Whether compiled by governments, UN agencies, nongovernmental organizations (NGOs), or other outside observers, these diagrams vary only slightly and are generally useful.

Therefore, one way for an outsider to observe that starvation is taking place, and to determine how far along it may be, is to identify and list the coping strategies being employed by those inside. The downward curve is also a measure of increasing desperation. Starvation and its defining social disintegration send characteristic signals: early signs, with a high possibility of reversing the conditions, include decreasing food supplies and rising prices in local markets, the eating of planting seeds and reserves, and the search for wild foods (famine foods). Later signals, with less possibility of reversal, include sales of large numbers of livestock or goods (such as housing materials). When people walk (migrate) out of their communities in search of food, as the chart illustrates, reversing conditions becomes very difficult; emergency interventions with food and medical relief may be the only viable response. Social disintegration is under way: families may break apart in search of work, or individual members engage in begging, stealing, prostitution, or other illegal activities to obtain food. In Ethiopia in 1973 the peasants who appeared outside Addis Ababa were engaged in a survival strategy: as hunger spread across the villages and districts back in the mountains, "the men reluctantly left their women and children

CHART 6.1

Coping Strategies: Reversibility and Time of Occurrence

more	○ Eating grain reserves/famine foods
	○ Borrowing food from neighbors, kin
REVERSIBILITY	○ Increasing labor inputs
	○ Selling livestock
	○ Selling household assets
	○ Selling land
	○ Disintegration of household/family
	○ Migrating for aid (males)
	○ Begging, prostitution, stealing/crime
less	○ Outbreaks of disease/excessive deaths
	earlier　　　　　TIME　　　　　*later*

Source: Adapted from House of Commons, 4 March 2003, 27.

and began a frightening search for food."[4] But by the time they had blocked the road and marched on their capital, this strategy was too late. As chart 6.1 makes clear, those peasant men were fleeing a starvation already well under way. "Abnormally high mortality may be the hallmark of famine," John Field reminds us, "but societal breakdown is its essence."[5]

Therefore, observing *coping strategies*—what people experiencing collapsing food supplies are likely to do and in what sequence—becomes a useful tool for analysis and response. In Ethiopia, Shepherd observed the starvation and used two primary resources: the U.S. Embassy's eyewitness "field reports" and the Ethiopian Ministry of Agriculture's crop-reporting system, "the best there was in a country with little statistical reporting,"[6] he wrote at the time. These, together with other first-hand accounts from Peace Corps volunteers, missionaries, relief aid workers and the UN Development Program (UNDP), enabled him to piece together the details of the starvation's progress that read almost like the list on chart 6.1: the borrowing of food, eating of reserves and seed stock; the selling of animals, tools, the wood from their huts, and their clothing. As reported in a 1974 publication of the Carnegie Endowment for International Peace,

> Sometime early in 1973 (no one will ever know exactly when), a mass migration of peasants began deep in the interior of Wollo and Tigre provinces. Almost 90 percent of the people's cattle had died. A few had been sold for grain, but grain prices were rising daily and cattle prices dropping, creating

what one UNDP report [later] called "an alarming downward spiral towards destitution." Men went out to search for food. Often they never returned. Some died; some deserted; some reached help but, too ill and malnourished themselves, couldn't get back. Women, children, and the elderly who were left behind starved in uncounted numbers. The same UNDP report grimly stated: "There are cases where whole communities simply died."[7]

Studies of coping strategies show the same pattern of behavior by other people in response to deepening threats to their survival. From the Great Irish Famine to more recent cases, the individual's rationing of consumption is a universal response to food shortages. The drive to preserve oneself, to avoid destitution and starvation, is powerful. Thus, those Irish peasants who were healthy and strong enough—and had money for the fare—emigrated to England and North America. Those left behind wandered the Irish countryside in large numbers in search of food,[8] not unlike the Ethiopian peasant farmers. And, in a classic profile of starvation, those who died in the Great Irish Famine and inside Ethiopia in the 1970s and 1980s were overwhelmingly those left behind: the children, pregnant or ill women, and the elderly.[9]

These observations of coping strategies come from *outside* a starvation. They are useful tools for generating donor responses. The outsider definition, writes Alexander de Waal in his eyewitness account[10] of famine in Darfur, Sudan, is "more of social philosophy than of social experience." Therefore, outsiders may look for four basic characteristics to define famine and tell us it is occurring: critical food shortages; widespread and observable hunger and starvation; extensive societal breakdown and disruption; and excess mortality. The outsider definition "focuses on extremity, notably on mass starvation unto death."[11] Mortality levels drive policy responses. If, for example, outsiders base their definition of starvation or famine on perceived conditions and mortality, then they will not act (respond) until suffering and deaths reach a certain level and meet that definition. Chart 6.1, a tool for outsiders, shows us that the outsider alarms increase on the descending line, and thus, response may be too late. Some people may starve because famine relief is dominated by the outsider definition. Those outside the starvation may wait too long to act.

How Do They Know? The "Insider" Observation

Do the definitions of starvation and famine, and the time and type of response, change if the observation comes from *inside*?

We find that those who *experience* chronic hunger and recurring starvation define and treat them differently from those outsiders who *observe* these conditions. Why is this distinction important? Alexander de Waal explains the differences between the outsider definition (above) and "the more subtle terms used by people who suffer famines in other parts of the world."[12] How do the victims themselves define "starvation" and "famine?"

In his analysis, de Waal tells of a herder in the Sahel, who, when asked in 1953 if there was a "famine" replied: "Yes. No one died, but the price of millet rose. When the sack of millet costs 6000 francs, isn't that a famine?"[13] In Darfur more recently, de Waal found that famine meant "not merely starvation, but also hunger (that is, all manner of suffering), destitution, and social breakdown. When people are dying, manifestly because of the hardship and disorder associated with a famine, it is a 'famine that kills.'"[14] But not all famines kill; de Waal offers an insightful account of famine names in the local dialect. These reflect the insider's view of the causes of famine: locusts, drought (the *Meliss* starvation in 1959, or "No Harvest"), or even people held responsible for conflict that caused famine (the *Salim* or the *Jano* famine). The word *maja'a*, which de Waal translates as "famine and/or dearth," contains the concepts of hunger, destitution, and death. Although all three terms taken together could serve as the outsider definition, with an emphasis on death, *maja'a* separates the definitions. The same word may indicate a famine of hunger only (like the herder's definition), or of social breakdown and destitution, or a "famine that kills."[15] From an insider's point of view, therefore, famine may include hunger, severe food shortages, societal breakdown, but not necessarily widespread mortality. It is seen as a process with the most feared outcome "not death by starvation, but destitution, a total deprivation of assets."[16]

Omar Mahmoud was eighteen when starvation first began seeping through his village of Tahoua, Niger, during the hunger season in 2004. He sold rice in his father's shop, and father and son, like de Waal's Sahel herder, could feel a societal shift taking place as fewer people, now desperately poor, came into their shop. "I know there is hunger," Omar said. "It is because there wasn't enough rain. The price of millet has gone up because there wasn't enough rain last year."[17]

The subtle complexities of the *maja'a* definition or the poverty-pricing sensitivity of the rice shopkeeper's son often identifies a hunger collapsing into starvation better than the outside definition. Whereas outsiders may define famine by food availability and mortality, those inside may see every other component *except* deaths as defining and important. Access to food may be blocked; various coping strategies such as eating famine food and migrating for help may occur; food may be available, but the starving cannot pay or barter for it. To these people, death does not define their circumstances. Access to food does: the cost of a bag of millet to a herder defines his community's starvation. If outside observers define starvation by the numbers who have died and they wait for mortality to reach a certain level, or they believe food costs or access are the defining elements, their policy responses will be delayed and may come far too late.

The "Moral Economy"

When we examine insider responses, we also have a better understanding of the tragic consequences of outsider interventions. Here, Malawi, Niger, and Mali require our attention. First we must examine precolonial relationships between peasant farmers and their leaders. We find that the terms of exchange between them often created a unique agreement and unusual bond designed to offset the insider definition of starvation. In China during the 1700s, for example, this concept produced the *ever-normal granaries*. Each region kept on hand enough grain to offset shortages during periods of crop failure, when demand would rise. Supply was thus "ever normal," stabilizing prices and protecting each community from starvation. In parts of Africa in the nineteenth century similar agreements formed part of the "moral economy,"[18] the establishment of food reserves to lessen the impact of hunger or the onset of starvation in times of shortage. Both are clear indicators of the resilience and skill of farmers and communities to design ways to survive severe food shortages. Both schemes were based on fairness, justice, mutual understanding, and obligation—but not individual gain. The way they worked was simple: peasant farmers donated to the government or its leaders a portion of their surplus food grains to be stored; chiefs or skilled local administrators protected and then, in times of shortage, redistributed these grains. This tradition took on the force of custom and, in some countries, of national law.

For example, during severe food shortages across rural China in 1743–1744, as Mike Davis writes, each locality immediately issued rations, even using the Grand Canal to bring millet and rice from storage depots in the south when supplies ran low in the north. In one case that Davis cites, "Two million peasants were maintained for eight months, until the return of the monsoon made agriculture possible again."[19] In Africa the "moral economy" often—but not universally—worked this way: in exchange for a food tax, the subsistence farmer received food insurance from the chief to whom it was paid. Thus, "the moral economy provided a degree of [food] security for the poor."[20] In a "moral economy," no one would starve.[21]

But colonialism changed the terms of Africa's traditional "moral economy." During the colonial period of the late eighteenth through the mid-twentieth centuries, the European colonial powers forced African farmers and their families into marginal agricultural lands with the least rainfall and poorest soils, weakening both the traditional means of production and community structures that upheld the "moral economy." The Europeans taxed these farmers and shifted their production from staple food crops to cash crops such as cotton and tobacco, tea and coffee.[22] Nutritious, drought-resistant crops like sorghum and millet were replaced by maize (corn). Over the course of the colonial era, Africa's agricultural practices evolved from the "moral economy" to dependency. Those terms of exchange continue today. In the postcolonial era, from the 1960s to the 1990s, Africa's emerging independent states remained locked in this commodity production and dependence on global markets. This dependency has in part created the foundation for Africa's chronic hunger, malnutrition, starvation, and famines. It has removed the protective structures of local food production and food-shortage strategies and replaced them with cash-crop production and dependencies on global markets. Today, many sub-Saharan African farmers are not producing food but flowers, coffee, tea, cocoa, tobacco, and horticultural products for export. As Peet writes, "The moral economy became a money economy."[23]

It is difficult not to be struck by parallels here with the Great Irish Famine. For example, as British settlement (or "colonialism") of Ireland took place in the form of the "plantation" structure, the traditional "moral economy"—in the form of public provision of food to lessen mortality during shortages— essential since the Irish starvations of the 1740s, "failed to prevent serious food crises." Instead, by the 1840s "market relations" became dominant[24] and food self-sufficiency gave way to the ideology of market economics and the exportation of grains and livestock, similar to what occurred a century later in sub-Saharan Africa, South Asia and India.

Our case studies of Malawi in 2001–2002 and Niger and Mali in 2004–2005 highlight several of these issues: (1) the destruction of indigenous food-reserve schemes (the moral economy) by international financial institutions; (2) the efforts by international financial institutions, however well-meaning, to apply popular economic theory to starvation in developing states that resulted in great human tragedy; (3) and, the slowness and delays by those institutions in engaging and mitigating starvation.

Malawi

Sometime after the harvest season ended, perhaps as early as April 2001, rumors of starvation began emerging from the farmlands of Malawi. That year "the hungry months" had proceeded beyond November–March, the growing season in this southern Africa nation. Even in normal years the previous harvest is consumed by March "while the next crop is still rising from the ground. Families often endure this hungry period on a single meal a day, sometimes nothing more than a foraged handful of greens."[25] By October 2001, six months later, two nongovernmental organizations, the Malawi Economic Justice Network

(MEJN) and the Catholic Commission for Justice—outside observers working on the ground—were frustrated from trying to push the government and donors to declare a "famine" in the country's rural areas. Their reports were "dismissed" as "lacking credibility."[26]

Perhaps this was because starvation rose slowly from Malawi's rural areas, and reports took on a classic outsider/insider dichotomy. In February 2002, almost a year after the first alerts, several hundred hunger-related deaths, or "perhaps several thousand," had been reported, making this "the worst famine in living memory, certainly worse than the drought of 1991–1992, and worse even more than the Nyasaland famine of 1949."[27] Traditional leaders were telling the president "that food shortages were becoming critical, particularly in rural areas."[28] Word arrived from the Kasungu region that more than 100 people had starved to death there during the "hunger months" alone, making it "the worst of Malawi's 27 districts."[29] On February 22, 2002, MEJN issued an urgent press release calling for action by the government and international donors: "The Government should acknowledge that there is hunger in Malawi. . . . government and civil society should provide food supplies to vulnerable groups."[30] By the end of February, 70 percent of the people—seven out of ten Malawians—were "reported to be on the verge of starvation."[31]

By then, of course, it was too late. No one will ever know exactly how many people died: "[I]n the nether regions of the developing world, famine is both less obvious and more complicated," Barry Bearak reported in Malawi for the *New York Times*. "Even small jolts to the regular food supply can jar open the trapdoor between what is normal, which is chronic malnutrition, and what is exceptional, which is outright starvation. Hunger and disease then malignly feed off each other, leaving the invisible poor to die in invisible numbers."[32]

How did this happen? There were several catalytic causes. Some, like the destruction of maize crops by flooding, visited Malawi as an act of nature. Others, like the sharp rise in the price of maize and the selling off of the country's grain reserves, occurred because of market fluctuations and fiscal interventions by people. The result was a nation "nudged into starvation" despite enough grain in the stores "if only the poor had the money to buy it." And this happened, "while well-meaning people were arguing about whether it was happening at all."[33]

We do know this: first, flooding of farmland and then erratic rainfall during the growing season caused maize production to drop from 2.5 million MT in 2000 to 1.7 million MT in 2001. In 2002 the maize harvest was down further to 1.4 million MT. The government hoped that farmers would cover this "food gap" by switching to cassava production but, when they didn't, the government blamed their countrymen for "inflexible food habits" that caused delays in emergency responses.[34] Second, the official price for maize jumped by 325 percent. On the ground, maize went for 40 kwacha a kilogram, about us50 cents—almost a full day's wage in a country where the average income is us$250 per person per year or about us68 cents a day.[35] People in the countryside ate "famine food" of leaves, small wild plants, or tubers if they could find them. The *Njala* (hunger) settled in. Third, even as starvation spread, the Strategic Grain Reserve was sold. By whom, and where it went, remain mysteries. But "Why?" is clearer.

During the late 1980s, the IMF (part of the World Bank) began encouraging selected developing states around the globe to address a broad range of obstacles to post–colonial state development by undertaking "economic structural adjustment programs" (ESAPS). The goal was to replace the colonial legacies of centrally planned and controlled economies—government interventions in markets, excessive state spending and ownership, and even corrupt and weak governance—seen by the IMF and others as barriers to economic stability and growth. Basically, the ESAPS were intended to liberalize markets and create free market economies. This policy came at a cost: to qualify for further loans or for lowered interest rates on existing debt, cooperating states would have to meet IMF-imposed conditions, or *conditionalities*. These included cutting jobs in government bureaucracies, removing price subsidies to farmers, privatizing state entities such as marketing boards and medical care, devaluing local currencies, and reducing state spending on social programs, "including social services to feed the poor and hungry populations."[36] Smita Narula, a New York University law professor and human rights researcher, wrote that the ESAPS "mandated the removal of food subsidies" and price supports for fertilizers and pesticides, "often resulting in substantial price hikes, with a disproportionate impact on the poorest and most vulnerable in the population."[37]

ESAPS have been highly controversial across the developing world. On the one hand in selected countries they have opened markets and brought about economic expansion and growth. Ghana may be Africa's best example. On the other hand they are accused of causing extreme social and economic hardship by collapsing some state economies, undermining state sovereignty, and favoring cash crops over food production. For some states, the results have been chronic hunger and entrenched poverty.[38] In Thailand, for example, 43 percent of the people fell below that country's poverty line as agricultural exports grew 65 percent. In the Philippines, farmland growing rice and corn declined when the fields for exported "cut flowers" were increased; more than 350,000 farm workers lost their jobs. In Mexico, Costa Rica, and Haiti, local farmers went unemployed when the IMF required open trade with the United States, which brought in subsidized corn and rice. The IMF reported that—before the earthquake in early 2010—half of all Haitian children under age 5 were malnourished and more than 50 percent of the population was living on less than US$1.25 a day;[39] both are barriers to Haiti's recovery.

Some African countries found the ESAPs onerous; there were strikes and even riots by angry citizens. "In several countries, governments were forced to adopt policies that were fundamentally opposed to their own long-established strategies and philosophies of development."[40] Food reserves, the "moral economy," became an early victim. By 1994, the World Bank was reporting that countries following ESAP conditions had much slower food production growth than those that did not. Tanzania, for example, started ESAP restructuring in 1986. Ten years later it was facing severe food shortages because fertilizer subsidies had been removed and their cost rose sharply. In Senegal IMF-imposed structural adjustments shattered the country's food security, causing production of maize and millet to collapse. By 1995 40 percent of Senegal's people were officially listed as chronically hungry.[41]

In 2003 the British House of Commons reported wider and more controversial impacts from ESAPs. During the 1980s and 1990s, as the IMF and the World Bank put ESAPs into play in many African countries, price controls and food subsidies were eliminated. Producers and buyers could no longer count on subsidized seeds and fertilizers, and the price of basic staples such as maize increased. As a result "price seasonality" became "a major cause of household food insecurity." Food prices in rural areas in many countries trace a predictable seasonal path, "with prices being lowest around the harvest period when supplies are abundant and market demand is low, then rising gradually through the dry season and into the next farming season, as granary stocks and market supplies dwindle."[42] Hence the emergence of *seasonal hunger*, the preharvest "hungry season" of diminishing food supplies and high rates of malnutrition. Moreover as Amartya Sen has shown, people in impoverished countries may die from starvation "simply because food prices rise to levels that are unaffordable for the poor, irrespective of the food availability situation at local or national levels." This was certainly the case in Malawi by 2001, where nutrition surveys "found clear evidence of deteriorating nutrition status—the outcome of acute food insecurity."[43]

Whatever the causes, by the year 2000, according to the House of Commons report and research by the International Food Policy Research Institute, sub-Saharan Africa was by several measures far poorer, more hungry, and more diseased than it had been during the 1960s, the first decade of independence. The number of malnourished Africans had jumped from 88 million in 1970 to more than 200 million by 2000.[44] Not all of this can be blamed on ESAPs, the IMF, the World Bank, or other international financial institutions. From the 1960s, and especially in the 1970s, through the turn of the century, sub-Saharan

African states had encountered major obstacles to state development. These included:

- Sharply rising population growth ("the most sudden and rapid population growth the world is ever likely to see").[45]
- Flat or declining per capita food output and an inability to disengage economically from commodity production (cash crops like tea, coffee, cocoa, tobacco) and shift to food security.
- Political destabilization (coups, war, corruption) that included eighty-five successful coups in thirty-five sub-Saharan Africa countries between 1960 and 2000, military rule in 60 percent of the region's states by the mid-1980s, and kleptocracies in Zaire (now the DRC), Kenya, and Zimbabwe, among others.
- Rising capital costs, especially for fuel (and thus fertilizer), multiplying sixfold in the 1970s, flattening global commodity prices, and resulting debt. Africa's public debt quadrupled between 1970 and 1976; by 1991 its external debt was greater than its annual GDP, and servicing payments exceeded inflow of foreign aid and investment. The result: "Africa's debt burdens are the new economy's chains of slavery."[46]

To their credit, the World Bank and IMF, along with other public institutions, sought to correct these colonial legacies: ESAPs were one measure of that effort. In Malawi, however, this went badly wrong.

In July 1999, Malawi established its National Food Reserve Agency (NFRA), an independent national trust with the mandate to create and hold emergency grain reserves.[47] This was a variation on the traditional "moral economy" pact between rural food producers and their government as a defense against extreme hunger and starvation. The NFRA's motto was: "Adequate Reserves for Malawi."[48]

By August 2000, following two good harvest years, the NFRA's Strategic Grain Reserve, as it came to be called, held 175,000 MT of maize as a hedge against food shortages. But during this period the IMF began imposing economic structural adjustment reforms on Malawi that included decreasing the size of its government, devaluing the kwacha (the state currency), and ending subsidies for fertilizer and seeds. The IMF, the EU, and other donors "increasingly counseled that national grain reserves should be run independently and on a cost-recovery basis." But this did not happen. The NFRA was undercapitalized and had borrowed money to purchase food stocks, "a crazy decision." By June 2000 it was in debt for 1 billion kwachas (about US$12 million)—but its granary was near full capacity.[49]

In 2001 the IMF directed the Malawi government to sell off 115,000 MT of its maize stocks, down to 60,000 MT, to reduce the cost of storage. This came despite the fact that the 2000–2001 maize harvest had a shortfall of 600,000 MT. The entire procedure was botched: instead of holding back even 60,000 MT, almost all of the reserve was sold, most to local markets. This happened despite the IMF's advice to export the maize rather than "dump" it on local markets, which might create "disincentives" to farmers to continue production and depress market prices. The sale was called "a major contributory factor to the food crisis."[50]

When the government tried to cover the resulting food gap by importing 220,000 MT, it proved too expensive and logistically difficult. Transport bottlenecks at the ports of Beira and Nacala in Mozambique, diversions of trucks to Zambia and Zimbabwe, and competing demands from neighboring states also suffering from food shortfalls "caused fatal delays and an escalation of maize prices to unaffordable levels." Not surprisingly, local traders inside Malawi, who had bought most of the maize reserves and stockpiled it, profiteered handsomely when prices rose up to 43 kwachas a kilo.[51]

"The IMF is to blame for the biting food crisis," said Bakili Muluzi, Malawi's president at the time. "They insisted the government sell maize from its strategic reserve and requested that the government abandon its starter pack agricultural subsidy program."[52] The IMF representative in Lilongwe denied this: "We have no expertise in food security policy and we did not instruct the Malawi Government or the National Food Reserve Agency to dispose of the reserves."[53]

This was literally true, but the IMF was deploying a semantic smokescreen. Although the financial institution's officers did not specifically "instruct" the Malawi government to sell maize in the Strategic Grain Reserve, it did indeed "advise" them to do so. Admitting later that its policy was based on "wrong information" about crop production in 2001, the Fund said: "We strongly advised the government to reduce the level of the grain reserve to between 30,000 and 60,000 tonnes, on cost-effectiveness grounds, but not to sell it all off."[54] But "sell it all off" they did, with horrific consequences.

Both the government and the donors hesitated in responding to the alarms about starvation. Malawian government misstatements about its people switching easily from maize to cassava probably caused the donors to delay emergency food responses. Certainly, the sale of the maize reserves and the corrupt profiteering "caused donors to vacillate for several months before responding to signals of distress with food assistance."[55] Four major donors—the EU, USAID, Britain, and Denmark—suspended all aid "citing widespread corruption and economic mismanagement."[56] Without the reserves as a safety net, delayed emergency food imports carried a high price. As a result, Barry Bearak reports,

"Hundreds, probably thousands, of Malawians succumbed to the scythe of a hunger-related death."[57]

Malawi offers one further example of the politics of starvation. It is a good one, an illustration of the resilience of Africa's smallholder farmers when given inputs and incentives. Elections in 2004–2005 brought Malawi a new government, and its president, Bingu wa Mutharika, promised a minimum price for maize surpluses, put a voucher system into play so that local farmers could obtain fertilizer at about 25 percent off the normal price, and made planting seeds more widely (and cheaply) available.[58] As a result, the 2006, 2007 and 2008 growing seasons were increasingly productive, helped by good rainfall. Total maize harvests jumped more than 30 percent in 2007, to 3.4 million MT. Family food production, higher rural wages, and lower food prices all benefited the poorer households, which self-reported their own economic well-being at 8 percent higher than in 2004.[59] The shift in government policies—away from the economic structural adjustment requirements of the 1990s—even brought the fiscally conservative *The Economist* to its editorial feet: Malawi's subsidies "enabled poor farmers to plant their crops more cheaply," *The Economist* wrote. "They [subsidies] have given them more to eat; and they have avoided the perverse outcome, in some other African countries, where farmers are reducing the amount of land they are planting at a time of high food prices because they cannot afford fertilizers."[60] Whether a return to food security is possible for Malawi remains to be seen. But as the *New York Times*'s Barry Bearak writes: "Families starve because families lack money. In most cases, it's that simple."[61]

Did the international institutions learn any lessons from Malawi? While Malawi was recovering, donor fatigue and delay, further market disruptions, and controversial economic policies continued to cost the African people dearly. Niger and Mali, two impoverished neighbors, also suffered starvation during 2004–2005, but with two very different outcomes.

Niger and Mali

In several ways, the countries of Niger and Mali mirror one another. Both are land-locked neighbors encapsulated inside colonial-era borders between the West African rain forest and the Sahara Desert. Both were colonized by the French and in time became part of the federation of French colonial territories, formally known as French West Africa. The northern halves of both countries are arid savannah or desert, part of the Sahel; gravel roads end at places with romantic names like Arlit and Timbuktu. Today, the people of Mali and Niger remain among the most poor: Mali is the fifth poorest country in the world and Niger the fourth, out of 177 countries measured.[62] The people of Mali, like those in Niger, have a "recurring" problem of "food shortages and associated malnutrition," the World Food Programme (WFP) warned, "especially at the height of the three-month annual lean season before the first harvest in October."[63] Yet when both countries faced severe food deficit problems beginning in October 2004, an illustrative and significant difference surfaced.

Drought visited Mali and Niger—it often does in the Sahel—just as the 2004 "lean season" entered its final months. Locusts, the worst in fifteen years, invaded and destroyed whatever meager crops had survived the drought. Then the familiar coping strategies took place: across the northern districts of both countries, at the height of the lean season, people ate their food stocks and planting seeds, and started selling off their animals and other assets. The cost of millet doubled, pricing the grain beyond the reach of most of the population. Those who could walked out of their communities searching for food.

In early 2005 WFP counted 2.5 million people in Niger "facing extreme hunger" along with another 4.2 million across the countries of the Sahel.[64] The WFP began a significant feeding operation that hauled food from West African ports overland by trucks. The agency borrowed from its own reserves and positioned food in critical areas; it even employed an Airbus 300 to fly in emergency food relief, an unusual and expensive action that signified the urgency of the situation.

In Mali next door the WFP counted 450,000 people—175,000 of them children—suffering from food shortages. Why the smaller numbers? Mali is also subject to food insecurity caused by cyclical drought, insect infestations, rudimentary farming techniques, and desertification. Poverty and precarious health and sanitation made the people of Mali vulnerable to a catalytic event: as in Niger, the locust invasion devastated Mali's ability to grow food and triggered severe hunger.

There was, however, one significant difference. In Niger, according to investigations by NYU's Smita Narula and Médecins Sans Frontières (MSF), economic policies "encouraged"[65] by the international financial institutions contributed to starvation there in 2004–2005. Drought and locusts, MSF reported, "do not fully explain the subsequent epidemic of hunger; despite the diminished yield, the country still produced sufficient food to feed its own population." But the government of Niger, MSF continued, had been "urged by the international financial institutions, key donor countries, and UN agencies to refrain from acting in a manner that would destabilize the local food market or drain resources from ongoing development projects."[66]

Niger relies heavily on the goodwill of the EU and France, its former colonial metropole, and their financial institutions, which "favour free-market solutions to African poverty."[67] (Niger contains about 8 percent of the world's uranium and has negotiated "lucrative mining contracts" with the EU countries and China.)[68] The MSF and other agencies urgently called for the distribution of free emergency food aid to those who were starving. But Niger's authorities, with support from the EU and international agencies, "declined to hand out free food to the starving."[69] Instead Niger started a series of "market-based" approaches. From September 2004 through June 2005, the government set up a system to sell millet "at moderate cost," and indeed some 42,000 tons were sold at below-market prices. But even the prime minister admitted that "hundreds of thousands of the 3.5 million people threatened by the food shortage were too poor to be able to purchase cereal, even at a low price." Many had already sold their livestock and other assets to feed themselves.[70]

Next, instead of distributing free emergency food, the Niger government proposed "cereal loans," to be repaid at the end of the harvest, when farmers presumably would have money. In effect, it was forcing those who were suffering to take loans to pay for their own relief aid. (The echo here of similar events during the Great Irish Famine is striking and painful.) Newspapers reported that "even as thousands perished by late June [2005], some donors praised the Nigerian government for respecting the market and not distributing free food."[71] Those donors applauded Niger's refusal to distribute free relief food. The reason, however absurd it now seems, "was that interfering with the free market could disrupt Niger's development out of poverty."[72] Médecins Sans Frontières, with its large presence inside both Niger and Mali, concluded that "economic policies encouraged by IFIs [international financial institutions] contributed to the famine that struck Niger in 2005." Drought and locusts played a smaller role but "do not fully explain the subsequent epidemic of hunger; despite the diminished yield, the country still produced sufficient food to feed its own population."[73]

Immediately to the west, Mali also suffered from drought and locusts. At the height of the lean season, October 2004, Mali's government also reported severe food shortages and increasing cases of acute malnutrition.[74] But Mali "escaped." How?

The Malian government tracked the starvation closely and reported the intensifying food shortages. In March 2005, government officials forecast that 1.2 million of its people would need help. Unlike the government of Niger, and unlike circumstances during the Great Irish Famine, Mali escaped the starvation by not conforming to "market-based" strategies. The government immediately released some 30,000 metric tons of food from its National Emergency Reserves to those suffering most; WFP quickly added 3700 tons.[75] In August the Malian government again drew down its reserves and distributed another 11,000 tons. "These timely interventions," reported the WFP, "averted a larger-scale crisis like the one facing Niger."[76]

The examples of Malawi, Mali, and Niger illustrate a number of points. First, poverty, hunger, and malnutrition in collaboration make communities vulnerable to starvation and disease. These conditions are, in turn, greatly worsened when an economic theory, formulated elsewhere and distant from on-the-ground realities, is pressed upon a people and their government. This was the case in the Irish Famine and, more recently, in southern Africa, the Horn, and the Sahel, where the same imposition of a rigid economic policy, this time *structural adjustment programs* as part of a free-market global economy, appears to have triggered starvation in several African states.

Second, in Malawi, Niger, and Mali, those suffering directly from severe food shortages used coping strategies far earlier than outsiders were able to observe. These strategies were known to NGOs on the ground and, along with satellite observations (discussed in chapter 7), should have triggered an accurate early warning system for international responses. Events in Malawi, Niger, and Mali sharply underscore the fundamental clash between insider and outsider definitions and responses to starvation. Mali especially offers an excellent example of *insiders* making an early alert to a consortium of *outsiders* in a central government and the international donor agencies, to good results.

Third, there were delays. The well-intended government of Mali waited as long as nine months (June 2004–March 2005) before responding. Other donors were unconscionably slow. By August 2005, for example, donations in response to WFP's March appeal for US$7.4 million in emergency food aid had reached just US$2.7 million—a 63 percent shortfall.[77]

Fourth, the IMF, World Bank, international financial institution lenders, and even UN member states have too quickly dismissed the potential of national food stockpiles. Could the people of Niger and Malawi have survived if their national food reserves had been left intact? Mali offers a resounding answer. First proposed at the World Food Congress in 1974, but with far deeper historic roots (as we have seen), stockpiles of food held in reserve should allow local governments to smooth out the spikes of food shortages, especially chronic seasonal hungers, and to maintain less volatility in food prices. They might also relieve some of the developing world's dependence on the goodwill of international donors. To date, a few African states, most notably Burkina Faso, Burundi, Gambia, and Malawi, are establishing food reserves—returning to "the moral economy"—as their responses to chronic hunger and threats of starvation.

7 Responses Government and International

Having looked at responses to the crisis of starvation by people on the ground, we now examine responses by governments and international agencies. We discuss the three forms of response—program, project, and emergency—but focus primarily on emergency food aid. This is because emergency food relief is by far the largest type of official "outsider" response, and it is also the most controversial. For one thing emergency food relief responds primarily to "loud emergencies." It does not address the long-term, systemic causes underlying the "silent emergencies." Even so, aid of either kind has engendered severe criticism and opposition. Another weakness of outsider intervention to emergencies, however well intended, is that the response is only as good as the information received and only as beneficial as the reaction generated. Both donor reaction and response often come too late. We suggest that this fundamental flaw in outsider response is caused by its heavy reliance—seen in the *outsider* definition of starvation—on "objective," quantifiable "evidence," especially large-scale mortality. Donors often ask: How many have died, and where? Denial and delay are inherent in the counting; yet the appeals and relief efforts are triggered primarily by these data.

In this chapter we briefly address the fundamentals of government and donor responses to starvation, the response mechanisms of the largest donor, the United States, and the ways in which it has used its emergency food aid as an instrument of its foreign policy. We also highlight two very different responses by outsiders to the Ethiopian famines of 1973–1974 and 1983–1986.

A series of questions and answers help us detail the complexities of government and agency emergency responses to starvation.

How Do Governments, Donors, and Relief Agencies Determine Starvation?

Data may be gathered on the ground by government or agency workers or more traditional outsider observers such as missionaries, journalists, embassy officials, field researchers, and others. Those observations are sometimes matched with global technologies such as FEWS satellites and GIEWS and then shared with international governmental and private agencies. This process has an interesting history relevant to our topic.

In November 1974, at the First World Food Conference, the delegates passed a Declaration on the Eradication of Hunger and Malnutrition and twenty-two resolutions to implement it.[1] Two of those resolutions have become significant in shaping governmental and nongovernmental organization (NGO) responses and in assisting the work of international food aid agencies. One resolution called for regional food stockpiles, discussed in chapter 6, and the second called for the building of a Global Information and Early Warning System (GIEWS) and a Famine Early Warning System (FEWS).

The GIEWS system, under the UN Food and Agricultural Organization (FAO), is an information database that uses real-time satellite images to monitor such things as weather assessments, insect migrations, animal and plant diseases, crop production, food aid, and grain export prices. Using that data, GIEWS creates a database incorporating global, regional, national, and subnational information. A forecasted drop in crop yields or outputs, for example, serves as an indicator of change in a region's vulnerability to starvation. GIEWS is primarily a food assessment and information-sharing resource; it issues special alerts and reports to the international community. It can measure world food production, the effects of monsoons in Asia or drought in Africa, which countries are food-insecure, and which need interventions. Today, GIEWS is used by 115 governments, 61 NGOS, and research centers, trade, and media organizations.

USAID (and other governmental agencies and NGOS) produce a FEWS for exchanging satellite data. USAID gathers global information from ground to satellites every ten days. Other satellite early warning systems also monitor the Earth's croplands and crop production every ten days. ARTEMIS (Africa Real-Time Environmental Monitoring Information System), operated by the European Space Agency, watches over global crop, weather, and rainfall or drought patterns with real-time satellites and reports to FAO's GIEWS. Japan's Meteorological Agency records rainfall over Southeast Asia, one of its principal sources of rice. NASA's polar orbiting satellites create eight-kilometer-resolution images of Africa, Latin America, and the Caribbean, while the VEGETATION instrument on board SPOT-4 covers the entire Earth at one-kilometer resolution every ten days and is suitable for monitoring crops down to subnational levels.[2] SPOT-4 is operated by the French space agency CNES (Centre National d'Études Spatiales).

In addition, GIEWS and FEWS are supplemented by reports from NGOS, journalists, local newspapers, missionaries, and others on the ground—especially in countries where international agencies are having difficulty operating or have been expelled. This reporting includes "risk-mapping" in some eighty low-income, food-insecure countries. Put together, this information measures local food crop production to determine the amount of food available in a given region. Information is also collected on indications of any coping strategies. Using these data, the World Food Programme (WFP) (and other agencies) cooperate on interventions with emergency relief food and longer-term nutrition programs.

Therefore, at no time anywhere on Earth is the food crop output of a geographical region unknown either to local communities, national governments, regional entities, or to global food donors. Food shortages and emergencies—rising hunger, starvation, famine—are now well identified and quickly and widely known. Ignorance, or denial, can no longer be a *catalytic cause* allowing starvation to take place, although donor fatigue or the lack of political will may be. Despite this technology, as Jacques Diouf, the director general of FAO, admits, "having an effective early warning system is no guarantee that interventions will follow." [3]

Where Do Donors Obtain Food Aid?

After the international community determines that emergency food aid should be sent to a country or region, or that long-term development program or project aid is needed, and the donors and recipients have agreed to the food aid amount, the commodities are then procured and shipped. For example, USAID submits commodity requests to the USDA, which purchases the food from commodity stockpiles or takes public bids, a process that may require several weeks. The United States no longer has large stockpiles of surplus grains; instead, these are purchased directly from producers or from grain-shipping corporations. High costs have shifted the U.S. government out of the grain storage business, but this has not deterred Congress from supporting U.S. farm subsidies by "raising food aid allocations as an appropriate response to industry and farmer demands for support in years of large crops and low prices." [4]

U.S. law requires that food aid be shipped by U.S. carriers and usually from U.S. ports. The purchase and shipping of all food aid in the United States are done so that the process does not cause disorder in domestic or international grain markets. Hence there are legal and market restraints on taking U.S. surplus food and feeding the world's hungry people. Where there may be risk of major market fluctuations, the Emergency Food Security reserve is drawn down to meet the immediate food aid need without upsetting global prices or markets.

What Is "Food Aid"?

As defined by international aid agreements, food aid must cross international borders, be free ("concessional") to recipients, and be actual food—known as direct transfers—or funds or goods that can be exchanged for food. Most food aid is in bulk form; it may be corn (corn flour), rice, wheat (wheat flour), or blended (corn-soy mix), dehydrated vegetables, powdered milk, and so forth.

It may also be high-energy nutritional aids like Plumpy'nut, a chewy bar made from peanuts, powdered milk, and sugar, with vitamins and minerals added, or BR-5, a high-vitamin-fortified and compressed dry food frequently used for emergency feeding.

What Types of Donor Responses Are Available?

There are three kinds of relief aid responses: program, project, and emergency food aid. The distinction sometimes blurs, but they serve fundamentally different purposes: long-term development support, nutrition assistance, and emergency relief. During the 1960s most food aid was in the form of *program aid* sold or donated government-to-government. But that has been steadily decreasing. In the 1990s program aid averaged 49 percent of all food aid; by 2000 it had dropped to 26 percent; and ten years later it was below 15 percent. Program aid disposes of surplus foods from donor nations. But surpluses among donor states "vary enormously from year to year," or no longer occur, making program aid highly volatile; between 2003 and 2004, for example, program aid fell from about 7 million tons to just above 4 million tons.[5]

Project food aid is primarily distributed through WFP, or NGOs, for nutrition programs, disaster, or emergency food relief. These include school lunch programs and food-for-work projects (similar in structure and intent to those used in the Great Irish Famine). Some project food aid, especially from the United States, is now also sold, and the funds are used for in-country development initiatives. Of the three categories, project food aid has remained steady at 2–3 million metric tons annually since about 1990.

Emergency food aid is free, short-term, and intended to be given directly to people struggling with starvation or sudden food shortages. Demands have risen sharply since 1990, from about 2 million metric tons to more than 6 million by 2003–2004, and remain high. As a proportion of all food aid, emergency food aid has sharp peaks and valleys. For example, it jumped from 49 percent of all food aid in 2000 to 67 percent in 2003, in response to starvation across southern Africa, but then fell back to about 59 percent by mid-decade.[6]

It is important to understand that food aid of all types forms a minuscule proportion of total world food production: about 0.015 percent.[7] Yet this aid plays a disproportionately significant role in the relationships between countries, and between the wealthy nations and the poorer ones.

Who Are the Leading Donors?

The United States provides the bulk of global food aid. Canada, the EU countries, Australia, Japan, and now China and South Africa are also significant providers. In 2007 for example, out of 5.9 million tons of emergency food aid, project aid, and program relief aid, the United States donated more than 2.6 million tons, or about 45 percent. The next closest donor was the EU (756,121 tons, or 13 percent), followed by two surprises, South Korea (431,432, or 7 percent) and China (307,141, about 5 percent).[8]

China is an excellent example of a food aid recipient turned donor. In April 2005 WFP made its last shipment of food aid assistance to China—43,450 tons of wheat for 400,000 poor farmers and their families in a WFP food-for-work scheme in four Chinese provinces. This ended twenty-five years of multilateral donations to China during which, by WFP's count, some 30 million Chinese had been fed. It was "a truly historic moment," said James Morris, WFP's executive director at the time. By 2009, China had become food-self-sufficient and was the world's fourth-largest food aid donor, according to Food Aid Monitor.

Who Are the Leading Recipients?

Although the food donors are changing, the recipients are not. More than half of all global food aid still goes to sub-Saharan Africa, as it has since the 1970s. The pattern of recipients is clear: all are impoverished states. Some become recipients because of natural disasters and then go off the list until the next drought, flood, earthquake, or insect infestation. Some need assistance because of continuing civil conflict or oppressive governments; they remain on the list for longer periods of time. Others are the world's poorest of the poor, and they form the core of the recipient list. In 2009–2010 Ethiopia topped the list of global food-aid recipients, followed by Sudan, Uganda, Eritrea, Kenya, and North Korea, which first appeared on the list more than fifteen years earlier.[9]

How Is Food Aid Distributed?

Some food relief gets funneled through NGOs; there are some 40,000 international NGOs. Aid monies come from grants, individual donors, as well as sponsors; some NGOs have retail fund-raising operations, such as Oxfam UK's donated clothing shops.

Food aid generally gets distributed through three sources: direct transfers, triangular purchases, and, as mentioned, purchases on the ground in local markets. *Direct transfers*, about 58 percent of all food-aid deliveries by 2007, are donations from the donor country. This is often "tied aid" with requirements such as purchase, processing, bagging, and even shipping handled inside the donor country; the United States requires that 75 percent of its direct aid have such ties, and Canada 90 percent.[10] *Triangular food aid* is purchased outside the donor country and sent to a third country. Most (perhaps 75 percent) is obtained in developing countries as part of a complex process. For example, one variation (commodity swaps) involves "the delivery of a food commodity to one country, where it is sold to buy a food commodity that gets shipped to a third country for use as aid." The European Commission (EC) is a major player here, with about 35 percent of triangular purchases in 2007.[11] Finally, in terms of local purchases, less than one-third of all food aid is purchased in the recipient country's markets.

How Does Food Aid Get to Those Who Are Starving?

Most food aid arrives by sea, is off-loaded through ports nearest the region suffering starvation, and is hauled by local road or railways to relief distribution points. It is often handled through the UN's World Food Programme or NGOS. To get relief food quickly into Niger and Mali in 2005, for example, WFP used every means at its disposal. "We're sending it to the ports," said a WFP logistics officer. "We're sending it by air; we have trucks ready at the ports and at the airports to deliver it to the warehouses. Once it's at the warehouses we log in the food and then we deliver it to the NGOS."[12]

Who Distributes the Food?

Supplying food to the world's poor and starving has become an immense global industry, assisted by available satellite technology and continuing food subsidies to wealthy country food producers. Moreover this is a narrowing field controlled by fewer and fewer large global distributors. All make a comfortable living from food shortages and emergencies and from the persistent continuation and spread of hunger and poverty.

There is a vast range of relief agencies, some with overlapping missions, that normally respond to international food crises, or engage in longer-term development work. These include an alphabet-soup of government donors (USAID, USDA), UN agencies (WFP, UNHCR, UNICEF), private volunteer organizations (PVOS), and nongovernmental organizations (NGOS). Government donors generally supply the majority of food aid in emergencies. They also contribute the largest portion of financial aid to NGOS for program and development work.

The biggest public agency is the UN's World Food Programme (WFP), part of the Food and Agriculture Organization, based in Rome. WFP describes itself as "the world's largest humanitarian agency and the UN's frontline agency for hunger solutions." As of this writing, WFP was feeding some 100 million of the world's hungriest people in seventy-seven countries.[13] While WFP provides bulk and blended food aid, other UN agencies are directly involved in other forms of nutrition: UNHCR supplies their refugee constituents with specialized food commodities; UNICEF distributes vitamins and food and nonfood items for feeding programs. The role of NGOS—World Vision, Oxfam UK, Catholic Relief Services, Lutheran World Relief, Save the Children, CARE, and so on—

varies one from the other. There are two major problems among NGOS: the lack of formal regulation and minimal technical standards; and, as we saw in Malawi, the sharing of information and coordination of relief efforts with the UN agencies. Rivalry among relief agencies has too often hindered sharing of information obtained on the ground, especially "shocks" like crop failures and price rises. This remains a serious problem. "The challenge," Save the Children's John Seaman warns, "is to find an effective institutional framework to ensure that these techniques are routinely applied. It is clear that the current involvement of multiple organizations, each with its own interests, cannot meet the basic challenge of early warning."[14]

It is helpful to look in detail at one example of agency response. Doing so will give us an insight into why that response is often slow, and why donors experience "donor fatigue" or seem to lack the will to respond. But the fact that aid is slow in arriving among those who need it does not mean that aid should not be given. It does, however, indicate that the entire process—identification of starvation, verification, response, distribution, local benefit, and impact— needs closer analysis and possible revision.

In 2003, drought across southern Africa was causing starvation among more than 8 million people. WFP set up a Logistic Advisory Centre (LAC) to coordinate port, road, and rail facilities to bring in emergency food aid. But access was difficult: five of the six countries facing the worst shortages are landlocked (Lesotho, Malawi, Swaziland, Zambia, and Zimbabwe); only Mozambique among them has seaports. Because the drought had started in 2001, little surplus grain was growing anywhere in the region by 2003, except in South Africa. USAID started a government-to-government food relief effort *inside* the region. Using funds from its basic legislative instrument (Public Law 480 Title III), USAID purchased surplus grains from farmers inside South Africa for distribution to neighboring landlocked states.

At the same time, WFP was urging donor governments worldwide to respond to southern Africa's crisis. WFP geared up for a massive logistics operation to distribute incoming emergency food aid. It noted the key ports of entry: Dar-es-Salaam in Tanzania; Durban and Cape Town, South Africa; Maputo, Beira, and Nacala, Mozambique. Beira and Nacala are good ports for entry into Malawi, Zambia, and Zimbabwe. Durban can reach Swaziland, whereas Cape Town is closest to Lesotho. Port captains could work with local authorities to offload the emergency food, store it, and move it by road or rail out of the ports into the countryside.

Right away, one problem—and a common one—became clear. This is called the "discharge rate"—the actual amount of food that can be offloaded per vessel per day. Ports, warehouses, railways, roads, and storage silos all need to be coordinated to move the relief food from a ship to the starving. Dar-es-Salaam, Maputo, and Durban could offload just 2000 MTS each per day. Beira and Nacala were actually slower because they lacked automatic bulk offloading facilities. Instead, relief grains—in this case, maize—would have to be bagged at the quayside. WFP estimated that it would take two weeks to move just 25,000–30,000 MTS from ship to warehouse. Then the maize would have to be hauled inland, usually by truck. But the need was for 1.5 million MTS of food aid. At this rate the emergency food aid moving from North America (Canada and the United States) would reach southern Africa's ports by ship in about two weeks. It would take at least another fifty days—almost two months—to offload the entire shipment in the ports. The trip upcountry, depending on the distances, might add another week. Getting relief food from source to the hungry—by ship to southern African ports and then inland to feed the starving—might take more than eighty-five days, almost three months. There are ways to do this faster, of course. As noted earlier, WFP sometimes flies emergency food aid into a country. This dramatic but expensive method can carry only very small amounts of aid. Bags of emergency grain also might be stored regionally, or, as with South Africa in 2003, donors may buy food locally for redistribution in the same country or to its neighbors.

However it is purchased, distributed, or maintained, emergency food aid remains highly controversial. Brought into a country or region, it may disrupt local markets and commodity prices despite the best of intentions. Providing free relief food may change local farming patterns and markets. There are other problems. Who is allowed into relief camps and who receives food aid may fracture traditional social structures and local communities. For example, relief camps can become "magnets" for impoverished people. Those inside relief camps receive medical care and regular meals; those outside do not. Those receiving emergency relief food obtain a special status, exclusive of others. Getting farmers out of relief camps and back into their fields may also be a significant struggle, as it was in Ethiopia in 1974 and again in 1986. In effect, relief camps may add to social dislocation and, as we have seen, even to the spread of disease. Yet they are essential in emergency situations.

Some efforts have been made to address these issues. Food-for-work projects may bring economic and nutritional gains to a community, although the work is often temporary and sometimes draws out farm labor. Direct food purchases from local markets may also stimulate increased farm production locally. But at their heart, emergency relief operations focus only on food availability and not on food entitlement. Immediate hunger is resolved temporarily for those who can reach the feeding stations or receive bags of food. Their underlying poverty is not.

The U.S. Example

The United States "remains the world's most generous food aid donor."[15] To dispense its food aid the United States engages six food distribution programs, all operating under the U.S. Departments of Agriculture and State. These include the Bill Emerson Humanitarian Trust,[16] the Food for Progress Act of 1985, Section 416(b) of the Agricultural Act of 1949, and the three Titles of the Agricultural Trade Development and Assistance Act (PL 480), passed in July 1954, and also later known as the "Food for Peace" Act.[17] Table 7.1 describes the programs, structures and methods of operation.

It is important to understand that in order to respond to international food needs the United States (and any government or agency) requires a legal instrument under which it can act. Public Law 480 is the primary U.S. legislative instrument designed for this purpose; Title II of PL 480 also reflects the shifting pattern of U.S. response to starvation since 1954. PL 480 was originally written during the Cold War with five principal objectives: (1) to help alleviate hunger and malnutrition; (2) to develop and expand foreign markets for U.S. agricultural products; (3) "to expand international trade"; (4) to encourage sustainable economic development in emerging states; and (5) "to foster and encourage the development of private enterprise and democratic participation in developing countries."[18] This law assumed that the United States would have increasing agricultural surpluses to dispense. It established the United States as the world's most generous source of food aid, a position it retains, and legislatively enabled the United States to give away its surplus food as aid or to sell it.

Public Law 480 has been amended several times, and its focus has also changed during the last several decades. Originally PL 480 was intended as a way to distribute U.S. surplus foods to parts of the world, principally Europe, still suffering from postwar shortages. In the 1960s, Congress shifted PL 480 toward a more humanitarian instrument and then redirected it again in the 1990s to promote food security in fragile states by using surplus U.S. relief food.

All three major U.S. programs—PL 480, "Food for Progress" (FFP) program, and "Section 416(b)" of the Agricultural Act of 1949—come with restrictions and conditions. There are limits placed on the amount of U.S. food available for distribution under PL 480 Title II; Food for Progress has a global cap of 500,000 MT and a $30 million transport limit. Commodities may not be shipped unless the recipient country has proper storage facilities—often difficult during a starvation. All three programs must meet the requirement that "at least 75 percent of the U.S. food aid tonnage be shipped on U.S.-flag vessels."[19] There are also restrictions on what countries are eligible. PL 480 Title I is limited to countries with a shortage of foreign exchange earnings that cannot fill "all of [their] food needs through commercial channels." Under Title III, a country must meet

TABLE 7.1

Aid Programs, Sources, Agencies

	Program		
	PL 480 Title I (Program Aid)	PL 480 Title II (Emergency and Project Aid)	Bill Emerson Humanitarian Trust (Emergency Aid)
Agency	USDA	USAID	USDA
Program Structure	Concessional sales of agricultural products, re-sold by developing states for budgetary purposes, etc.	Commodity donations for emergency and long-term needs; sold by recipient for development assistance	Private firms paid by US government to store commodities in US for drawdown during emergencies in developing countries
Operating Agencies	Governments; private	Governments, PVOs, NGOs, intergovernmental (WFP), public/ private	Governments, NGOs, intergovernmental, public/private

Source: Sophia Murphy and Kathy McAfee, *U.S. Food Aid: Time to Get It Right* (Minneapolis: Institute for Agriculture and Trade Policy, 2005), 13.

poverty conditions and all of the indicators of being food deficient and malnourished: per capita caloric intake of less than 2300 calories, a child mortality rate for children under 5 years in excess of 100 per 1000 births, and an inability to produce enough food or import food needs because of a lack of foreign exchange earnings. Food for Progress is restricted to "developing countries and emerging democracies that have made commitments to introduce or expand free enterprise elements in their agricultural economies." This was broadened in 1992 to include the newly independent states of the former Soviet Union.[20]

Public Law 480 and the other programs are adequate for the short term. Countries like China, Greece, and South Korea, for example, were PL 480 recipients who "graduated" to food self-sufficiency. Central Europe and parts of Central and South America, at one time large recipients, have stabilized and are experiencing economic growth and democracy. But little in the law's history indicates that it has expanded export markets or international trade. (Some opponents of U.S. food aid argue that it has reversed these objectives.) Without

Program		
Food for Progress (Project Aid)	Food for Education and Child Nutrition (Project Aid)	Section 416(b) Agricultural Act of 1949 (Project Aid)
USDA	USDA	USDA
Donations of food from CCC stocks, 416(b), PL 480 Title I to eligible countries	Donations of food and financial or technical aid for educational and nutritional projects in poor countries	Donations of CCC surplus commodities for PL 480 Titles II and III or Food for Progress
Governments, NGOs, intergovernmental, public/private	Governments, private, intergovernmental	Governments, NGOs, intergovernmental, public/private

food surpluses, as previously noted, the United States must buy most of its food aid,[21] thus supporting a large and growing industry *inside* the United States with taxpayer dollars, while continuing to put farmers in developing states at risk by distributing inexpensive and subsidized U.S. food in those countries. Their poverty and our food aid are now locked together in a very large and controversial business.

Is U.S. food aid helpful? This important topic gets aired in Congress each time the U.S. Farm Bill comes up for renewal. It also requires extensive discussion and analysis that is largely outside the boundaries of this book, although we will return to its central points as they shape our narrative.[22] We must bear in mind that, as Sophia Murphy and Kathy McAfee remind us, "even poorly designed and badly managed food aid saves lives, at least in the short term."[23]

One model may be the way in which the United States and the international community respond to nutritional and health emergencies. Public health officials and medical doctors have improved sanitation and clinical conditions in relief camps. Mortality among malnourished children has declined, although diarrhea, malaria, measles, and dysentery remain persistent afflictions. Coordination, accountability, and the positioning of NGO response teams and UN agencies have all improved. Perhaps most important, overt medical and nutritional response reactions based on political considerations have diminished.[24] The perfect food aid program, Murphy and McAfee suggest, would prevent deaths now from food emergencies and construct sustainable food production systems in the developing world for the long term. This forms one of the recommendations in this book (chapter 14). None of these legislative devices is currently doing that.

Recurring arguments about the value and impacts of U.S. (and other donor) relief food aid, however, include concerns about disincentives to producers when free food aid lowers prices too sharply or the impacts on those people who are not starving and remain outside relief camps or feeding stations. Often commodity aid does not arrive at the time of most critical need. Sometimes the surplus food aid is culturally inappropriate: cheese to West Africa, or genetically modified corn to Zimbabwe—both rejected when they arrived because cultural or nutritional concerns of the recipient were ignored. Other times, commitment reflects global prices. During the famines in the Sahel and Ethiopia in the 1970s and 1980s, PL 480 surpluses varied in any given year between 19 million MT and 3.5 million MT, in part because of declining U.S. government commitment to the program and in part because of high global prices and demand for surplus grains. Funding also fluctuates. For example in 1983, as the second Ethiopian famine was spreading across the highlands, Congressional appropriations under Ronald Reagan were at the lowest ever in the history of the program.[25]

Beyond these issues, there are more substantive concerns about food aid delivery instruments. One is that U.S. food aid programs make it possible for private voluntary organizations (PVOS) to sell U.S. food aid in the recipient country and redirect those funds to PVO development projects. In addition, export credits—actually taxpayer dollars—are being used to facilitate concessional sales of program food aid. Together, the commercialization of food aid is thought to be displacing sales by local producers, thus weakening developing economies and agriculture. Only South Korea and the United States are both food aid donors *and* sellers.

Moreover U.S. food relief operations have expanded, created, and supported an enormous U.S. agribusiness, to the detriment of U.S. and global smallholder and organic farmers. Four corporations now run more than 60 percent of the grain-handling facilities in the United States (Cargill, Cenex, ADM, and General Mills). Three companies export 82 percent of the corn—the principal PL 480

Title I and II food aid—from the United States (Cargill, ADM, and Zen-Noh). This concentration has also encouraged large-scale production of a small list of food crops, primarily wheat, corn, soybeans, and rice. There is further a narrowing of competition "to a small-group of multinational corporations" with accompanying accusations of "kickbacks" and other forms of irregularity in the U.S. government agencies that have had "a good-old-boy attitude" toward the export companies.[26] Today the ten largest food corporations control 60 percent of the food and beverages sold in the United States.

To assure continuing subsidies from the Farm Bills, grain producers and suppliers spend more than $100 million a year lobbying Congress.[27] It pays off. The top three crops receiving taxpayer subsidies are corn, wheat, and cotton. Those subsidies go to just 30 of the 435 U.S. Congressional districts, but those 30 U.S. Representatives also form the majority on the House agricultural committees; the Senators from these states also comprise the majority of the Senate Agriculture Committee. This might be tolerable if it benefited rural farming in America. But the U.S. Census in 2000, the most recent as we write, shows that three out of four rural counties in the United States had below-average economic growth "despite the record level of farm subsidies."[28] And in 2005, 46 percent of those subsidies went to agribusiness corn farmers, and, as we know, corn is a principal foreign aid commodity.[29]

Corn has become our staple (with its own commercial film, *King Corn*). Taxpayers pay U.S. farmers through the U.S. Farm Bill more than $4 billion a year to grow 45 percent of the total global corn production. That crop covers more than 125,000 square miles of North America. Cheap corn now sprouts up in more than 90 percent of the U.S. diet, much of it in the form of high-fructose corn syrup in soft drinks, snacks, and breakfast foods, and as feed for the animals we eat (cows, chickens, pigs, and even fish). "Our entire food supply," writes Michael Pollan, the U.S. food watchdog, "has undergone a process of 'cornification' in recent years, without our even noticing it." With it has come rising obesity and associated diseases. "It is probably no coincidence," Pollan continues, "that the wholesale switch to corn sweeteners in the 1980s marks the beginning of the epidemic of obesity and type 2 diabetes in this country."[30] More recently agribusinesses and the large grain companies are redirecting corn into ethanol, vitamin C, and biodegradable plastics.[31]

Use of Food as a Political Instrument

Perhaps the largest problem of food aid is found in the intrusion of ideology and politics into the response process. Too often the international community has made highly selective and morally inconsistent decisions about when, where, and how to intervene in the domestic food crises of developing countries. Although kindness, generosity, and concern for the well-being of others are frequently present, too often denial, hesitation, accusation, and manipulation are also among the donors' responses.

For example between 1917 and the end of the Cold War in about 1990, emergency food aid was often used as a tool or instrument by the food-rich West in support of its struggles against the East or Communism. The history of U.S. food aid in the twentieth century contains two basic themes: the ambiguity of deploying U.S. food relief both as a humanitarian tool and as a political instrument; and the persistent deployment of U.S. food aid as a foreign policy weapon. Over the last century, beginning with U.S. responses to starvation in the new Soviet Union in 1921, U.S. food aid was used to further the interests of the state, to bind relations between states, to win support in international organizations like the UN, and to subvert foreign governments—as well as an instrument of peace and stability. Here are a few examples:

○ On May 16, 1945, President Harry S. Truman met with his secretary of war, Henry Stimson. Truman later wrote that Stimson had voiced concern about "pestilence and famine" in Europe after the war, followed by "revolution and communistic infiltration." Both agreed that the best defense would be stabilizing the European governments. "It was vital," Truman wrote, "to keep these countries from being driven to revolution or communism by famine."[32] Within three years, the United States implemented political action wrapped inside a humanitarian policy: the Marshall Plan—The Foreign Assistance Act of 1948—to help stabilize, feed, and rebuild a Europe devastated by war. From 1948 to 1952, the United States sent more than $13.3 billion in food aid, equipment, machinery, and technical expertise to seventeen countries in Europe. Long-term results from this foreign aid included the stabilization of Western Europe, the creation of the Organization of Economic Cooperation and Development (OECD), NATO (a major anti–Soviet Union organization that remains today, long after the end of the USSR), and the European Common Market, precursor of the European Union. All became buffers against Soviet advancement in Europe and the Mediterranean.

○ In 1977 the Carter Administration amended PL 480 to deny U.S. relief food to any country engaged "in a consistent pattern of gross violations of internationally recognized human rights."[33] This added the element of humanitarian concern to the law's list of conditions. In 1978 President Carter offered U.S. food aid to Egypt's Anwar Sadat in exchange for a peace agreement with Israel. U.S. food aid to Egypt increased sharply after Sadat signed the Camp David Accords. By 1980 Egypt had become the single largest recipient of U.S. food aid, and within four years, by the end of the first Reagan Administration, Egypt was still the number one U.S. food aid recipient.[34] During the mid-1980s, as famine spread across sub-Saharan Africa, Egypt received as much as ten times more direct food aid as the next recipient country. The pattern continued throughout the 1980s, when Egypt took in three times the amount of all U.S. food aid sent to leading sub-Saharan recipients *combined*.[35]

o No such generosity reached the Ethiopians, just 1500 miles up the Nile River from Cairo. The tragedy that swept the Horn of Africa in 1973–1974 and again in 1984–1986 helps us to understand the complex relationship among food, starvation, and politics—in this case, the use of food as a foreign policy weapon.

In 1973–1974 the international community, donors included, knew that starvation was under way in Ethiopia. But for more than a year they chose to remain silent. Why? First, Ethiopia was an important ally in the Cold War. The Ethiopian military was funded, trained, and equipped by the United States in exchange for strategic CIA "listening posts" around the country pointed deep into the Middle East. Next door, the Soviet Union supported Somalia and had constructed a navy base at Berbera, on the Indian Ocean at the mouth of the Red Sea. Second, Haile Selassie was an old friend and ally, a popular figure in the West, who was hosting the tenth anniversary of the Organization of African Unity in early 1974. He did not want his country to appear to be "just another starving African nation," *embarrassed* by the sight of large-scale emergency aid activities. Most important, the donors were not *asked* to intervene. They decided to honor a *diplomatic nicety* that donors do not enter a country to feed starving people unless, and until, the government invites them in. For these reasons, the starvation of peasants in the mountainous interior remained a minor irritant, their protesting march on the capital ignored as long as possible.

But in August 1974 Selassie's government collapsed in a military coup. The Emperor was eventually replaced by Mengistu Haile Mariam, a brutal dictator[36] whose military government (The Derg) terrorized Ethiopians until 1991, when he was then forced to resign and fled into exile.[37] Under Mengistu, Ethiopia turned to the Soviet Union, and—completing the flip-flop—Somalia became pro-West. The United States was now welcomed in Mogadishu, the Soviets in Addis Ababa. Starvation, however, remained the condition of the Ethiopian peasants.

As drought and starvation continued through the 1970s, Mengistu and the Marxist Ethiopian government raised alarms and called for food aid. They announced in the press and at the UN that perhaps as many as 7.9 million Ethiopians out of 42 million people were starving.[38] Ethiopian medical teams found "widespread" malnutrition, marasmus, and kwashiorkor among the children. By October 1980 UNHCR reported that Ethiopia had the largest number of disaster victims in Africa.[39] But as the starvation continued, the Ethiopians found—unlike 1974—a very unreceptive international response.

The early warning system, put into play after the 1974 World Food Conference, tracked starvation in Ethiopia and the Horn. The U.S. government knew what was happening. But this starvation was occurring under a Marxist government, and despite the warnings and public calls for assistance, the United Kingdom and the United States (headed by Margaret Thatcher and Ronald Reagan, respectively) refused to send food aid to the Mengistu government. At least one independent account[40] suspects that the United States, in particular, was attempting to stoke the continuing civil war between Ethiopia and its runaway province, Eritrea (today a separate country), in an effort to topple Mengistu. The U.S. and British attitude was "let the peasants vote with their feet" and move to the Eritrean guerrilla side.

Once again national sovereignty was a core issue during starvation. Should the donors violate Ethiopia's sovereignty and feed starving peasants who walked over to the guerrilla side? In 1985, the United States decided to violate Ethiopia's sovereignty with a "back-door" feeding scheme through Port Sudan and, by truck, into the Eritrean side of Ethiopia. This unlocked a massive outpouring of international emergency aid; it stimulated an unprecedented generosity that reached its pinnacle with the fund-raising global telecast, "We Are the World." But the controversy between national sovereignty and the obligation to feed starving people continues today.

To us the "predisposing cause" of the two Ethiopian starvations was the entrenched poverty of the rural Ethiopian peasant. The profile is similar to that of the Irish peasants during the Great Famine and remains familiar today. In Ethiopia of the 1970s and 1980s, nine out of ten Ethiopian peasants lived in the remote and mountainous rural areas; eight out of ten were a full day's walk from *any* road. They scratched out an existence as subsistence farmers dependent entirely on rain-fed agriculture. They survived on a single crop, *teff*, used to make their staple food.

They also farmed under Ethiopia's ancient feudal land tenure system. Before the coup in 1974, the peasant farmers owned only 5 percent of the land in the most stricken provinces, Tigre and Wollo. Across Ethiopia, 27 percent of the landowners were absentees; almost all of the arable land belonged to the State, the Crown (the Imperial Ethiopian Government of Haile Selassie), and the Ethiopian Orthodox Church. One survey showed that a single Ethiopian landlord owned 2 million acres of land and received three-quarters of the produce grown on it by peasant tenant farmers. Ethiopia's peasants earned an average of US$82 a year—about 22 cents a day.[41] This system of land tenancy, the onerous payment of crops to owners, single-crop dependency, and the resulting abject poverty, meant these people were easily "tipped" into starvation. Under Mengistu, the system shifted to one of coerced collectives. Whatever the political system, the peasants always starved.

In both decades, the weight of poverty—with hunger, malnutrition, disease—made the peasant farmers vulnerable to the persistent droughts that visited the Sahel and eastward into the Horn of Africa. There are no reliable figures for how many people lived in Ethiopia during this period, how many starved, and how many died. Ethiopian sources, however, estimated that during the fifteen-year period between 1972 and 1987, more than half of all Ethiopians suffered from starvation. In 1972–1974, perhaps 250,000 Ethiopians died from starvation-related causes.[42] In 1984 the U.S. House Select Committee on Hunger said that more than 300,000 Ethiopian men, women, and children had starved to death by that point in that famine.[43]

The Ethiopian starvations are interesting for at least two reasons. One is the willingness of President Reagan to violate Ethiopia's sovereignty by entering the country without permission through the "back door" of Port Sudan, and to haul in emergency food aid by truck convoy. The other is the denial, delay, and then a slow response by the donors. This remains a significant concern as we write. For example the wfp regularly reports that people may starve to death or have rations cut because international donors "lack the political will" to act. Across southern Africa, for example, where in 2003 some 8.3 million people were facing starvation, wfp collected less than 30 percent of pledges from international food donors.[44] The relief agency had to cut emergency food for 2.8 million people in the region following "a decline in contributions from donors who are beset by compelling demands for numerous crises." When wfp geared up a three-year appeal for help in the region, donors responded with just 2.5 percent of the requested aid.[45] It is worth repeating the anguished statement of wfp's Morris, cited earlier, that "Hunger today is a creation of politics. And it demands political solutions. There are no obstacles—other than lack of political will—that would prevent us from ending hunger tomorrow."[46]

In the post–Cold War era, the United States and other donors have shifted away from using food aid as an instrument of foreign policy. To be sure concerns remain about countries seen as enemies or targets of armed conflict. How should donors respond, for example, to conditions in Iran, Afghanistan, the Democratic Republic of the Congo, Zimbabwe, and North Korea? All have experienced severe food shortages. Zimbabwe and North Korea remain nettlesome political problems, largely because of self-inflicted (or "artificial") food shortages and starvation caused by their own government policies.

Between 2000 and 2007, as many as 6 million people in Zimbabwe faced starvation—more than half of a population that was already declining from

12 million to about 8 million because of hunger-related deaths, violence, and emigration. The government of Robert Mugabe denied Zimbabweans the chance to move surplus foods around their country to diminish the impact shortages, and either ordered the agency to leave the country or refused to allow WFP permission to enter.

In North Korea by 2004 more than 6 to 7 million people (out of 23 million) repeatedly suffered starvation, largely the result of extreme poverty, drought, and diversion of the country's food production to its armed forces. In the late 1990s between 500,000 and 1 million North Koreans died from starvation and its associated diseases. People were publicly executed for stealing food; others, according to Amnesty International, reportedly died in labor camps from malnutrition.[47] Foreign donors voiced alarm about the diversions and political favoritism in distributions. At one point in 2004 WFP briefly suspended its feeding operations for 4.2 million North Koreans because of low donor response and contributions.[48] By 2008, however, WFP was expanding its work in North Korea, and perhaps in response to negotiations with that country over its nuclear program, the United States was shipping in food to the port of Nampo, near Pyongyang, while U.S. NGOs distributed it in two North Korean provinces.[49]

As we write, Ethiopia, Somalia, and Kenya are afflicted with deepening hunger and starvation. The WFP warns that 17 million people need emergency food assistance. "We are knocking on the door of a major regional crisis," the WFP special envoy said. The causes: drought, poor seasonal rains, civil conflict, and rising costs of food. Only half the arable land has been sown as farmers wait for the rains. The WFP sees a shortfall of almost $450 million for its operations over the coming months. "We appreciate that the global financial crisis is squeezing resources everywhere," said the envoy, "but we are urging donors to step forward quickly and generously, before it is too late."[50]

Breaking this pattern will require reexamination of government and international responses and not only emergency food aid but also long-term development aid and social, economic, and political change. Only then, as Timothy Shaw writes, if we are willing, can we "deny famine a future."[51]

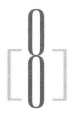

Responses to Malnutrition

A hungry man is not a free man.
—Adlai Stevenson (1900–1965)

The man who has bread has many problems.
The man who has no bread has one.
—folk wisdom

The Pathophysiology of Starvation:
Protein-Energy Malnutrition

In chapters 3 and 4 we discussed the basics of the biochemistry and physiology of nutrition. We learned that the three macronutrients carbohydrates, fats, and proteins are generally treated similarly by the processes of digestion via chemical reactions that hydrolyze the bonds that hold their constituent building blocks together. The simpler sugars, fatty acids, and amino acids are then transported across cell membranes, internalized, and used for immediate energy requirements, storage for future energy requirements, or growth via biosynthesis.

We are now prepared to discuss the mechanisms by which our bodies defend this process and what happens when access to nutrients becomes inadequate. In order that we might fully understand the abnormal states of malnutrition, semistarvation, and eventual starvation, it will be helpful for us to answer some basic questions. What are the biological mechanisms that regulate our intake of macronutrients? What causes us to seek food; that is, what is hunger? What happens when we do not get enough food to fill either our requirements for energy or our need for essential nutrients to maintain our bodies? Answers to these questions will help us understand hunger as a primary driver of human behavior. It will also demonstrate how the complexities and needs of our biological systems compel us to seek adequate nutrition. It additionally enables us to understand the deterioration of our minds and bodies when we fail to obtain food, when we become malnourished, or when we suffer from chronic hunger.

Hunger—the Physiology of Food-Seeking Behavior

Webster defines hunger as "a craving or urgent need for food or specific nutrient, an uneasy sensation occasioned by the lack of food, a weakened condition brought about by the prolonged lack of food." In chapter 2 we advanced the definition used by investigators in the fields of the social sciences. Although these definitions are grammatically accurate and useful for the purpose of scientific study, they do not do justice to the human sensation of hunger. Kamala Purnaiya Taylor (1924–2004), an Indian novelist who wrote under the pseudonym Kamala Markandaya, described hunger in more evocative, experiential terms in her defining novel *Nectar in a Sieve*:

> For hunger is a curious thing; at first it is with you all the time, waking and sleeping and in your dreams, and your belly cries out insistently, and there is a gnawing and a pain as if your very vitals were being devoured, and you must stop it at any cost and you buy a moment's respite even while you know and fear the sequel. Then the pain is no longer sharp but dull, and this too is with you always, so that you think of food many times a day and each time a terrible sickness assails you, and because you know this you try to avoid the thought, but you cannot, it is with you. Then that too is gone, all pain, all desire, only a great emptiness is left, like the sky, like a well in drought, and it is now that the strength drains from your limbs and you try to rise and find you cannot, or to swallow water and your throat is powerless, and both the swallow and the effort of retaining the liquid tax you to the uttermost.[1]

However we might define it, hunger is the basic driving force of human behavior. Abraham Maslow (1908–1970), considered the father of humanistic psychology, first published his Theory of Human Motivation in 1943.[2] In his model, known as Maslow's hierarchy of needs, he defined five levels of human needs: physiological, safety, love/belonging, esteem, and self-actualization. Maslow pointed out that the more basic, primitive needs have to be fulfilled before any attention is paid to those higher in the hierarchy. The basic or more primitive physiological needs include food, water, homeostasis (including maintenance of body temperature), and as Maslow quite correctly points out,

> For the man who is extremely and dangerously hungry, no other interests exist but food. He dreams food, he remembers food, he thinks about food, he emotes only about food, he perceives only food and he wants only food. The more subtle determinants that ordinarily fuse with the physiological drives in organizing even feeding, drinking or sexual behavior, may now be so completely overwhelmed as to allow us to speak at this time (but only at this time) of pure hunger drive and behavior, with the one unqualified aim of relief.

To paraphrase his succinct summary of the situation: man does indeed live by bread alone, when there is no bread.

The psychological aspect of hunger as a prime driver of human behavior seems simple, especially for anyone who has ever really been hungry. The physiological drivers of hunger, however, turn out to be extraordinarily complex. Our nutritional status is of such crucial importance that it is defended by multiple complex systems; nothing is left to chance.

On a minute-to-minute, day-to-day time scale, our metabolisms are closely regulated to exquisitely maintain our blood glucose levels, whether or not a person's hunger can be abated by access to food. The hormones primarily responsible for this regulation are the polypeptide hormones insulin and glucagon and, to a lesser extent, the catecholamine epinephrine and the glucocorticoid cortisol. (Polypeptides are chains of amino acids and include the proteins.) The discovery of the most famous of these, insulin, began with an accidental observation reported in 1889 by Oskar Minkowski and Joseph von Mering at the Hoppe-Seyler Institute in Strasbourg, Germany.[3] In trying to determine whether or not the pancreas was involved in fat digestion in the dog, they surgically removed the pancreas from an experimental animal. Before they could begin their experiment on fat digestion, however, the dog developed copious urination (polyuria) and very high glucose levels in the urine (glycosuria), both cardinal symptoms of diabetes mellitus. (In fact the name of that metabolic disease comes from the Greek and Latin roots for "flow" [*diabetes*] and "sweet" [*mellitus*]. The reason it was called this is that physicians initially made their diagnosis by tasting the patient's urine—if it was sweet, then there was sugar in it, a cardinal manifestation of diabetes.) Minkowski and von Mering realized there must be a factor in the pancreas the lack of which caused diabetes, but they were unable to isolate it. It was not until 1921 that Frederick Banting and Charles Best at the University of Toronto isolated a pancreatic protein that was able to cure the symptoms of diabetes in dogs.[4] They named it insulin, since it was known to be produced in nests of cells in the pancreas called the islets of Langerhans (Latin *insula*: island) as we noted in chapter 4.

As we discussed in chapter 4, glucose homeostasis (maintenance of a stable, constant level) is tightly controlled, despite the fact that our intake of nutrients is intermittent, depending on the timing, content, and interval between meals. Our daily metabolic state can be divided into a fed state (anabolic, or storage and biosynthesis), an intraprandial state (between meals—catabolic, using stored energy), and a fasting state (catabolic—using stored energy and making new glucose from other sources). During the fed or anabolic state, the major hormonal regulation comes from insulin, which is released by the β *islet cells* of the pancreas. Insulin is the major anabolic hormone; its secretion is stimulated by increases in blood glucose concentration, and its main function is to drive glucose into the body's cells where it can be metabolized to create ATP or stored (mostly in the liver, but also in skeletal muscle) as the animal starch glycogen. Insulin also has major effects on fat metabolism, causing the synthesis of fatty acids from excess ingested glucose and the synthesis of glycerol, which is used to form the triglycerides that are then stored in the adipose tissue. Insulin also has critical but less well-understood functions in protein metabolism. It acts to stimulate amino acid uptake by the cells. It stimulates the synthesis of new protein from the ingested amino acids as well as new ones formed from excess glucose by stimulating DNA transcription of selected genes (especially those coding for enzymes involved in the anabolic process), increasing translation of RNA into new protein, and it also inhibits protein catabolism (to a large extent by depressing the rate of gluconeogenesis or the rate of new glucose formation, the substrate of which is mostly the amino acids derived from breakdown of skeletal muscle protein).

During the intervals between meals insulin secretion is suppressed, and the major hormonal activity is from glucagon, which is similar to insulin in that it is a polypeptide hormone secreted by the pancreas, although glucagon is secreted by the *α cells* of the islets of Langerhans. Glucagon, a major catabolic hormone, has opposite physiological effects of insulin in that its secretion is stimulated by dropping blood glucose concentrations, and the end result of its effect is to increase blood glucose concentration.

There are two major metabolic mechanisms by which glucagon does this. The first is by causing glycogen to be broken down into glucose in the liver (*glycogenolysis*), thereby releasing glucose into the bloodstream for use by other organs, especially the brain (in the case of muscle glycogen, it allows the glucose to be used by the muscle itself for energy). Glucagon also stimulates the liver to produce glucose de novo via the biosynthetic pathway called *gluconeogenesis* (literally "new glucose creation"), using lactic acid, amino acids, and the glycerol from triglycerides as substrate. During more prolonged fasting, in addition to more active gluconeogenesis driven by glucagon (and other catabolic hormones such as epinephrine and cortisol), there is progressive production of the ketone bodies we described in chapter 4, to make sure that the brain has adequate access to energy sources. Although the hormonal interactions during these various stages of nutrient availability are far more complex and interactive than we describe, the important point here is that the events they control occur on a short time scale (seconds to minutes to hours), and the ultimate purpose is strict homeostasis of blood glucose level between narrowly defined limits over each twenty-four-hour period. Although blood sugars will vary during any twenty-four-hour period between, for example, 70 to 200 milligrams per deciliter, blood glucose levels greater than 200 milligrams per deciliter for any prolonged period of time would be considered consistent with a diagnosis of diabetes, with all of its attendant complications. What is more alarming for the purposes of this discussion, however, is the fact that a blood glucose level much below 70 milligrams per deciliter can cause significant and progressive organ dysfunction, specifically of the central nervous system, and can quickly lead to coma and death within minutes if it is low enough, occurs abruptly, or is not quickly reversed. For this reason, when all is said and done, the body's physiology defends its blood sugar levels.

Whereas blood glucose concentration is what the body carefully regulates on a minute-to-minute, hour-to-hour time span, over the long haul the biological metric that is carefully regulated by our body's homeostatic mechanisms is the body mass index (BMI). For medical and scientific purposes it is best to describe weight not in terms of the weight alone but as an index of weight versus height. The metric conventionally accepted as the standard is the body mass index (BMI) and is defined as weight (in kilograms) divided by height (in meters) squared (kg/m^2). In this way normative values can be determined and defined, with a BMI less than 18.5 considered underweight, 18.5–24.9 normal, 25–29.9 overweight, 30–39.9 defined as obesity, and equal to or greater than 40 morbid obesity.

The diseases of people in the resource-rich countries of the world are much more associated with BMIs at the higher end of the spectrum than the lower, a subject we do not address in this book. The problems of diabetes, obesity, and a complex of abnormalities called the metabolic syndrome are diseases of affluence and overconsumption, and they are epidemic in the resource-rich countries. For the purposes of this volume, it will suffice to say that people with a BMI over 28 have a threefold to fourfold greater risk of diabetes, stroke, and heart attack when compared to their slimmer cohorts. On average obesity shortens life-expectancy by five to seven years, morbid obesity by twenty years.[5]

(You might want to calculate your own BMI, but brace yourself. A calculator can be found at the National Heart, Lung, and Blood Institute's website at http://www.nhlbisupport.com/bmi/). Table 8.1 lists the accepted categories for each body mass index class.

Body mass index, for people with access to adequate nutrition, is remarkably well maintained for any one individual. Although failure to maintain blood sugar can result in death within minutes, failure to maintain an adequate body mass index will result in failure of the ability to reproduce (from the perspective of genetic fitness this is the evolutionary equivalent of death), and if this failure is severe and prolonged enough, it will lead to premature death within the longer time span of months to years. In addition to the hormones involved in the minute-to-minute regulation of blood glucose concentration, which themselves have direct and indirect effects on the sensations we feel as

TABLE 8.I
Classification of Nutritional Status Defined by Body Mass Index

BMI	Classification
underweight	less than 18.5
normal weight	18.5–24.9
overweight	25–29.9
obesity	greater than or equal to 30
morbid obesity	greater than 40

hunger and satiety, there are other, exceedingly complex interactions among them, other more recently discovered hormones, anatomic or physical inputs (such as gastric stretching, the sense of smell), and neurohormonal processes involving hormones with *orexigenic* effects (appetite-stimulating) and *anorexigenic* effects (appetite-depressing).

In the 1950s the British scientist Gordon Kennedy theorized such a system in the lipostat theory to explain the relative constancy of body weight. He reasoned that there must be some mechanism by which the centers in the brain that controlled food-seeking behavior, eating, and satiety (known to be located in the hypothalamus, a central portion of the brain between the upper centers and the brain stem) would be informed by some feedback loop of the amount of stored energy in the form of adipose tissue mass in the body. He theorized a substance produced by adipose tissue that would provide this feedback and inhibit eating (anorexigenic stimulus). Forty years later, a substance was identified in a strain of mice that was the product of a gene called *Ob* (for obese). Normal mice had two functional copies of this gene, but mice with two defective copies behaved physically and physiologically as if they were perpetually starving and became severely obese, up to three or four times as heavy as their normal siblings. This gene product was found to be a polypeptide hormone that was named leptin (from the Greek *leptos*: thin). It is produced by adipose tissue, and its receptors are found in the arcuate, ventromedial, and dorsomedial nuclei in the hypothalamus—areas known to regulate feeding behavior. Among other messages, leptin "tells" the brain that fat stores are sufficient and causes the hypothalamic centers to send signals that decrease appetite (or hunger) and increase energy utilization, for example, increasing blood pressure, increasing heart rate, or increasing heat production by uncoupling electron transfer from ATP synthesis in the mitochondria of adipocytes. Insulin has a similar effect on appetite, and a number of other anorexigenic neuropeptides have been described: cholecystokinin (CCK), α-melanocyte-stimulating hormone (α-MSH), corticotrophin-releasing hormone (CRH), and cocaine- and amphetamine-regulated transcript (CART). All of these are produced in the hypothalamus, although CCK is also produced in the duodenum and has major local effects in the production and excretion of bile. Countering the effects of these appetite-suppressing or anorexigenic hormones are a group of appetite-stimulating or orexigenic polypeptides such as neuropeptide Y (NPY) and ghrelin. Neuropeptide Y is produced in the hypothalamus and is an extremely potent appetite stimulant. Ghrelin (from the Greek: to grow) is another potent orexigenic hormone produced (among other places) in the wall of the stomach. Its release is stimulated when the stomach is empty, and its two major biological activities are the regulation of energy balance and stimulation of growth hormone secretion by activating receptors in the hypothalamus.

The important point to take away from this big picture is this: our nutritional homeostasis is exquisitely monitored and maintained by intricate, elaborate, and redundant pathways. If we consider the inordinate amount of evolutionary pressure and biological investment that resulted in the evolution of these mechanisms, we can then truly begin to understand just how central this concept is to life. Although the specific details of these mechanisms might be fascinating, they are of less importance to our discussion than the central fact that body mass index is regulated and maintained by a complex, interacting, multi-sited, and multifunctional array of physical and biochemical functions that provide feedback and fail-safes to ensure the homeostasis necessary for long-term survival and reproductive success, very much like the regulation of blood glucose concentration that is necessary for short-term functionality and survival. Maintenance of our nutritional status is fundamental to our biological success, and it is therefore defended at all costs. It is fair to say that the science relating to the regulation and control of hunger and metabolism is not rocket science—it is much more complex than that. The other important fact to consider is this: when access to nutritional resources is inadequate, body mass index is sacrificed to maintain blood glucose concentration (long-term survival is potentially forfeited to preserve short-term survival), we begin to cannibalize our internal resources, and slowly but surely, we begin to die.

Macronutrient Deficiency—Protein-Energy Malnutrition

Malnutrition due to inadequate access to one or more macronutrients is termed protein-energy malnutrition.[6] Why should protein be singled out as a specific case in macronutrient deficiency? As we learned in chapter 3, both carbohydrates and proteins provide a potential 4 kilocalories per gram, whereas fats provide 9 kilocalories per gram. Carbohydrates act as a basic source of energy as well as immediately available stored energy in the form of glycogen, which can be used in the short term by muscle and which the liver breaks down into glucose to be released immediately to the bloodstream in order to maintain blood glucose concentration within a very tight range. Fat, in addition to being the most energy-dense macronutrient, acts as an effective long-term storage of energy both because it is energy-dense and also because it can be stored without excess water.

Protein, on the other hand, is a very special case. Although both carbohydrates and fats are necessary as immediate and stored energy sources, and to some extent function as structural and functional elements of cells, it is proteins that perform life's functions. This is a critical point. If DNA, the genetic material that encodes our very being, is the informational code for life, proteins, as translated from the genetic message via the intermediary RNA, are the actualization of life. The functional elements of our internal organs, muscles, intracellular mechanisms, mediators of biochemical reactions (in the form of enzymes), intra- and intercellular signalers, are all, for the very most part, peptides or polypeptides (proteins). As such, proteins are critical to life's functions and for that reason are conserved and maintained preferentially. They are used as stored fuels under only the direst of circumstances. Under normal conditions, 75 percent of our body's protein is recycled in order to ensure the availability of the essential amino acids for protein synthesis. Only 25 percent of our internal amino acids are used for metabolic purposes.

As we shall see, however, in a circumstance of continued nutritional energy deficit, our bodies adapt so that 95 percent of our amino acids are recycled, allowing for continued synthesis of the proteins critical to the performance of life's functions. This adaptation cannot occur in kwashiorkor as a result of the absence of adequate essential amino acids. For this reason kwashiorkor is a particularly damaging syndrome, wreaking havoc with the physical and mental development, and eventually the lives, of the people most likely to suffer from it—the children.

Protein-energy malnutrition (PEM) can be either a primary problem, that is, due to inadequate food intake, or a secondary problem, as the result of a disease that leads to decreased food intake, decreased nutrient absorption from the GI tract, or increased nutrient requirements as is the case with AIDS, tuberculosis, or cancer. PEM can also occur as either a primary energy deficiency (*marasmus*) or a primary protein deficiency (*kwashiorkor*). Marasmus and kwashiorkor share a number of manifestations, such as decreased physical activity and anemia (low blood count), that are both partly due to adaptive mechanisms. Other shared features include an impaired immune response, impairment of growth (in both body and mind) in children, and emotional damage in both the child and adult. There are also distinct metabolic differences between the two. Although most people suffering from chronic malnutrition experience a mixed deficit of both caloric deficiency and protein deficiency, it is helpful to describe the two pure forms of protein-energy malnutrition in order to understand the resultant physiological effects.

Marasmus

Marasmus (from the Greek: withering) is the condition caused by primary energy deficiency, that is, inadequate caloric intake to maintain appropriate growth and body maintenance. In the case of early or mild to moderate energy deficiency, the observer would note sedentary behavior—lack of work in adults and lack of playing in children. This, of course, is an adaptive response to inadequate energy supplies—the body does only what it has to in order to maintain homeostasis. The following is a quote from Fania Fenelon, one of the few survivors of Bergen-Belsen concentration camp, recalling the liberation of the camp by the British Army at the end of World War II. It describes this "interesting medical fact" with an eloquent clarity that does not allow clinical detachment.[7]

> A new life breathed in the camp. . . . Our liberators were well-fed and bursting with health, and they moved among our skeletal, tenuous silhouettes like a surge of life. . . . They called to one another, whistled cheerfully, then suddenly fell silent, faced with eyes too large, or too intense a gaze. How alive they were; they walked quickly, they ran, they leapt. All these movements were so easy for them, while a single one of them would have taken away our last breath of life! These men seemed not to know that one could live in slow motion, that energy was something you saved.

People suffering from poor caloric intake appear apathetic, with a deficit of attention to their surroundings. Physically, as this becomes increasingly severe, one sees a "skin and bones" appearance. There is generalized muscle wasting and an absence of subcutaneous fat. Children suffering from prolonged chronic primary energy deficiency are generally 60 percent or less of the normal weight-for-height (known as wasting), and they will have significantly lower height-for-age (stunting). Their hair is sparse, thin, dry, and easily pulled out; their skin is dry and wrinkled. Both children and adults suffering from this severe degree of chronic primary energy deficiency will have an anxious appearance, with sunken cheeks manifesting the loss of the cheek pads, a late sign in starvation. Medical examination would reveal a slow pulse (bradycardia), low blood pressure (hypotension), and low body temperature (hypothermia). Chronically starving individuals may be anorectic (lacking appetite) or ravenous, but they all vomit easily. Refeeding must be done carefully by trained personnel experienced in determining the extent and composition of the nutritional deficiencies and any co-morbidities that may exist, since inappropriate nutrition, either in amount or composition, can lead to progressive morbidity and death.

Kwashiorkor

Kwashiorkor is a condition caused by primary protein deficiency, with or without adequate caloric intake. For decades physicians and scientists interested in chronic malnutrition recognized a form of malnutrition, more common in young children but not infants, that was associated with weight loss and growth retardation but also with the formation of diffuse edema (retention of fluid in the body's tissues), and that could also be found in children who were not starving in regard to caloric intake or who were from families in good socioeconomic position with adequate access to energy-rich foods. Because of the dermatologic manifestations associated with this condition, investigators theorized a possible link to vitamin deficiency or tropical parasites. In the 1930s the pediatrician Cicely Williams, working with the Ga people in Ghana, noted that the native name for this disease, kwashiorkor, translated to "first-second" or "displaced or rejected one," and meant "the disease the first child gets when the second child is born." She noted the association with the weaning of the older child from breast milk with the birth of the next child, and the replacement of this high-protein diet with a carbohydrate-rich, protein-poor diet—in the case as she reported in The Lancet, with maize,[8] although kwashiorkor has since been associated more with diets heavily weighted toward the carbohydrate-rich, protein-poor tuber cassava (also known as manioc, the flour of which is tapioca).

Although it was the physical manifestations of kwashiorkor, the diffuse swelling or puffiness caused by the edema and the dermatologic manifestations that first differentiated this type of malnutrition from marasmus, it is the physiological differences caused by the primary protein deficiency that distinguish kwashiorkor as particularly insidious and debilitating.

As discussed earlier, all people suffering from chronic malnutrition manifest adaptive responses, including physical ones such as inactivity and anemia. How is anemia an adaptive response to chronic malnutrition? As there is a decrease in lean body mass and resultant physical activity, there is a concomitant decrease in the body's total oxygen demand. Coupled with this and a decrease in dietary amino acids, there is a decrease in hematopoiesis (production of the formed elements of the blood such as red blood cells, which contain the oxygen-carrying protein hemoglobin), and the recycled amino acids can then be used for the synthesis of other proteins. This is an adaptive response as long as the body's tissues decreased oxygen demands are met. This is one of the areas in which uninformed refeeding can lead to serious problems. Refeeding leads to increased muscle mass, increased physical activity, and increased tissue oxygen demands. The resultant increased demand for blood oxygen-carrying capacity causes a marked increase in hematopoiesis. If there is not simultaneous replacement in the diet of hematinics (micronutrients necessary for the synthesis of hemoglobin such as iron, folic acid, etc.), serious secondary anemia and debility can be created.

In addition to the adaptive response above, we mentioned the fact that, in the fed state 75 percent of amino acids are normally recycled, whereas in the chronically malnourished state, there is an adaptive response causing up to 95 percent recycling of amino acids so that critical protein synthesis can be maintained. This is true unless there is a significant, persistent deficit of high-quality protein in the diet (high quality being defined as protein containing adequate amounts of the essential amino acids). Under those circumstances, needed protein synthesis is limited, and protein stores necessary for vital functions begin to be depleted. Probably the best way to bring this into focus is to consider the difference between what happens to basal oxygen consumption per kilogram body weight in marasmus versus kwashiorkor (basal oxygen consumption per kilogram body weight, a metric that measures oxygen consumption at rest indexed to the weight of the individual and dependent on the "mix" of active versus resting tissues in any one individual's body, is different from total body oxygen demand and should not be confused with the example above).

Patients with marasmus suffer skeletal muscle wasting, but visceral protein is spared. If we think about this teleologically, this makes perfect sense. The skeletal muscles are important for physical activity, but this is "optional" and can be (and is) decreased in situations of inadequate nutrition. Visceral function, on the other hand, is "mandatory" or vital to survival, and must be maintained regardless of the availability of adequate nutrition (much like the blood glucose level). Since the viscera must remain active, their oxygen consumption at rest continues despite the lack of physical activity. Because of this biochemical adaptation to caloric deficiency, the basal oxygen consumption per kilogram body mass in marasmus actually increases compared to the fed state, as more of the lean body mass is now made up of fully functioning and therefore oxygen-consuming visceral tissue and less is made up of resting skeletal muscle (which has minimal oxygen consumption at rest). The opposite occurs in kwashiorkor. Because of the underlying severe protein deficiency, visceral protein cannot be spared. Both skeletal muscle and visceral protein are cannibalized, and the basal oxygen consumption per kilogram body mass falls, as the viscera begin to malfunction and use less oxygen at rest. One does not need a medical degree to understand why this situation is maladaptive and particularly dangerous.

Why is it important that we understand the biochemical and physiological differences between the caloric or energy deficiency of marasmus on the one hand and the specific syndrome associated with the protein deficiency of kwashiorkor on the other? Although this distinction may not be of importance in our overall understanding of the physical and mental damage that hunger and chronic malnutrition cause in general, it is of great importance, if we are to rectify this situation, that we understand that our dietary needs are complex; that even in the presence of adequate caloric intake, we can "starve to death" if other essential nutrients are not present—in this case, the macronutrient protein. We address this point further in the ensuing sections on micronutrients. We shall see that the inadequate intake of just one essential nutrient, needed in only microgram amounts, is enough to cause disability and death. At this point it is important to recognize the following: although it is true that man *does not* live by bread alone (as long as there is bread), it is also true that man *cannot* live by bread alone.

Micronutrient Deficiencies

Although macronutrient deficiency is by far the major nutritional problem facing us today, there are a number of micronutrient deficiencies that historically and to the present day affect the quality of life and longevity of millions if not billions of people.[9] The term *micronutrients* refers to dietary requirements that are necessary in only relatively small amounts to support life's processes and includes the vitamins and minerals. These nutrients serve either functional or structural roles as opposed to providing a source of energy in the form of calories.

Vitamins

Mankind has always been plagued with unexplained diseases, some of which were clearly contagious, whereas others did not seem to be. Many of these were documented in the medical literature dating back to the ancient Egyptians and Greeks. The Egyptians recommended the use of liver for the relief of night blindness. This is actually a very plausible remedy in that the most frequent cause of night blindness is vitamin A deficiency, and liver is a very rich and potent source of vitamin A. Unfortunately, the records suggest that the liver was to be placed on the eyes rather than eaten. Perhaps it worked because, protein sources being in short supply, it was also eaten once it had served as a topical remedy. Scurvy-like illness is described in Egyptian records dating back to 1500 BCE and was described by Hippocrates in the fifth century

BCE. The devastating effects of scurvy played a major role in human history until the mid-eighteenth century, when the Scottish physician James Lind definitively demonstrated the cure (if not the cause) in what was probably the first randomized, clinical human study.

It was not until the early twentieth century when a Polish biochemist, Casimir Funk, fascinated by an article he had read by the Dutch physician-scientist Christiaan Eijkman describing the incidence of beri-beri in people who ate polished rice as opposed to unmilled brown rice, looked for and was able to isolate what he thought was the responsible substance (he was apparently incorrect). As we discussed in chapter 3, because this substance was vital to health, and was a nitrogen-containing compound (an amine), he called the substance a vitamine (vital amine). It was only later, when it was realized that not all of these substances were amines (vitamin C is an acid, ascorbic acid, [a: without; scorbic: referring to scurvy]), that the e was removed. His work led to further investigation by Frederick Gowland Hopkins and Dr. Eijkman, who later shared the 1929 Nobel Prize in Physiology or Medicine for their discovery of the role of vitamins, using the model of the role of vitamin B_1 (thiamine) deficiency in the causation of beri-beri. Five other Nobel prizes were subsequently awarded for discoveries related to vitamin structure and function including: the 1934 prize in physiology or medicine awarded to George Whipple, George Minot, and William Murphy for their work on pernicious anemia (not recognized to be due to vitamin B_{12} deficiency until 1948); the 1937 prize in physiology or medicine awarded to Albert Szent-Györgyi for his work on vitamin C; the 1937 prize in chemistry awarded to Walter Haworth and Paul Karrer for their work on the structure of ascorbic acid and other vitamins; the 1943 prize in physiology or medicine awarded to Carl Peter Henrik Dam and Edward Adelbert Doisy for their work in the discovery of and chemical nature of vitamin K; and the 1967 prize in physiology or medicine given to George Wald for his work on the relationship between vision and vitamin A.

Vitamins are divided into two groups based on a specific physical characteristic, that is, whether they are water soluble or fat soluble. The water-soluble vitamins—all of the B complex of vitamins and vitamin C—tend to act as cofactors in the enzymatic reactions of metabolism as noted in chapter 3. The fat-soluble vitamins A, D, E, and K tend more to behave as regulators of cellular function: they behave like hormones. They also have antioxidant properties (vitamins A and E) as well as very specific physiological functions such as the role of vitamin A in vision, vitamin D in bone metabolism, and vitamin K in blood clotting.

Vitamin E deficiency is extremely rare in humans and is generally found in only three situations: in patients with an underlying disease process that limits

TABLE 8.2

Vitamins and Human Nutrition

Vitamin	Function	Deficiency
Fat soluble		
A	maintain healthy epithelium, vision	night blindness, permanent blindness, increased susceptibility to infection
D	growth and maintenance of bone	rickets
E	anti-oxidant, role in blood development and clotting	very rare
K	blood clotting	bleeding disorder
Water soluble		
B_1 (thiamine)	metabolic coenzyme	beri-beri
B_2 (riboflavin)	coenzyme in metabolism, energy transport	breakdown of skin, mucous membranes
B_3 (niacin)	energy transport in metabolism, DNA repair, steroid hormone synthesis	pellagra
B_5 (pantothenic acid)	critical to formation of coA (metabolism)	rare and poorly defined
B_6 (pyridoxine)	neurotransmitter synthesis	neurological disorder, very rare
B_7 (biotin)	fat, glucose, amino acid metabolism	very rare
B_9 (folic acid/folate)	DNA synthesis	anemia, neurological deficits, and congenital abnormalities
B_{12} (cyanocobalamine)	blood formation, nerve function	pernicious anemia
C (ascorbic acid)	anti-oxidant, maintains healthy tissues, wound healing	scurvy

their ability to digest and absorb fats; in individuals with a very rare, specific genetic abnormality in a protein necessary for the transportation and transfer of vitamin E; and in premature, very low-birth-weight infants. Although clinically apparent vitamin E deficiency may develop under catastrophic circumstances, such as ecological disasters, famine, and in war, it is not felt to be an important specific factor in chronic malnutrition. Vitamin D deficiency can be medically important, but the factor can be produced by humans if exposure to sunlight is adequate. Even though intermittent and isolated cases of clinically significant vitamin D deficiency are still reported, mostly in northern latitudes, severe vitamin D deficiency of large populations associated with concurrent chronic malnutrition does not seem to be a significant problem. Vitamin K, although an important element in the diet, is also produced by the bacteria in our large intestine (although there is some controversy as to this source's bioavailability and contribution to total body stores). Dietary vitamin K deficiency is rare, although it can be of significant consequence in the newborn and up to the age of six months. Clinical deficiency in the adult as a result of dietary inadequacy is essentially unknown. Table 8.2 lists the functions of the major vitamins, along with the symptoms or diseases associated with deficiency.

Most will recognize the names of the diseases associated with the vitamin deficiencies: scurvy and vitamin C deficiency, pellagra and niacin (B_3) deficiency, beri-beri and thiamine (B_1) deficiency, rickets and vitamin D deficiency. Less well known is the fact that vitamin A deficiency remains the number-one cause of preventable blindness in children in the world and a critical cofactor in the increased morbidity and mortality in infectious diseases that ultimately kill children who are chronically malnourished. Many of the vitamin deficiencies— scurvy, beri-beri, pellagra—are fascinating in regard to their medical presentations and histories, but they are thankfully only intermittently seen in modern times and not presently of major importance demographically. Unfortunately the same cannot be said for vitamin A deficiency.

VITAMIN A. Vitamin A deficiency remains a significant factor in the morbidity and mortality of large portions of the world's population, especially in children less than five years of age.[10]

Vitamin A is found in nature as the active compound retinol and as inactive, provitamin A carotenoids that must be cleaved during digestion or assimilation to form active retinol.

Vitamin A is found in both animal (the active vitamin A retinol) and plant sources (precursor or provitamin A carotenoids). Animal sources high in vitamin A include liver, egg yolks, and high-fat dairy products such as butter and whole milk. It is found in plant sources as a group of provitamins called carotenoids (after the yellow pigments originally extracted from carrots). There is a misconception in regard to the richness of vitamin A availability found in plant sources as opposed to animal sources. The animal sources, found in high amounts in relatively high-fat animal products such as eggs and dairy products, are in the form of active vitamin A (retinol). It is very well absorbed from the digestive tract as the high fat content of the accompanying meal facilitates its absorption, and it is immediately bioavailable as the active vitamin. Plant sources, however, are only present as the vitamin precursor or provitamin carotenoids, which are bioavailable depending on the conversion rate of the specific carotenoid and the presence or absence of accompanying fat in the diet. Vitamin A deficiency is most common in areas where people obtain most of this nutrient from vegetable (provitamin carotenoid) sources and with minimal concurrent dietary fat. Vitamin A deficiency is highly dependent on a number of complex dietary factors. These are coupled with other environmental factors such as seasonal variation in food availability (for example, absence of vitamin A–rich mangoes for much of the year versus a glut of mangoes during harvest time), or timing of common childhood diseases that are worsened by vitamin A deficiency (diarrhea, respiratory infections, measles) and that coincide with periods of dietary vitamin A insufficiency.

VITAMIN A AS A VISUAL PIGMENT. Vitamin A, in its chemical form as retinal (an aldehyde), has an interesting property called stereoisomerism—that is, it exists in two forms that are identical in their molecular formulas and sequence of atoms bound one to the other, but they differ in their three-dimensional spatial orientation. There are different types of stereoisomers, but in this form the difference is related to the configuration of side-chain functional groups (in this case methyl [CH_3] groups) and their placement in relation to double bonds in the molecule. If the methyl groups are situated on the same side of the molecule in relation to the double bond, the configuration is called *cis* (pronounced "sis"). If they are on opposite side, the configuration is called *trans*. In the *cis* configuration, the retinal molecule is bent, but in the *trans* configuration it straightens out. As is true of many stereoisomers, retinal is photoreactive; in this case transforming from the *cis* configuration to the *trans* configuration when it absorbs a photon.

In the retina of the eye, specifically in the photosensitive cells called rods (responsible for vision in dim light and in detecting motion) and cones (responsible for color vision) the retinal molecule in the *cis* configuration is bound to a protein called *opsin*. The type of opsin involved differs depending on the cell type (rod vs. cone) or species (different organisms will have different visual needs depending on their environment). Of some interest, however, is that the retinal form of vitamin A is the photoreactive element of all visual pigments regardless of the taxonomic classification of the organism, that is, the basic molecular function of light reception and translation to neural input is the same whether you are human or a squid.

In human rod cells, one type of opsin associates with *cis*-retinal to form the visual pigment *rhodopsin*. When light of the appropriate wavelength strikes the retina, it is absorbed by the visual pigment and causes a transformation of the bound *cis*-retinal into the *trans*-retinal configuration. This causes the retinal to straighten, dissociate from the opsin, and, through a process called signal transduction, generate an impulse in an associated neuron, which then carries the impulse through the optic nerve to the visual cortex of the brain. The *trans*-retinal is subsequently reconverted to *cis*-retinal, which reassociates with an opsin molecule. Dietary deficiency of vitamin A depletes the retina of adequate visual pigment, impairing visual acuity in low-light situations. This is the cause of night blindness in people with vitamin A deficiency.

A more disabling and permanent effect on vision can occur due to the effect of vitamin A deficiency on epithelial cell growth and maintenance. In its forms as retinal and retinoic acid, vitamin A is essential for synthesis of glycoproteins and mucopolysaccharides, and as such it is necessary for the normal growth regulation and mucus production that ensures epithelial tissue integrity. Remember from our discussions in chapter 4 that epithelial tissues make up our skin, mucous membranes, and internal tissues such as intestinal epithelium that act as a barrier and transportation device between us and our external environments. As vitamin A deficiency progresses, the lack of normal epithelial tissue growth and lack of normal mucous and tear production especially affects the corneal tissue of the eye, which thickens and develops fissures, allowing frequent infections to occur. This condition, called *xerophthalmia*, leads to progressive scarring and eventual permanent loss of vision. This devastating outcome, seen in children between six months and six years of age, is considered the number one cause of avoidable blindness in children in the world and is reported to cause between 500,000 and a million cases of blindness every year.[11]

There is yet another consequence of vitamin A deficiency that has a more devastating effect on the health of children in resource-poor countries. It is estimated (quite possibly underestimated) that 10 million children under the age of five die unnecessarily each year. As we discuss more fully in chapter 10, they are not dying of relatively high-profile diseases such as malaria, HIV/AIDS, or tuberculosis but of the rather ordinary diseases of diarrhea, pneumonia, and measles. These are the disease analogies of the "silent emergency." Vitamin A is necessary to maintain the health of our first defense against invading organisms, the epithelial tissues of our skin and mucous membranes. In addition vitamin A deficiency weakens the immune system's ability to fight off invading organisms once they are established. Although these avoidable deaths are multifactorial, in part due to chronic malnutrition on a macronutrient level, inadequate vaccination programs, and inadequate access to safe drinking water and sanitation (among other issues), there exists sufficient scientific evidence to validly estimate that correction of vitamin A deficiency alone could prevent between 180,000 and 230,000 of these deaths, specifically some of the deaths that result from diarrhea and measles.[12]

Minerals

In addition to the vitamin deficiencies, there are deficiencies of minerals such as iron and iodine. Defined as naturally occurring substances, minerals generally are found in the solid state and have a defined chemical composition and crystalline structure; they are most familiar to us as the substances that make up rocks and certain types of soils. Familiar examples include the silicates (various oxides of silica that make up to 60 percent of the Earth's crust), such as quartz and the igneous rock feldspar. Others include carbonates (limestone), sulfates (gypsum), and the oxide ores such as the iron ores hematite and magnetite. Biologically necessary minerals include all of the inorganic elements and compounds necessary for the structure and function of our bodies. Chemically the term *mineral* is something of a misnomer, as these substances exist as ionized *salts* in biological systems—salts being defined as inorganic substances that ionize or dissociate into positive (cationic) and negative (anionic) ions in solution—the common example being sodium chloride (NaCl) or table salt (Na^+ and Cl^- in solution). For our purposes the term *mineral* is useful as it is commonly understood to represent the inorganic substances necessary for normal life functions, that is, elements other than carbon, hydrogen, nitrogen, and oxygen.

Dietary minerals can be divided into the major minerals (those required in relatively large amounts) and the trace minerals (required in small amounts, but critically important nonetheless). The mineral that makes up the largest proportion by weight in our bodies is calcium, necessary functionally as a cofactor in cellular function and as a major structural element in bone. The next most common is phosphorus, structurally the anionic complement to calcium in bone and critically important functionally because of its ability to form high-energy bonds in the cellular energy source ATP (adenosine triphosphate). Phosphorus is also a vital component of the nucleic acids deoxyribonucleic acid (DNA) and ribonucleic acid (RNA). Other major minerals include potassium, sodium, and chloride, all of which are critical components of our internal "sea," both inside our cells and in the fluids bathing our cells (such as blood).

The trace minerals include zinc, iron, manganese, copper, iodine, selenium, and molybdenum (in order of their recommended daily allowances or RDA).

Of these, dietary deficiency leading to significant negative health effects in individuals or large populations are extremely rare for all of them except iodine and iron.

A lack of biologically available iodine in the diet leads to an inability of the thyroid gland to produce adequate thyroid hormone (an iodine-containing hormone necessary for the body to maintain normal metabolism and for normal growth and development in children). This is generally seen in remote inland areas where there is little marine food available in the diet, especially in areas where the soil has been depleted of iodine due to leaching of the soil on a geologic scale by water runoff (such as melting glaciers). When this iodine deficiency occurs in pregnant women, it can lead to a condition known as cretinism in the infant. In addition to other associated birth defects, cretinism is a leading cause of preventable mental retardation worldwide.[13] According to the World Health Organization (WHO), up to 2 billion people, over 30 percent of the world's population, suffer from some degree of iodine deficiency, with many millions of children suffering irreversible damage to their cognitive function. The treatment for this is preventative—addition of trace amounts of iodine as a dietary supplement in the form of iodized salt. A great deal of progress has been made in making iodine deficiency a medical curiosity of the past, but there is still work to be done in seeing to it that iodized salt is easily available to all.

Although there is no doubt that protein energy malnutrition, food insecurity, and the associated physical and mental suffering are the most pressing areas of concern in regard to the gross inequities in access to resources between the haves and the have-nots of the world, according to WHO the most common and globally prevalent nutritional deficiency in the world is iron deficiency.[14]

Iron is an abundant element in the Earth's crust, making up about 5 percent of the crust by weight, but it has little to no bioavailability because it is present as either the oxide or metallic form, both of which are insoluble. Much as we saw with the fixation of inorganic nitrogen into organic compounds by microorganisms, making the nitrogen available to other life forms, many microorganisms have developed the ability to access the inorganic iron in the environment. They do this by secreting peptides (small chains of amino acids) called *siderophores* (Greek: iron carriers) into the environment. These siderophores have very high affinity for atomic iron, forming special bonds called *chelation* bonds (Greek: claw)—each atom of iron forming multiple bonds within the siderophore. The iron-rich siderophore complexes can then be reabsorbed making the iron atom available for metabolic purposes.

Iron is a critical component of a number of basic biochemical processes, generally as an element of a "prosthetic group" of two types of iron-containing proteins; the iron-sulfur complexes or clusters and the heme proteins. (A prosthetic group is a molecular structure tightly bound to the protein base of an enzyme necessary for enzymatic function.)

Iron-sulfur proteins are a diverse group of proteins that have complex iron-sulfur molecular constructs as their active prosthetic groups. They take advantage of the chemical reactivity of these two inorganic elements to catalyze reactions involving the transfer of electrons between substances in various roles such as photosynthesis, nitrogen fixation, the cytochrome system, the tricarboxylic (Krebs) cycle, and oxidative phosphorylation. Note that most of these processes have to do with either the transformation of energy (light) into nutrient (sugar) or the transformation of nutrient (sugar) into energy (ATP), the basic mechanisms of which entail transferring electrons from high-energy states to low-energy states and capturing the resultant "residual energy" as a chemical bond that can then be stored for later use (as a nutrient) or directly used to maintain life (as ATP).

The *heme* proteins are the other major group of proteins requiring atomic iron as part of their prosthetic group. The most familiar of these proteins are the proteins involved in oxygen transport and storage. It is the iron-containing heme group that allows the binding of oxygen and its subsequent transport in the blood by *hemoglobin*, and oxygen uptake and short-term storage in muscle by *myoglobin*.

The average human body contains 3 to 4 grams of iron, 2 grams of which circulates in the red blood cells as hemoglobin, 0.5 to 1 gram is stored in the liver, and the rest is distributed in prosthetic groups in the other various enzymes that require iron to function. Dietary sources of iron include animal and plant sources. Animal sources are mostly in the form of heme, which is easily absorbed and incorporated into our bodies. Plant sources of iron are less bioavailable, to a large extent because of coexisting inhibitors of absorption such as phytates and polyphenols, found in high concentration in many plants (spinach included).[15]

Deficiency of iron can be caused both by inadequate dietary intake, more common in mostly vegetarian diets as the iron in vegetables is either in a less absorbable form or is accompanied by inhibitors of absorption, and by blood loss. The average adult man loses about 1 milligram of iron a day through various processes, including minute (and undetectable) gastrointestinal blood loss as well as sloughing of cells in the GI tract, skin, and other mucous membranes. In addition, women of reproductive age lose additional iron through their monthly menstrual cycles. An additional cause of significant blood loss (not including the losses experienced in pathological situations such as bleeding ulcers or tumors) is the presence of certain intestinal parasites, such as hookworm, or urinary parasites, such as schistosomiasis, which in some resource-poor parts of the world cause substantial morbidity and contribute to preventable mortality, especially in women and children.[16]

The major result of chronic iron deficiency is iron-deficiency anemia. Because iron is necessary for the body to make functional hemoglobin, inadequate iron stores limit hemoglobin production, the red blood cells produced carry decreased amounts of hemoglobin (and therefore are small [microcytic] and pale [hypochromic]) and cannot transport adequate oxygen to the body's tissues. This results in weakness, fatigue, and, in children, stunted development both in physical and mental growth. Large-scale epidemiologic studies of chronic iron-deficiency anemia are difficult to perform, in part because the cause of anemia is frequently multifactorial—for example, falciparum malaria is a frequent cause of anemia in the areas of Africa where large segments of the population also suffer from iron deficiency. In an extensive review of the available literature, Stoltzfus, Mullany, and Black have conservatively estimated that, considering direct sequelae of iron deficiency as well as increased risk of mortality and morbidity from other causes, iron deficiency anemia is responsible for over 800,000 deaths annually and 35 million disability-adjusted life years globally.[17] As the deaths and disability are primarily due to anemia in pregnancy and early infancy, it follows that the vast majority of the burden falls on women and children, specifically in Asia and Africa.

It is appropriate to include a few words about the unusual eating disorder known as pica, as it has been associated with iron deficiency anemia. The word itself comes from the Latin word for magpie, a bird known to have a large and indiscriminate appetite. *Pica*, as defined medically, is an eating disorder characterized by a compulsive need to eat nonfood items such as clay, dirt, paint chips, and even feces. It is generally not applied to children between the ages of six months and two years (who will put anything in their mouths) and is not considered abnormal behavior until it has lasted at least one month. Pica in iron-deficiency anemia has been associated with a craving for eating ice cubes, in pregnant women with eating clay or dirt, but there is general disagreement as to whether or not the nonfood item craved actually contains the missing micronutrient. Pica appears to be quite common in some cultures, but is otherwise considered to be an eating disorder, and has been linked to serious risk of toxicity, especially in children with access to lead-based paint.

Summary

In this chapter we have reviewed the homeostatic mechanisms that enable us to maintain a healthy nutritional status when we have access to adequate caloric intake and essential micronutrients. We have touched briefly on the pathophysiology, the abnormal functions, associated with the inadequate access to calories seen in marasmus; the inadequate access to protein seen in kwashiorkor; and the debility and disease associated with some of the micronutrient deficiencies. What we have not been able to impart is the profound nature of the human suffering, the despair and desolation felt by millions of people every day as they go to bed with their stomachs empty, listen to their children cry inconsolably, and watch them die before they reach the age of five.

Lessons from the Great Irish Famine [1845–1850]
Nineteenth-century Ireland and Modern Africa

There are subtle lessons to be found in comparing the Great Famine with colonial and postcolonial Africa. These include, as we have discussed in chapters 6 and 7, echoes from the Great Famine found in both the predisposing and catalytic factors that have caused the more recent starvations in Ethiopia, Malawi, and Niger. We also find some commonalities between the plights of the Irish and of Africans. And we learn that chronic hunger, malnutrition, starvation, and famine are equal opportunity killers, particularly of children. Starvation and famine may be unpredictable, however; they may strike those who are not only poor, but also (in Cormac Ó Gráda's words), "desperately unlucky."[1] But the fundamental commonality of the politics of starvation is not age or gender, or the color of someone's skin, or even the ethnicity or geography of one's community. It is the depth and persistence of poverty.

Poverty, along with its attendant chronic hunger, malnutrition, and disease, seeps quietly into the farthest corners of the world. In Europe today Italy has the highest rate of child poverty, followed by Great Britain, where one child in four lives below that nation's poverty line; half the children in Inner London live in poverty.[2] In the United States, at this writing, one child in every fifty (1,555,360 American children) is homeless;[3] 17 million children—more than one in five—live in families where food is scarce;[4] one person in every eight goes to bed hungry each night.[5]

The Great Irish Famine teaches us about assumptions, the concept of "the other," and about racism. One might argue that there are no connections— indeed, that there are fundamental dissimilarities—between the Irish Famine and the famines of the twentieth and twenty-first centuries addressed in this book. After all, the Irish Famine was "Europe's last famine," whereas starvation and famine continue today across the developing world. But it would be super-ficial to say that the Irish Famine struck down "Europeans" (that is, "white" people), whereas contemporary starvations and famines afflict only "people of color."

Closer examination indicates a universality of suffering. We may start with the trans-Atlantic trade in human beings. For two centuries, in addition to African slaves, Europeans—mostly Irish, Scots, English, and Germans—were taken to the Caribbean, Brazil, and the British colonies in substantial numbers. They shared a common experience. Perhaps as many as two-thirds of all white immigrants to the British colonies during the seventeenth and eighteenth centuries were indentured servants; in some colonies, they made up 75 percent of the people living there. Just ten years after the Great Irish Famine, the 1860 U.S. Census identified 393,975 individuals who owned 3,950,528 slaves. Enough of them were *not* Africans to cause W. E. B. Du Bois, himself a famous African American, to look at the wider framework of the Atlantic trade in human beings and write: "Any attempt to consider the attitude of the English colonies toward the African slave-trade must be prefaced by a word as to the attitude of England herself and the development of the trade in her hands."[6]

The British played a major role in the Atlantic slave trade, starting in 1562 and continuing into the nineteenth century. That shameful history is well documented,[7] but what concerns us here is British colonization of Ireland and the West Indies, the so-called "white Atlantic slave trade." In 1649, Oliver Cromwell took an army of 20,000 into Ireland and drove Irish landowners from several million acres of arable land. He installed his soldiers on large estates and his son, Henry, in command of the English soldiers. The system of "plantations" linked Ireland with the West Indies island colonies of Barbados, Jamaica, St. Kitts, and Trinidad, and then with the North American mainland. Both the Irish and West Indies plantations demanded labor, however obtained. To meet this demand, large numbers of African slaves were sent to the New World, averaging 50,000 annually from about 1680 to 1786. Some scholars estimate that more than 2 million African slaves were shipped into the British West Indies alone.

Joining them were enslaved Irish peasants. Under Henry Cromwell's command, any Irish man, woman, or child found east of the river Shannon was arrested and sold into slavery in the West Indies; when that happened, the person was said to have been "barbado'ed." This soon expanded to mass kidnappings throughout Ireland; the unlucky were sold and shipped across the Atlantic to the Caribbean. W. E. B. Du Bois wrote that, "Even young Irish peasants, some younger than 12 years, were 'hunted down as men hunt down game, and were forcibly put on board ship, and sold to the planters in Barbados.'"[8]

The exact number may never be known, but between 1648 and 1655 alone more than 12,000 Irish (some reports say 60,000 to 100,000)[9] were involuntarily shipped to the West Indies to work on tobacco and sugar cane plantations as slave labor. This served several purposes: it removed political prisoners and displaced peasant laborers from Ireland; it decreased the Irish Catholic population of the United Kingdom; and it supplied British plantation owners with free peasant labor in the Caribbean colonies. It also brought African and Irish closer together in a shared history.

Those who commit immoral acts often seek justification for them. The capture of Irish men, women, and children and their enslavement in the West Indies was pardoned by the British government as a "measure beneficial to the people removed, who might thus be made English and Christians; and a great benefit to the West India sugar planters, who desired the men and boys for their bondsmen, and the women and Irish girls in a country where they had only Maroon women and Negresses to solace them."[10]

Thus, the Irish peasant joined the captured African as slaves in the New World. Through the late seventeenth century they were further united by the "custom" of plantation owners to "marry" their white indentured servants to African slaves to increase their labor force. Both also "suffered in harsh conditions and joined together in revolt against British settlers."[11] Although it is true that the Irish, mostly indentured servants, were freed long before the Africans, their treatment and length of indentured slavery was often equal to that of the Africans. And, as mentioned in our second comment on the Irish Famine, their later passage across the Atlantic in "coffin ships," although on a far smaller scale, was also marked by high mortality. Moreover Africans and Irish shared the experience of population collapse: much as sub-Saharan Africa's population declined for almost a century because of slavery, the Irish Famine "was remarkable for the fact that the population of Ireland as a whole never recovered in number, remaining to this day [1997] at half the pre-famine level."[12]

There is another, often overlooked, connection: racism. To conquer, subjugate, and colonize a people, a government needs to mythologize and stereotype them. European mapmakers during the thirteenth and fourteenth centuries portrayed Africa as inhabited by people with one leg, three faces, and the heads of lions. A Benedictine monk named Ranulf Higden, for example, drew a map of the world as he saw it around 1350 with Africa inhabited by one-eyed people who covered their heads with their feet. During the Age of Navigation in the fifteenth century, as Europeans lead by the Portuguese ventured farther south, they were warned that when they sailed beyond the Canary Islands in the Atlantic they would enter the Sea of Darkness, "where the heavens fling down liquid sheets of flame and the waters boil . . . where serpent rocks and ogre islands lie in wait." If they dared press onward, they encountered the Sea of Obscurity where they might be "lost forever in the vapors and slime at the edge of the world."[13]

At the time, no European had actually penetrated Africa's interior nor had a conversation with an African person there. Yet Africa was portrayed with certainty as a place reached through dangerous seas and slime, inhabited by strange creatures different from civilized Europeans. This made exploration of Africa, and then enslavement and colonization of its people, acceptable, even justified. Europeans would bring and give to Africans the three C's: Christianity, Civilization, and Commerce.

Similar myths were created about the Irish—and for the same purposes. To attack and defeat the Irish, the conqueror needed to demonize them. As early as the twelfth century, Gerald of Wales described the Irish in a widely read document as "a wild and inhospitable people . . . a barbarous people."[14] He called them "a filthy people, wallowing in vice." They were heathens. "Of all peoples it is the least instructed in the rudiments of the faith. They do not pay tithes or first fruits or contract marriages. They do not avoid incest."[15]

These descriptions, by a Welsh Celtic observer, influenced English views toward the Irish for several centuries. The distinction between Celt and Anglo-Saxon in the British Isles had long standing, and by the time of the Great Famine the British image of the Irish was firmly "recast in biological racial terms."[16] The colonization of Ireland did little to change this view in the nineteenth century, much as the myth of Africa as "The Heart of Darkness" persists to this day.[17] As the Great Famine began "the standard image of the good-natured Irish peasant was revised, becoming that of a repulsive ape-like creature" placed somewhere between a monkey and the racial caricature of the African.[18] English observers characterized Irish peasants as "white negroes" and "apes."[19] The British press routinely called the Irish "the missing link" and the popular satirical magazine *Punch* regularly drew or described the Irish as beneath the English, on the same level as Africans: "You to Sambo I compare . . ." went one verse.[20] Such descriptions were acceptable even among the country's elite and well-educated. Ten years *after* the Great Famine, Charles Kingsley, recently appointed to the distinguished academic post of Regius Professor of Modern History at the University of Cambridge, traveled through Ireland and wrote to his wife that "I am haunted by the human chimpanzees I saw . . . I don't believe they are our fault. . . . But to see white chimpanzees is dreadful; if they were black, one would not feel it so much."[21]

In addition to racism and ethnic hatred therefore, we suggest that the Great Irish Famine and contemporary famines share five other "commonalities."

1. Emigration and slavery. As we have noted, both Ireland and sub-Saharan Africa experienced large-scale forced removals of their people. "The Irish outflow was so great—removing one-third to one-half of each rising generation—that it provoked repeated warnings of de-population."[22] This trend continued into the twentieth century. Both emigration and the slave trade created profound social and economic disruption and transformation.

2. Colonization. Both regions were colonized, and many Africans lived under the same colonial power as the Irish.[23] Colonialism created divisions

and dependencies within its colonies. These tied Ireland and the colonies of sub-Saharan Africa to their colonial metropole's own social, financial, and educational institutions. These strictures contributed significantly to Irish and African underdevelopment.

3. Forced movement of labor. The Great Famine was also marked by the colonization of the Irish farmland. Native Irish peasant farmers were forced from more than 500,000 acres of arable land and replaced with settlers from Scotland and England in a system known as "planting." The property was consolidated into large estates, or "plantations." During the Great Famine, as mentioned earlier, plantation owners undertook mass evictions or "clearances" of Irish tenant farmers so they could cultivate grain or livestock for export. Perhaps as many as 750,000 to 1 million Irish were forced from their lands and 200,000 smallholder farms lost to consolidation. "These helpless creatures are not only unhoused, but often driven off the land, no one remaining on the lands being allowed to lodge or harbor them."[24] They built shelters along stonewalls, lived in ditches or bog-holes. "There were hoards of poor on the roads every day."[25]

Similarly, in sub-Saharan Africa the European colonial powers forcibly evicted Africans from arable land into the margins of those colonies. Settlers from Europe were then encouraged to come out to the colonies and establish large commercial farms to raise crops for export back to Europe. For example, Uganda, Kenya, Tanganyika (Tanzania), German South-West Africa (Namibia), the two Rhodesias (Zambia and Zimbabwe), Nyasaland (Malawi), Angola, Mozambique, and South Africa all experienced forced clearances similar to Ireland's. Two examples: In South Africa, the Natives' Land Act of 1913 was used to evict black Africans from arable land into just 7 percent of the colony (later 13 percent), all of it in rural semi-arid regions with low rainfall. These later became the locations for the notorious Bantustans during the *apartheid* period (1948–1992). In Southern Rhodesia (Zimbabwe), the 1930 Land Apportionment Act removed native Africans from the fertile central highlands and Chimanimani Mountains to the margins of the country where low rainfall permitted only maize production and the raising of livestock.

4. Wealth extraction; commodity agriculture. Externally created colonial economies were forced upon Ireland beginning in the eighteenth century and on much of sub-Saharan Africa during its colonial period. Both regions exported agricultural products to Great Britain and other European metropoles. As we have detailed, with the potato as its staple food, Ireland redirected much of its arable land to corn and livestock production for export. It became, even during the Great Famine, "a kind of granary for the rest of the United Kingdom."[26] Sub-Saharan Africa's British colonies sent raw materials (minerals and ore) and agricultural commodities in the form of cash crops (grains, tea, coffee,

cocoa, cotton, and tobacco). Britain benefited economically at the cost to all of its colonies and required them to trade exclusively with its own companies. Thus, one theory of underdevelopment identifies the wealth of Ireland and the African colonies—in manpower (slaves), minerals, natural resources, and agricultural products—as the fuel that powered Great Britain's and Europe's Industrial Revolution.

Unlike Ireland, however, postcolonial African states exchanged political independence for economic dependencies and some remain tied today to mineral extraction (oil, minerals, diamonds, gold, and ores) and cash crops (flowers, tobacco, tea, coffee, and cocoa). These producers are vulnerable to off-continent market forces such as "globalization" and "free-market" economics espoused by international financial institutions. (The impact of off-continent consumers on sub-Saharan Africa is more fully discussed in chapter 9.) The Republic of Ireland, on the other hand, is today an economically viable member of the European Union.

5. Economic systems. Irish and Africans have had imposed on them financial structures and restrictions, detailed in chapters 6 and 7, based on prevailing economic theories and policies at the time. Ireland suffered under *laissez-faire* economics and the absence of government intervention in "the free market." More recently the World Bank and the International Monetary Fund (IMF) pressed Economic Structural Adjustment Programs (ESAPS)—part of a "free market" economic theory—on selected African states during the last two decades of the twentieth century. Much as the British government has been criticized for its economic role in the Great Irish Famine, so are the World Bank and IMF seen today as imposing an economic system on Africans tantamount to a new form of colonialism, often termed "neo-colonialism." The IMF has become one of the most significant influences in the economic and political life of most Africans.

Ireland of the mid-nineteenth century and modern Africa share other characteristics, among them patterns of chronic hunger striking a vast and poor majority; relief aid schemes, such as food-for-work projects; even armed conflict against the same colonial power (Northern Ireland; Southern Rhodesia/ Zimbabwe and Kenya, for example). "Donor fatigue," a significant factor in weak responses to starvation in Africa, was during the Great Irish Famine "indicated by the ebbing of private charity in 1848 and later."[27]

There is another, and perhaps most important, lesson to be learned from comparing the Great Irish Famine with modern African starvations. This is about humanitarian concern and how peril and suffering connect all of us. It is "a way of seeing the world," Adam Hochschild writes, "a human capacity for outrage at pain inflicted on another human being, no matter whether that pain is inflicted on someone of another color, in another country, at another end of the earth."[28]

This lesson starts on March 23, 1847, at the height of the Great Irish Famine, when a Native American group of Choctaws gathered in Scullyville, Oklahoma, to put together a famine relief fund. In 1830, President Andrew Jackson—whose parents had emigrated from Antrim, a county in northernmost Ireland—had signed the Indian Removal Act as part of U.S. government policy to force the Native American people from their traditional homes. In 1831, the government seized the fertile lands of the Chickasaw, Cherokee, Creek, Seminole, and Choctaw and forced them to march westward even as they died from exposure, starvation, and disease.[29] By 1846, through letters, newspaper accounts, and first-hand reports from refugees, the Irish in North America had learned of the famine underway in Ireland. Individuals donated money and ship tickets, formed relief committees, or solicited charitable societies, businesses, churches, and synagogues. Thus, the Choctaws learned of the expulsions of the Irish poor from their native land, of the starvation and deaths, and of the long journey of Irish survivors to a new homeland. In March 1847, just sixteen years after their own "removal," when they were forced to walk up to 500 miles from Alabama, Mississippi, and Louisiana into Indian Territory (now Oklahoma), the Choctaw people took up a collection. Despite their own poverty, and in part because at least 2500 to 6000 of the Native Americans had died from starvation, disease, and exhaustion along "The Trail of Tears," the Choctaw Nation donated $710 to a U.S. famine relief organization[30] to ease the suffering of the Irish people.[31]

Today Choctaw and Irish continue to recite the similarities of their experiences: the destruction of their traditional lives and eviction from their homes by a colonial foreign government; the forced migrations and exile that scattered and killed many of their people; the starvation of their men, women and children; the suppression of their culture and language. In 1990, a delegation of Choctaws joined the annual walk in County Mayo that commemorates a "death march" that took place during the Great Famine. In their honor, the Irish renamed the County Mayo route "The Trail of Tears." In 1992, twenty-four Irish retraced the Choctaw's journey from Mississippi to Oklahoma. Mary Robinson, Ireland's first woman president, was made an honorary Choctaw chief. Looking beyond their similar histories, she told the Native American audience: "I believe we have in common that bond of humanity and it should be an additional reason why we should particularly reach out now to countries who suffer from poverty and hunger. . . . [T]here are people today who need the support that the Choctaw Nation gave 150 years ago to the Irish people."[32]

Ms. Robinson, who later served as the UN High Commissioner for Human Rights, was echoing the words on a small plaque posted at Mansion House, the official residence of the Lord Mayor of Dublin. The plaque honors the Choctaw Nation's contribution to the Great Irish Famine. It also gives voice to another bridge between the Irish and Choctaw people and to those suffering hunger now in the developing world: "Their humanity calls us to remember the millions of human beings throughout our world today who die of hunger-related illness in a world of plenty."[33]

PART IV

Why People Starve and Die

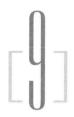

Why Do Some People Starve?

Is it possible that starvation and famine across sub-Saharan Africa may be caused by conditions that originate *outside* of Africa?

In this chapter we explore the possibility that there may be at least three *outside* causes of this continent's recurring starvation and famines: persistent and widespread violence and conflict (funded and armed from outside), particularly over Africa's natural resources; the impacts of climate change—especially drought and El Niño and La Niña effects—caused by off-continent pollution; and shortages in global grain markets created by purchases from large, wealthy buyers. Three investigators guide us in our examination:

o Paul Collier has contributed seminal work on the rising international demands for the rich natural resources of Africa—oil, diamonds, gold, and *columbite-tantalite* (nicknamed "col-tan"), for example.[1] These natural deposits precipitate conflict, or "resource wars," in such impoverished states as Ethiopia, Nigeria, and the Democratic Republic of the Congo. Does Africa's vast natural resource wealth actually fund the violence and conflicts that in turn perpetuate the continent's chronic malnutrition, starvation, and poverty?

o Mike Davis argues that, beginning in the Victorian era, the major causes of starvation in the developing world should include the effects of El Niño/La Niña and global climate change.[2] Research by other scholars suggests that pollution from wealthy nations may also contribute to unusual weather changes that in turn result in chronic hunger and starvation in developing states. Therefore, we next ask: Are global environmental changes causing "environmental accidents" leading to "ecological poverty" in sub-Saharan Africa?

o Lester Brown, the environmental activist, warns that if a large grain purchaser—China or India, for example—enters the global market, it might rapidly buy up most of the available grain supply on that market.[3] China has recently become self-sufficient in terms of food production but, as we describe here, struggles with serious internal stresses as the result of its successful economic development. Its population and industry continue to grow and expand onto its finite arable land, and both are redirecting water out of agriculture to industrial and household uses.

If China were to suffer domestic food shortages, the country would go on the international grain market to make up the shortfall. There, the large amounts of grain China would buy might create global shortages and divert or prevent emergency food relief needed in regions experiencing hunger or starvation. History offers us an example, in this case a large and powerful country (the Soviet Union) buying global surplus grains in 1972–1974 to devastating effect on food-short Africans in the Sahel and Horn. Could emergency food relief supplies suddenly become unavailable because of global purchases by a large and wealthy individual state?

Collier, Davis, and Brown suggest three significant, non-African threats to the continent's ability to feed itself and rise out of poverty. Together they reconfigure the way we think about the causes of starvation and famine and warrant a closer examination.

The Paradox of Wealth

In the 1960s as the individual colonies of the European countries began securing their independence, Dr. René Dumont made a simple proposition. He suggested that the most secure path to self-reliance by the newly independent former colonies was not to follow the economic model of their old colonial powers toward industrial development but, rather, to become self-sufficient in agriculture.[4] Being food secure, he proposed, would make these new states truly free from outside economic and political forces and allow them time to modernize and grow.

Many developing states, however, pursued the colonial model of capitalism; others adapted a Marxist ideology. Neither worked well for them. Gaining political freedom, former colonial states soon found themselves locked into one form or another of economic colonialism that linked them to their wealthy former colonial power and/or to international financial institutions. Some were also absorbed as ideological surrogates. Their young economies stagnated under burdens of cash crop exports, global pricing structures, rising costs of energy and modernization, and debt. Many states found it expedient to assign their natural resources to multinational corporations that were accountable to no one. By the 1970s most of these new African states had exchanged political freedom for economic neocolonialism.

Taking back full ownership of their natural resources, developing food security, and restoring peace to areas troubled by persistent conflict would go far toward ending chronic hunger and malnutrition and averting starvation and famine. Researchers at the International Food Policy Research Institute (IFPRI) write: "Food security can help prevent conflict and is essential for sustained and peaceful recovery after wars have ended."[5] The connection between conflict and starvation is clear. Robert Stock notes: "Most of the countries with the greatest food deficits and highest rates of under-nutrition—Somalia, the

Democratic Republic of the Congo, Ethiopia, Angola, Mozambique, and Sierra Leone—share a common history of bitter, protracted wars that undermined the productive capacity of the country."[6]

Paul Collier, an economist with the World Bank, argues that countries with valuable natural resources are predisposed to violence and conflict. In the twenty-five years between 1970 and 1995, sub-Saharan African states experienced more than thirty wars. This included more than 200 coups or attempted coups between 1950 and 2000, or about four coups a year. By 2000, when Collier did his initial research, eighteen sub-Saharan African countries were experiencing conflict or recovering from recent conflict.[7] Ellen Messer et al. at IFPRI show that conflict reduces food production and causes food insecurity; prolonged conflicts prevent farming and marketing from taking place: "Conflict-related destitution thus creates conditions of chronic food insecurity and shortages for households that otherwise may have been temporarily or seasonally short of food."[8] Overall, armed conflicts "put at least 80 million people at risk of hunger and malnutrition" inside Africa alone.[9]

Conflict also creates social disintegration, a key element in our definition of starvation. For example, in the 1980s more than 5 million Africans were displaced by war; in the 1990s, more than 23 million refugees fled conflicts, up from 2.5 million in the 1970s.[10] Most recently, United Nations agencies calculated that more than 37 million Africans (out of 45 million people worldwide) who had experienced or recovered from conflict needed food and other humanitarian assistance. Another 198 million Africans (out of 842 million people globally) were without reliable food resources.[11] In fact, civil conflict has been "the single most significant factor explaining the persistence of famine" across sub-Saharan Africa since independence began in the late 1950s.[12]

Early warning systems and more efficient emergency aid responses have largely prevented famines *except* in areas of conflict or deliberate starvation by national governments. Mozambique and Ethiopia are examples of the former; North Korea and Zimbabwe of the latter. As the IFPRI report states, "Conflict-linked food shortages thus set the stage for years of food emergencies, even after fighting has officially ceased."[13] In addition according to the World Health Organization (WHO), "Emergency situations caused by wars, civil strife and natural disasters, constitute some of the most serious threats to health in Africa."[14]

As Devereux points out, militarization of the developing world has drawn off a disproportionate amount of foreign exchange reserves. For example, during the 1970s and 1980s Ethiopia had the highest military spending per person of all sub-Saharan African states. By 1978 Mengistu was diverting most of that country's export earnings, largely from coffee, to the Soviet Union and East

Germany in payment for weapons and military equipment.[15] In 1984, at the height of another Ethiopian famine, "an incredible 46 percent of the national budget was spent on arms." Spending for rural development and agriculture dropped to record lows during the same period.[16] Conscription into the Ethiopian army added to this burden by taking young men out of the agricultural sector and increasing the dependency on that sector for food supplies to the military. A growing population and a worsening balance of trade payment meant that Ethiopia needed more food but could not pay for importing it.[17] By 2010, as we have seen, Ethiopia remained the world's leading recipient of international food aid.

Two immediate observations come to mind:

1. Most conflicts in developing states occur within those states. That is, of the twenty-five conflicts globally in 2000, twenty-three were intrastate conflicts occurring within national borders. In Africa, of 103 conflicts between 1989 and 1997, only six were fought between countries. One major example was the long war in the Democratic Republic of the Congo, which was an interstate conflict with Rwanda, Burundi, Uganda, Zimbabwe, and Angola all engaged.

2. Internal conflicts and economic exploitation are closely linked. In Africa, "local elites and trans-national corporations increasingly use war as a cover to generate wealth through natural resource extraction."[18]

Collier offers strong supporting analysis and evidence for these observations. His analysis emerges from a fundamental reality: global demand for basic natural resources will continue to grow as global population grows. As we write, there are about 6.7 billion people living on the earth; we will grow to almost 8 billion by 2020 and 10 billion by 2040. Thus, three contributing factors are coming together:

○ The expansion of global resource demands.
○ The emergence of global resource shortages.
○ The proliferation of what Michael Klare calls "ownership contests." These are "resource wars" or "Conflicts that revolve, to a certain degree, over the pursuit or possession of critical resources."[19]

Collier's initial work studied the global causes of civil war (intrastate conflict) from 1965–1999.[20] His conclusions are shocking. "The most powerful risk factor" for civil war in a developing state, Collier found, occurs where "a substantial share of [state] income (GDP)" comes from "the export of primary commodities."[21] Commodities like timber, coffee, gold, diamonds, or oil are vulnerable to looting; their production relies on assets that are long lasting and basically immobile (mines, forests, and fields). Rebel groups may also attempt to secede with the land on which the primary commodities are grown or mined—for example, Katanga Province (copper, diamonds) in the Democratic Republic of the Congo and the Niger delta region (oil) of Nigeria.

Nigeria, for example, is one of the world's richest oil states and poorest countries. It has pumped hundreds of billions of dollars of petroleum out of its Niger delta region. International oil corporations and the Nigerian government split oil revenues, 60 percent (government) and 40 percent (companies). The extraction of oil and its sale have generated great wealth, but also, paradoxically, created conflict in Nigeria and extensive poverty.

There is a long history of conflict over resources in Nigeria. In 1967 the people of the eastern region tried to secede and form the Republic of Biafra; oil in the region drove demands for economic and political freedom. The resulting armed conflict lasted almost three years, until January 1970. A military blockade and civil war created a humanitarian disaster followed by accusations of deliberate starvation of the delta Nigerians. Perhaps as many as 100,000 people died from starvation-related causes; war casualties pushed the number even higher. Sporadic protests and fighting continue to this day, the result of protests about pollution of the region's environment and the loss of income, freedom, and rights for the delta's people. In 1994, Ken Saro-Wiwa, president of the Movement for the Survival of the Ogoni People (MOSOP), and eight others who had been campaigning against pollution and for human rights, were arrested, tried, and executed by the Nigerian government. In June 2009, Shell Oil agreed to pay US$15.5 million to relatives of nine anti-oil protestors for human-rights violations. As of this writing, the armed Movement for the Emancipation of the Niger Delta (MEND) still operated out of thirty camps in the delta region with attacks on pipelines and oil production facilities and occasional kidnappings of foreign oil workers.

Although many Nigerians—not to mention oil executives—have gotten rich, USAID reports that more than 70 percent of the country's people live on less than US$1 a day. Nigeria's own corruption watchdog estimates that since the 1960s between US$300 billion and US$400 billion have been stolen or wasted. The people of the delta, who exist by fishing and farming, have endured more than 6000 oil spills since 1970 that have covered their land and waterways in sludge. "To most Nigerians," an observer noted, "oil is a curse."[22]

Like Nigeria, the Democratic Republic of the Congo (DRC) should be among the world's richest countries. Instead, the DRC is a worst-case example of the "wealth paradox." Its riches are matched by its poverty, corruption, and violence. The country is covered with tropical forests containing valuable hardwoods and endangered African animals and plants found on the CITES list;[23] its provinces offer rich seams of copper, diamonds, gold, manganese, uranium, zinc, cobalt, and "col-tan." Yet the DRC's people are poor: per capita income is estimated at US$714 a year, less than US$2 a day, which puts the DRC third from the bottom of the UN global rankings. Transparency International ranks the country 168th out of 179 nations in terms of freedom from corruption; mining contracts with multinational corporations are especially suspect.

Extensive violence and looting of resources have been the norm in the Congo basin almost from the moment in 1874 when Henry Morton Stanley set off leading an expedition of porters and guards "heading for the biggest blank space on the map, the equatorial heart of the continent."[24] Following the Berlin Conference in 1884–1885, King Leopold II with his agents and private companies began a systematic looting of the Congo basin's resources. First they extracted human beings as slaves, then slaughtered elephants for their ivory. In the 1890s, they forced Africans to extract the coagulated sap from vines to make rubber for the tires of the bicycle and auto industries just emerging in Europe and the United States. The African gatherer had to cut the vine and dry the sap, Adam Hochschild writes in King Leopold's Ghost, "and often the only way to do so was to spread the substance on his arms, legs and chest."[25] This was extremely painful, and, as a Belgian agent wrote in his journal in 1892, "The native doesn't like making rubber. He must be compelled to do it."[26] Violence became the essence of this resource extraction. Belgian agents and military officers seized women, children, even the elderly as hostages. They chopped off hands, ears, and noses of Africans who would not work. If an entire village refused to gather rubber, "state or company troops or their allies sometimes shot everyone in sight, so that nearby villages would get the message."[27] By the 1920s, early human rights advocates estimated that half the people of the Congo had been killed—about 10 million men, women, and children—in the frenzy to extract their region's natural resources. More conservative figures have put the number at 5 to 8 million lives. "Even half as high," writes Hochschild, "the Congo would have been one of the major killing grounds of modern times . . . a death toll of Holocaust dimensions."[28]

News of this brutality caused an international outcry, and Leopold ceded control of his colony to his country, Belgium. The Congo Free State became The Belgian Congo. Although its name changed, the extraction of the Congo's resources continued apace, as did the killing and mutilation of the Congolese people. At independence, June 1960, The Belgian Congo became Zaire, under the dictator Col. Joseph Mobutu, whose kleptocracy further looted the region of copper, diamonds, gold, timber—taking great wealth for himself. Civil war included efforts of the rebellious (and copper-rich) Katanga province to secede from Mobutu's government, an event that featured Belgian paratroopers protecting European access to the Congo's wealth. In October 1996

Laurent-Désiré Kabila overthrew Mobutu. The region became the Democratic Republic of the Congo, or DRC. By 1997 a brutal civil war churned through the country, and the world discovered child soldiers. The fighting soon covered the eastern regions of the DRC, drawing Zimbabwe, Angola, Rwanda, and Uganda into what was called "Africa's First World War." Often portrayed as a struggle for "independence" and "justice," this conflict hardly distracted international agencies from the two-century-long frenzy over the Congo basin's natural resources and wealth.

We gain an insight to this greed from a United Nations report, published on April 21, 2001. It is a uniquely candid and detailed account[29] that unlike the standard UN document names the specific men and women, regional and international companies, army officers and diplomats active in the current stealing of the DRC's resources. It helps us to understand why, and for what purposes, conflict and resource extraction continue apace in the Congo region.

Like previous resource extractions, the violence in the 1990s began as a crude "smash and grab" country-wide mugging that accelerated. Between September 1998 and August 1999 soldiers from various African states and the DRC itself looted livestock, storage facilities containing coffee beans, timber, and other forest products. When those stockpiles were exhausted, "the exploitation evolved to an active extraction phase," the UN report states. "Both Congolese (civilians and soldiers) and foreigners (civilians and soldiers) became engaged in the extraction of natural resources." For example, more than half of the Congo's gorilla population was killed or exported; elephants and rhinos were shot for their ivory tusks and horns.[30]

Some eighty-five multinational corporations—the UN names twenty-nine companies and fifty-four individuals, mostly African and Belgian—began scrambling for gold, diamonds, copper, and cobalt. These included DeBeers, Anglo-American, and Barclays. The looting focused not only on gold and diamonds, but also on the obscure mineral col-tan (columbite-tantalite).[31] This rare ore is used in capacitors essential to our mobile phones, laptops, antilock braking systems, video and digital cameras, GPS and ignition systems, hearing aids, and pacemakers—the twenty-first-century equivalent of King Leopold's extraction of rubber for bicycle and car tires.

Everyone had a muzzle in the trough: government officials, military officers and enlisted men, wives and in-laws, desperately poor laborers in the rural areas, even children, who became soldiers or worked in the gold and diamond mines.[32] Government ministry officials from Rwanda and Uganda, army officers and their wives, all elbowed in. The Central Bank of Uganda reported that the country exported gold valued at $105 million in 1997, almost five times the exports of $23 million just two years earlier. IMF officials told the UN that "the volume of Uganda gold exports does not reflect this country's production levels but rather [what] might be 'leaking over the borders' from the Democratic Republic of the Congo." In addition, despite no known diamond production, Uganda nonetheless exported diamonds in the late 1990s, which coincided "surprisingly with the occupation of the eastern [DRC]."[33]

As the fighting ebbed and flowed in the late 1990s, Zimbabwe jumped in (by invitation) and used the war as a cover to join in the looting. Kabila cut a deal with Robert Mugabe, Zimbabwe's president, to send 11,000 Zimbabwean troops into the civil war in the DRC's Kasais and Katanga provinces—areas rich in diamonds, cobalt, copper, and gold—in exchange for access to diamond concessions, valued at $1 billion. It was a soldiers-for-diamonds deal.[34] But the Zimbabwe army used diamond mining as a cover for other operations.[35] Three stand out: to extract and sell timber, plants, and animals (many on the CITES endangered list, such as the African grey parrot and rare Congo rainforest orchids); to mix DRC-mined diamonds with illegally obtained diamonds elsewhere on the continent—"blood diamonds"—used to fund other African conflicts, and then pass them through diamond markets in South Africa and Brussels; and to engage in "money laundering," primarily U.S. dollars obtained from the diamond sales.

None of this benefited the people of Zimbabwe. While the Mugabe government was growing rich on diamonds (and other resource assets), between 6 and 7 million people in Zimbabwe experienced recurring chronic hunger and starvation, in part because of drought and the destruction of Zimbabwe's commercial farming sector by President Mugabe. Once southern Africa's regional breadbasket, beginning in 2001, Zimbabwe failed to produce enough food to feed its own people for almost a decade.[36] By 2009, the WFP reported that half the people in Zimbabwe would need emergency food assistance.[37] At the same time Médecins Sans Frontières, the international medical NGO, reported that Zimbabwe's entire health system had "collapsed," and WHO warned that all ten provinces of that country were suffering the worst outbreak of cholera in its history.

In the DRC, although the UN instilled a semblance of order that allowed elections in 2006, between 1998 and 2008 more than 5.4 million Congolese were killed. Those who managed to survive the protracted conflict and violence continue their precarious lives. Today more than half of the DRC's people have no access to clean water; the capital, Kinshasa, houses some 15 million with no sewage system. People living in the DRC suffer the full range of diseases: malaria, diarrhea, pneumonia, and persistent malnutrition. The country ranks tenth on the list of twenty-two states with "high-burden tuberculosis." Some 47 percent of those deaths are among children. For a baby born in the DRC in

2010, life expectancy was less than forty-six years.[38] At this writing, the WFP was continuing relief food for 3 million people. In 2009, the situation in north-eastern DRC was so desperate that WFP started airdrops to more than 130,000 people cut off by conflict and heavy seasonal rains.[39]

Using Collier's research model we find that 90 percent of sub-Saharan African states rely on commodity production for some 70 percent of their exports. Foreign mining companies have increased investment in the same region by more than 54 percent. In addition to the more traditional wealth in minerals, precious gems, petroleum, and natural gas, other valuable resources today include arable farmland, crops and crop residues, forests, water. ("Land-grabbing" of such assets, now accelerating, is discussed in chapter 13.) Since 2002 coffee has become the second-largest export commodity in developing countries, after petroleum. It accounts for a significant share of export earnings in countries experiencing conflict: for example, 50 percent in Ethiopia and more than 60 percent in Burundi. Coffee revenue supported Idi Amin in Uganda, rebel forces in Sierra Leone, and Ethiopia's Haile Selassie and Mengistu Haile Mariam. In Central America coffee is closely linked to violent conflict, according to an IFPRI study.[40]

There are measurable connections between conflict and food production, and thus hunger, malnutrition, and even starvation. Messer et al. noted that between 1970 and 1993—a period when sub-Saharan Africa was undergoing rapid transformation from colonialism (and, by 1992, *apartheid*)—African countries experiencing conflict produced on average about 12.4 percent less food. Since 1980, "Peace would have added 2 to 5 percent to Africa's food production per capita per year. In the 1990s, war reduced growth rates of food production per capita by 3.9 to 5.3 percent."[41] By 2010, the United Nations was juggling nine different peacekeeping operations across Africa in partnership with the Africa Union, including the DRC and hybrid peacekeeping missions in Darfur in the Sudan. UN peacemaking efforts have been successful in Angola, Mozambique, Namibia, and more recently, in Liberia and Sierra Leone.

As Collier, Messer, and others make clear, conflict over Africa's wealth is also causing Africa's intractable poverty. A 2003 study by WHO linked natural disasters, war, "civil strife," and "emergency situations" with "some of the most serious threats to health in Africa." These "result in several hundreds of thousands of deaths, especially of children and women; vast population movements; malnutrition; and the wider propagation of diseases such as HIV/AIDS, tuberculosis, malaria, acute respiratory infections and intestinal disorders, not to mention sheer human suffering and several other communicable and non-communicable diseases, including mental illness." At the time of the WHO report, conflict or violence was occurring in twenty-three of forty-six African countries, displacing some 35 million people across the region. "It is imperative," WHO concluded, "for lasting solutions to be found to Africa's wars and civil strife if the health of the people is to be protected and promoted in any meaningful way."[42] But to reach those "lasting solutions" will require creating a more equitable distribution of Africa's natural resources.

The Impacts of Global Climate Change

As we mentioned in chapter 1, James Morris, of WFP, told the UN Security Council in 2002 that weather "is the largest threat we face . . . The scale of WFP's activities has tracked closely with the occurrence of abnormal weather phenomena."[43] Weather-caused conditions of drought and floods disproportionately impact on the vulnerable. In addition there is increasing concern about a "climate gap" between the rich (and mostly northern) countries and the equatorial poor states.

Mike Davis asks: How did the developing world come into being? He tracks the connection between weather change—especially prolonged and severe drought—and starvation and poverty by examining drought and famine in the late nineteenth century. He finds that three global droughts brought famine to India, Brazil, and Russia that killed millions of human beings in 1876–1879 and 1889–1891; in Ethiopia and Sudan "perhaps one-third of the population died." In 1896–1902, monsoon rains repeatedly failed across the tropics and in northern China. Malaria, bubonic plague, dysentery, smallpox, and cholera "culled millions of victims from the ranks of the famine weakened." Davis estimates "the total human toll" at between 30 and 50 million dead.[44]

He details "the famine children of 1876 and 1899 [who] have disappeared," forgotten by modern historians. "At issue," Davis writes, "is not simply that tens of millions of poor rural people died appallingly, but that they died in a manner, and for reasons, that contradict much of the conventional understanding of the economic history of the nineteenth century."[45] He asks a troubling question: "How do we explain the fact that in the very half-century when peacetime famine permanently disappeared from Western Europe, it increased so devastatingly throughout much of the colonial world?"[46]

Could these repeating, erratic weather patterns, which caused so much human suffering more than a century ago, be occurring again? And could we argue that a principal, or predisposing, cause of chronic hunger and starvation in these regions is the combination of global climate change and household poverty, or what we might call "ecological poverty"?

El Niño and La Niña oscillations, unknown scientifically in the nineteenth century and not modeled by scientists until the 1970s, are two extremes of a cyclical weather pattern caused by shifts in the ocean temperature in the southern Pacific. Normally, surface winds blow westward from the coast of

South America to the western equatorial Pacific and cause an up-welling of cool, nutrient-rich water off Peru. Every few years a climate shift known as El Niño-Southern Oscillation (ENSO) disrupts this pattern. Westward surface winds weaken, which depresses the upward movement of cool coastal water and warms the surface of the ocean off South America. ENSOs typically last from several months to more than a year and occur about every three to four years, although the interval has been as long as seven years. When an ENSO lasts twelve months or longer, it severely disrupts populations of plankton, fish, and seabirds in the upwelling areas and can trigger extreme weather changes over much of the globe. The results are seasonal variations in tropical weather systems and erratic patterns of global rainfall.

The impact of El Niño/La Niña oscillations, and of global climate change more generally, on sub-Saharan Africa has been severe. When ENSO-dominant rainfall patterns shift toward Asia and the Pacific, this causes drought in Central America, Brazil, Australia, Indonesia, and Southeast Asia, and destructive flooding in South America. It also creates extremely dry conditions in southern Africa, but higher than normal rains in East Africa and the Horn. Recent El Niño (ENSO) events have occurred in sub-Saharan Africa in 1986–1987, 1991–1992, 1993, 1994, 1997–1998, 2001–2002, and 2006. The repetition of the pattern of the 1990s ENSOs is unusual and coincides with other dramatic climatic changes such as temperature extremes. The worst El Niño in the region to date, 1997–1998, caused widespread drought and food shortages.

La Niña, on the other hand, is marked by yet another shifting pattern in wind and sea temperatures across the southern Pacific. It is common for La Niña to follow El Niño. Its effects in sub-Saharan Africa, for example, include above-average rainfall across southern Africa with dryer than normal conditions in East Africa and the Horn. The impacts can be devastating. For example, in 2000 Mozambique experienced severe flooding from heavy La Niña rainfall and an accompanying cyclone with winds up to 125 miles per hour. Tropical trees were uprooted and propelled along the Olifants River scouring wide swaths on either side of its banks. Several thousand people died. Similar cyclones and flooding returned in 2003, 2006, and 2008.[47] Between 2000 and 2008, WFP alone sent more than 100,000 metric tons of emergency food aid to some 250,000 people in Mozambique at a cost of $20 million.[48] But the real devastation was to the country's agriculture. FEWS reports in 2009—nine years later—showed that Mozambique, while recovering slowly, was still experiencing food production shortfalls caused by these "poor agroclimatological conditions." Impoverished households could not overcome repeated production losses. "Given their low cash incomes, these populations are further constrained by the current above-average food prices."[49]

Davis asks whether or not the power of weather events, recorded since the late nineteenth century, might have caused the famines of the 1870s, 1890s, or even the 1970s. He finds that the most prolonged and widespread droughts in sub-Saharan Africa, as measured by SPOT satellite, have occurred in 1973, 1984, 1992, and most recently in 2001–2002, 2006, and 2007, which match up well with ENSO occurrences.[50] But is there cause and effect here? As the FEWS statement above makes clear, poverty is often the predisposing factor, not weather. Does blaming starvation and famine on an ENSO event, as Davis writes about the nineteenth century ENSOs, merely echo the official British position at the time that in Victorian India "millions were killed by extreme weather, not imperialism"? Weather or poverty? Or, as the Chinese put it: "bad climate" versus "bad system"?[51]

Davis makes a clear choice. He argues that weak governance ("state decapacitation"), "household poverty," and "ecological poverty"—defined as the "depletion or loss of entitlement to the natural resource base of traditional agriculture"—together explain the emergence of a developing world "and its vulnerability to extreme climate events."[52] That is, poverty and vulnerability make it possible for a La Niña-El Niño event to have devastating effect. The poor in nineteenth-century India, created by British imperialism, had little resilience to severe weather when it struck them. We saw a similar effect among the U.S. urban poor in New Orleans when Hurricane Katrina devastated that city in 2005.[53] Wealthier areas and people in Louisiana suffered far less and recovered more quickly.

Today, global climate change is already striking two specific populations: the poorest of the poor and those living in island states or coastal regions that are easily flooded. They number about 1 billion people in one hundred countries. Poverty is also their common denominator. Many of them depend on rain-fed agriculture, tropical forests, and subsistence fishing to survive. But global warming will erode coastlines, spread pests and disease, and produce erratic weather patterns, making their livelihoods even more difficult.[54]

Climate change is already having real effects on them. According to a United Nations report, for example, some 40 million Africans now at risk of starvation "may be among the first victims of climate change worldwide."[55] A conference paper from the Brookings Institute estimates that African farmers dependent on rain-fed agriculture will lose US$28 in income per hectare per year for every 1 degree Celsius rise in global temperatures,[56] thus increasing their poverty. According to another research paper from the John F. Kennedy School at Harvard, eleven of the twelve warmest years on record have occurred since 1995.[57]

These 1 billion people share two other important characteristics. First, they are the voiceless who suffer inside "a silent crisis";[58] they are too poor to defend themselves or articulate their own plight. A 2008 report by the Global Humanitarian Forum (GHF) estimated that climate change was already causing more than 300,000 deaths annually across the developing world, and that number will reach 500,000 by 2030. Nine in ten of those deaths are the result of "environmental degradation due to climate change." Second, "their own carbon footprints are tiny."[59] As the GHF report states, "Those who suffer most from climate change have done the least to cause it." They consume little, yet are the recipients of pollution from wealthy states at great distance from them. "Developing countries bear over nine-tenths of the climate change burden: 98 percent of the [people are] seriously affected [by climate change]," the report continues, "and [it causes] 99 percent of all deaths from weather-related disasters, along with over 90 percent of the total economic losses." But while the largest carbon footprints and amounts of pollution come from people living in the developed world, "The 50 least developed countries contribute less than 1 percent of global carbon emissions."[60]

Are people in the wealthy developed states inadvertently causing starvation and poverty in the developing world? As we have already noted, from about 1970 until 1985 Africans in the Sahel and the Horn experienced repeated episodes of searing drought. During those fifteen years, perhaps as many as 1.2 million people in that region died from starvation and other drought-related causes. Research in 1977 indicated that "insoluble mineral aerosols" in the lower atmosphere over the North Atlantic Ocean had in fact increased "by a factor of 3" during the decade before the long drought began. Further, that pollution generated by high-energy consumption in North America might be "related" to the drought then continuing across the Sahel and Horn.[61]

In 2002 Australian and Canadian scientists corroborated that early assessment by using atmospheric global climate and mixed-layer ocean models that analyzed rainfall trends over land from 1900 to 1998. Both models found a drying pattern across the Sahel with an accompanying drought, which suggested "that the indirect effects of anthropogenic sulfate may have contributed to the Sahelian drying trend."[62] That is, tiny particles of sulfur dioxide from energy sources (burning fossil fuels) likely drifted with the prevailing winds from the North American continent over the North Atlantic, where they created more condensation nuclei for cloud formation. Aerosol particles can drift in the air for five to twenty days. It is thought that these remained suspended in clouds, rather than falling as part of the rain into the ocean. The aerosols in these clouds may have been brighter than normal, reflecting sunlight away from the ocean surface, which in turn cooled the North Atlantic and reduced normal rainfall as far away as sub-Saharan Africa by as much as 50 percent.[63] Dr. Leon Rotstayn, an atmospheric scientist at Australia's Commonwealth Scientific and Industrial Research Organization, which led the study, warned that "The Sahelian drought may be due to a combination of natural variability and atmospheric aerosols. . . . Global climate change is not solely being caused by rising levels of greenhouse gases. Atmospheric pollution is also having an effect."[64] Thus, aerosols from North America may have been partially responsible for environmental events such as drought across the equator of Africa.

Other studies have confirmed that aerosol pollutions—including black carbon or "soot"—are altering regional atmospheres. In China, for example, "black soot" from industrial expansion has produced increasing summer rainfalls and floods in the south and drought in the north.[65] Another piece of evidence comes from further studies of the North American aerosols. During the 1990s, while climate change shifted El Niño/La Niña effects in East and southern Africa, normal patterns of rainfall returned to the Sahel and Horn. One possibility posed by researchers is that stricter emission standards in industrialized North America had successfully reduced aerosol pollution.

Challenges of the "Nutritional Transition"

Our third example of outside actors triggering hunger and famine in developing states asks: Is it possible that Africans have starved in the past—and may starve in the future—because of purchases in the global grain markets by other, distant, actors and states? In this chapter we explore modern China, and then return to the starvation across the Sahel and Horn during 1973–1974. Is there a warning from that history?

It is important to begin any discussion of China with one about population. No other single factor directs and influences the future of China more than the size and growth of its population. In 1960 the world's population was 3 billion. In forty years it doubled. By 2020 it is expected to reach 7.5 billion. During this period global food production has often increased even faster than global population; yet at least one person out of every six remains chronically hungry. Among the impoverished states of sub-Saharan Africa the number of continuously malnourished people remains at about one African out of every three.[66]

Between 1995 and 2020, more than 73 million people will be added to the world population each year. More than 97 percent of that increase will occur in the developing world. The overall growth will be most rapid in Africa. But one-third of the total global population increase is expected to take place in just two countries: India and China. Three significant trends are already under way:

Rapid urban population growth. Most of the population growth globally will take place in the cities of the developing world, which are projected to double from 1.7 billion to 3.4 billion in 2020. This means that more than half of the developing world's people (52 percent) will be living in urban areas by 2020, up from 38 percent in 2000.[67]

Rising incomes. With urbanization comes rising incomes, and total income in the developing world will increase about 4.3 percent annually by 2020. This may double the average annual per capita incomes to US$2200 per person per year.[68] Rising urban growth is also under way in sub-Saharan Africa, but it is not being accompanied by rising incomes. In fact by 2020 per capita income in sub-Saharan Africa is projected to be less than US$1 per day (US$359 per capita per year). The International Food Policy Research Institute, looking at rising incomes elsewhere, writes of sub-Saharan Africa, "Poverty of this magnitude will condemn many people in this region to food insecurity."[69] Thus we are seeing a further dichotomy in wealth distribution within the developing world.

Nutritional transition. With rising urban populations and increasing incomes will come a dramatic change in eating preferences and food demands. What does this mean? A significant "nutritional transition" is already under way in the developing world. Rapid urbanization and rising incomes are shifting diets from coarse grains (corn, sorghum, and millet) to rice, wheat, fruits, vegetables, and processed foods.[70] Consumption of meat is also increasing, creating a parallel rise in demand for grains. As discussed briefly in chapter 1, this "nutritional transition" generated by urbanization and a parallel expansion of wealth is already placing pressure on global grain supplies.

Pull this together. There are, therefore, two profound claims being placed on the finite global grain supply. One comes from *rising wealth* among the developing world's urban and educated (creating a nutritional transition), and the other from *increasing poverty* among the "bottom billion" of very poor people (creating a nutritional crisis). In the first instance, rapid population shifts into the cities of developing states and rising urban incomes are causing the "nutritional transition" by redirecting food demand and production. More grains are going into meat and processed foods and beverages (beer, for example) than into direct grain consumption. On the other hand, for many of the poorest people of the developing world, the gap between food production and need will continue to be wider than the gap between production and demand "because many of these people are priced out of the market, even at low food prices, and their market demand fails to reflect fully their food needs."[71] They are thus chronically hungry and malnourished, and trapped in an intransigent nutritional crisis. It will take very little to tip them into starvation, and when this occurs, the donor states and agencies will need to go into the global grain market for emergency relief food. But given the rising claims of the "nutritional transition," will the grain be available?

China's population and its growth magnify these issues. China's domestic problems are actually the result of its development success. Between 1995 and 2007, for example, China's economy expanded by 93 percent and ranked among the top globally. Although its economy slowed greatly during the more recent global recession, and China struggled, the size, pace, and thrust of the country's economy continues to make China a consumer of large amounts of oil, copper, nickel, tin, coal, timber, agricultural products, and other resources.[72] During the boom years China's consumption of energy expanded 4.3 percent annually, four times the rate of Western Europe; oil consumption jumped 150 percent and natural gas, 1100 percent.

By the end of the first decade of the twenty-first century, China's population had moved beyond 1.4 billion people. During the same period its domestic "floating populations" continued to migrate into its cities by the tens of thousands. By 2005 the country was "orchestrating an industrial revolution, hoping to telescope into a few decades what it took Western countries a century or two to accomplish." To transition from an agrarian to an urban society, Chinese officials announced plans to move more than 400 million people—about half the rural population—into its cities by 2030.[73] Can China balance industrial growth and the rising numbers of urban inhabitants and still shift from an economy based on agriculture to one based on industrial development? If not, how will China feed its people?

For one thing, the country faces enormous environmental problems: pollution of air and water, shortages of clean water for its cities and for its agriculture in the North. The Great Leap Forward and the Cultural Revolution were "disastrous for the modernization of Chinese agriculture." The Chinese famine of 1959–1961 may have killed more than 25 million people (and perhaps as many as 40 million) under the guise of an agriculture success.[74] In the 1970s Deng Xiaoping restored incentives to family-sized farms and unleashed "the genius of the traditional [Chinese] farmer." China's agriculture by 1994 was producing four times the amount of grains harvested during the previous two decades, "a phenomenal achievement." The rapid growth of China's agriculture was "one of the major events on our planet."[75] By 2010, China was food self-sufficient, feeding all of its citizens (about 20 percent of the world's population), although only 7 percent of the country's land is arable farmland.[76]

But in parallel with the "phenomenal" growth of China's agriculture was the country's unmatched industrial development. And with that transition have come some systemic problems. Water is increasingly scarce and polluted. By 2008 in Northern China desertification had consumed some 36,000 square kilometers of arable land, and the region's water supply had fallen to just 30 percent of requirements. Ground water is being pumped out faster than it is replenished.[77] Most Chinese cities treat none of their sewage; the World Bank reports that more than half of the water in China's seven largest river basins is "unfit for consumption."[78] The Intergovernmental Panel on Climate Change warns that the Himalayan glaciers that feed China's largest rivers and its agricultural system are melting, and, at the current rate, that water will disappear by 2035.

For every degree of global temperature rise, rice yields in China are projected to *decrease* by 10 percent. China is also losing its arable land to rapid development, especially in the central and northern provinces and around the urban areas on the coast. In 1952, when the first modern census was completed in China, about 583 million Chinese were living on the output of 260 million acres of cultivated arable land. Between 1988 and 1995, as population and industry expanded rapidly, China lost 1.7 million hectares of arable land.[79] By 1998 China's population growth and industrial expansion (plus widespread pump irrigation that made 5 million acres of soil alkaline) had reduced that arable land to 225 million acres, but now feeding some 1.2 billion people. Today the country is losing about 1.5 percent of its arable land annually.[80] By 2006 farmers were battling local officials over the confiscation of farmland for industrial expansion.[81] Climate change will make this worse: rising sea levels along China's coast may further reduce much of that region's rice production.

Despite the "tremendous efforts" of China's farmers, says one former diplomat, "sometime in the twenty-first century China will become the world's largest food importer."[82] As of this writing China was already aggressively outsourcing some of its domestic problems and needs. Before the economic downturn in 2008, the country, according to Lester Brown, was "importing vast quantities of grain, soybeans, iron ore, aluminum, copper, platinum, potash, oil, and natural gas, forest products for lumber and paper, cotton for the world's largest textile industry." For example, in 2009 some ninety large freighters loaded with raw materials (iron ore, copper, nickel, tin, and zinc) and commodities (soybeans and canola) were idling off Chinese ports, waiting to offload.[83] Its "voracious appetite for materials [was] driving up not only commodity prices, but ocean shipping rates as well."[84] If domestic development continues, by 2020 China will be a major oil importer from six sub-Saharan Africa countries and a consumer of one-third of the world's global rubber supply.

In terms of food resources the "nutritional transition" under way in China "is forecast to account for one-quarter of the global increase in demand for cereals and for two-fifths of the increase in demand for meat."[85] And while India's population is projected to increase faster than China's, and its resilient economy is sustaining demand for commodities despite the global recession that began in 2008, "its share of the global increase in demand for meat is expected to be only one-tenth that of China" largely because of continuing widespread poverty in India and "culturally-based food preferences."[86] With that increase in China's demand for meat will come, of course, a far larger demand for grains; it takes 16 pounds of grain and 5000 gallons of water to produce one pound of beef.[87]

Perhaps anticipating this dilemma, China continues to redirect funds and resources to its agricultural initiatives overseas. Chinese civilians are themselves operating farms from Southeast Asia to sub-Saharan Africa to grow and export palm oil, rubber, teak, eucalyptus, maize, cassava, sugar cane, and other crops to meet their country's demands. In Zimbabwe, for example, the China International Water and Electric Corporation is reportedly farming some 250,000 acres of maize on former commercial farms seized and redistributed by the Mugabe regime.[88]

What if China cannot continue to feed its own people and comes into the global grain market to offset shortfalls in domestic food requirements? Lester Brown asks: "Who will feed China?" His answer is worth our attention, especially given former U.S. diplomat Albert Ravenholt's clear warning that by midcentury "a much more affluent China will necessarily become a major grain importer."[89] Brown's argument goes like this:

China's record in agriculture had been exceptional through the 1990s. After Deng restored incentives to small farmers and incorporated other agricultural reforms, by 1978 output climbed from 200 million tons to 300 million tons, which put China ahead of the United States as the world's leading grain producer. By the mid-1990s, grain production had increased fourfold, "a phenomenal achievement," and China had attained overall food self-sufficiency. However, Brown writes, in 1994 a 60 percent rise in grain prices led the Chinese government to purchase a record 6 million tons of grain from the global market during a single month, mostly from the United States. In March 1995, the National People's Congress stated candidly: "China is facing a looming grain crisis, with a hike in imports the only apparent solution to the demands of a growing population on a shrinking farmland."[90]

Brown then issued his warning. A significant demand by China for grains on the world market would be unprecedented and perhaps catastrophic. He wrote: "[I]t will quickly overwhelm the export capacity of the United States and other countries, driving food prices upward everywhere."[91] Brown worried: "China's emergence as a massive grain importer will be the wake-up call that will signal trouble in the relationship between ourselves, now numbering 5.7 billion, and the natural systems and resources on which we depend."[92] But Brown's "wake up call" roused few people. The Chinese denied it and distributed statistics showing how well their agriculture was doing.

In March 2004, however, the Chinese announced an "emergency appropriation" increasing China's agriculture budget by 25 percent in order to raise subsidies for wheat and rice, the country's primary food staples. Why? After "a remarkable expansion of grain output" to 392 million tons in 1998, China's grain production had declined in four of the next five years and fell by 2004 to 322 million tons. That 70-million-ton shortfall was at the time greater than Canada's entire grain harvest. As a result, the Chinese went on the global market for 5 million tons of grains, and world grain prices rose sharply.[93] Brown warned of "early tremors before the quake." China was covering shortfalls by drawing down its "once massive stocks of grain." Its wheat harvest was short of consumption by 19 million tons. The rice shortfall of 20 million tons equaled almost the total world annual rice exports (26 million tons at the time). Maize (corn) was short 15 million tons, and stocks "largely depleted."[94]

What caused this? In part, the addition of 11 million people annually every year along with "fast-rising incomes" encouraged the "nutritional transition" from basic grains to grain-fed livestock products (pork, poultry, eggs, beef, and milk). The arable land devoted to grain was also shrinking, as we noted earlier, from 90 million acres in 1998 to 76 million in 2003. This was caused by water shortages that increased aridity, the expansion of desert, and by industrial and highway construction devouring farmland. China's economy was booming and, with every twenty cars added to China's fleet, the country lost about 1 acre of land (0.4 hectares) to parking lots, streets, and highway construction. In 2003 the 2 million new cars sold in China meant paving over another 100,000 acres of land.[95]

Putting these statistics together, Brown issued a new wake-up call: "When China turns to the world market, it will necessarily turn to the United States, which controls nearly half of world grain exports. This presents an unprecedented geopolitical situation in which 1.3 billion Chinese consumers who have a $120-billion trade surplus with the United States—enough to buy the entire U.S. grain harvest twice over—will compete with Americans for food, likely driving up food prices for the United States and the world." Even shipping grain on this scale from the United States to China could divert the equivalent of as many as two to three ships per day, every day. This might "become one of the major U.S. foreign policy challenges of this new century," Brown concluded.[96] Far-fetched? As of January 2009, China held more than $730 billion worth of U.S. Treasury Securities.[97] This provides the Chinese with enormous financial and political leverage with which to negotiate with the United States concerning grain supplies.

China illustrates the change in eating patterns that is taking place as states develop, the increase in demand for grains from a "nutritional transition," and the potentially significant impacts on the global grain market if food shortages occurred in the world's largest population. If starvation continues across the developing world, as it is predicted to do, what might be the impact if China needed the U.S. grain production? We have a "distant mirror" that helps us answer this question. During the 1972–1974 famines in Africa's Sahel and Horn regions, the Soviet Union (USSR) entered the global grain market in what has come to be called "The Great Grain Robbery."

In 1971 and continuing through the summer of 1972 the people of the USSR suffered from widespread and severe drought. The seriousness and impact of this were not fully disclosed. The Soviets had experienced grain production shortfalls before and largely managed to keep them hidden. During those periods they had cut back on consumption while importing what was needed to cover losses. But although the 1971–1973 drought in the USSR was known outside the country, the extent of the Soviet need and their "buying intentions" remained a secret.

In July and August 1972 the Soviets quietly began making separate, but large, purchases of grain on the global market. The total amount soon proved to be enormous. That July and August, for example, they contracted for 440 million bushels of wheat from the United States for $700 million, "more than the total U.S. commercial wheat exports for the year." That demand was unprecedented, "equivalent to 30 percent of average annual U.S. wheat production during the previous five years and more than 80 percent of the wheat used for domestic food during that period."[98]

Moreover, the Soviet grain-buying agency cut deals with several different companies to "conceal its order book from the trade while it was actively in the market."[99] In the late 1960s and early 1970s the international grain trade had been challenged by low prices and substantial surpluses. The sales between the United States and USSR involved a series of subsidized contracts in which the U.S. government, perhaps too eager to draw down its grain surpluses and increase exports, made available a line of credit for $750 million to the Soviets for the purchase of grain over a three-year period.[100] In effect, the United States allowed the Soviets to "bet"—using U.S. taxpayer dollars—that the price of grain would increase, to their profit. Shortly after the sales were publicly announced, "the domestic price of wheat began to rise, and within a few months the prices of feed and food grain, soybeans, and livestock turned upward and all continued to rise at a high rate during most of the next twelve months."[101] By the end of 1972, food prices were also up "sharply." The price of wheat almost tripled by August 1973, while corn and soybeans doubled. An add-on effect followed: steer prices up 55 percent, hogs up 102 percent, chickens up 153 percent. The wholesale price index for all farm products also jumped 66 percent; the wholesale price of food rose 29 percent, and retail food prices "generally continued upward."[102]

Later, when the General Accounting Office (GAO), the "watchdog" of Congress, reviewed the U.S. agreements with the Soviet Union, it "questioned" the U.S. Department of Agriculture's (USDA) management of the wheat export subsidy program. The GAO concluded "that the export subsidies were excessive and that the sales caused a dramatic rise in the price of wheat and higher consumer prices for bread and most livestock products."[103]

In fact "The Great Grain" had met "the great farm subsidy"—an issue relevant today. Through subsidies to its farmers, the United States (and the EU and other countries) can stimulate production. During the early 1970s, and continuing into the 1980s, U.S. government subsidies to its farmers created unprecedented surpluses, which then required further subsidies to grain exporters to haul off those surpluses. The mountains of wheat that attracted the Russian's interest had accrued "as the result of a national policy of maintaining high price supports to wheat producers." This was not a new food policy: for more than two decades before the 1972 Soviet Union wheat purchases, the United States had used subsidies to create large surpluses, and the USDA had then used export subsidies to reduce those surplus stocks. But this time the grain export companies joined the farmers and "reaped large Federal subsidy payments at the same time they were making windfall profits from the export sales, and the transactions drained the United States of wheat supplies, contributing to sharply rising food prices."[104] Since the objective of such programs is higher farm prices and incomes,[105] the sale to the USSR was, in effect, a very embarrassing success. In 1972–1973, U.S. agricultural policy worked for everyone— except the small U.S. farmer and the American taxpayer.

Three lessons emerge from "The Great Grain Robbery." First, the United States had rapidly expanding food surpluses, which it could use as a foreign policy instrument. The USDA was holding in storage a large excess of "carryover stocks" of all feed grains (wheat, corn, oats, barley, and grain sorghum) at taxpayers' expense. Thus since the early 1950s when farm subsidies began in earnest, "a major problem of the Government farm programs, given the level of price supports, [was] the disposal of accumulated surpluses."[106] Wheat stocks carried over into the 1972–1973 marketing year totaled 865 million bushels, which when added to the 1972 production of 1551 million bushels, resulted in a total surplus of 2417 million bushels. Drawdown in the past had averaged 1426 million bushels over the previous five years.[107] In 1972 the United States had a Mount Everest of surplus food grains.

Second, the global grain market was further jolted by drought in Australia, one of the five major surplus food-producing nations at the time. This sharply decreased production in that country, with a ripple effect globally. In 1972 India also came into the global grain market for sizable quantities of wheat. Supply and demand were shifting.

Third, the comptroller general of the United States in a GAO report to Congress found the capitalist economists of the USDA no match for the centrally planned economy of the Soviet Communist government and its equivalent agency. The Americans got snookered. "Trading rules and procedures of the USDA," the comptroller scolded, "are not adequate for dealing with the bargaining power of a foreign state trading monopoly."[108] The media howled about "The Great Grain Robbery" pulled off by the Russians.

The result was a windfall for a lot of people. The subsidies enriched some large commercial grain producers and food exporters. The Russians contracted for wheat at US$62 a ton, paid that amount, and took possession as the price hit $214 a ton.[109] The USDA crowed that "the Russian transactions resulted in a net saving to the [U.S.] Treasury of $457 million" which was, Clifton Luttrell writes, "consistent with the farm program objectives during a two-decade period of excessive wheat stocks." Such stocks had been seen as liabilities. If the basic U.S. farm policy was to pay U.S. farmers to produce more, and to give them a subsidized price for their wheat, it was a huge success. The transaction with the Russians increased the prices that U.S. farmers received, "creating new jobs," and "improving the balance of trade."[110]

True, the subsidized transactions caused domestic food prices to rise, "and reduced the well-being of U.S. consumers."[111] Between 1972 and 1973 prices jumped 140 percent for wheat, 165 percent for corn, and 210 percent for soybeans. This was helped along by an unforeseen decline in global production of wheat, rice, corn, and peanuts as the result of spreading drought that increased global demand for U.S. wheat, feed grains, and soybeans. Rising demand caused rising prices, and a 40 percent increase in the consumer price index for meat, poultry, and fish during the first six months of 1973—all of which "was likewise unforeseen."[112]

In 1972–1974 there was a further unforeseen cost, but to other people. Drought followed by starvation was spreading across the Sahel and Horn of Africa. While the developed countries could insulate their domestic markets from these price rises, the developing world became residual buyers in the international export markets. As a result, they were obliged to pay much higher prices for the food they imported—and so were their people. And so, too, were the public and private agencies attempting to gather emergency grains to feed starving Africans during this same period.

We cannot blame the USDA or the U.S. government, or the governments of the USSR, or India for what happened. The results were indeed unanticipated.

In 1972–1974 there was no accurate early warning system yet in place. As the Russians started negotiations, who among us knew of the drought that was already winnowing through Africa's farms and villages, cracking the topsoil and lifting swirls of dust into the dry air, pulling behind it "a famine that kills." As global grain prices rose, peasant farmers ate their planting seeds, sold whatever possessions they had, and walked (if they could) away from their families and communities in a desperate search of food. When alarms elsewhere finally sounded about a famine striking millions of Africans from the Atlantic Ocean to the Red Sea, donors found global supplies of wheat and maize scarce, and prices high. These grains were very slow in reaching those who truly needed them. The result was what one observer called a "Disaster in the Desert."[113]

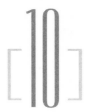

Why Do Some People Die?

Humanity has but three great enemies: fever, famine, and war;
of these by far the greatest, by far the most terrible, is fever.
—Sir William Osler (1849–1919)

And I saw when the Lamb opened one of the seals, and I heard, as it
were the noise of thunder, one of the four beasts saying, Come and see.
   And I saw, and behold a white horse: and he that sat on him had
a bow; and a crown was given unto him: and he went forth conquering,
and to conquer.
—Book of Revelation 6:1–2

William Osler is considered to be the father of modern medicine. A human-ist, teacher, and extremely astute clinician, he is credited (among other things) with the development of bedside teaching as a critical means of training new physicians. A man of great intelligence and insight, his meaning in the above quote is not intuitively obvious—one would expect most fatalities in war to be due to combat-related injury; most deaths from chronic malnutrition due to organ dysfunction and eventual organ failure.

In the quote below, Thomas Malthus seems to have considered the Third Horseman of the Apocalypse, famine, to be the final arbiter of death.

Famine seems to be the last, the most dreadful resource of nature. The power of the population is so superior to the power of the earth to produce subsistence for man, that premature death must in some shape or other visit the human race. The vices of mankind are active and able ministers of depopulation. They are the precursors in the great army of destruction; and often finish the dreadful work themselves. But should they fail in this war of extermination, sickly seasons, epidemics, pestilence, and plague, advance in terrific array, and sweep off their thousands and tens of thousands. Should success be still incomplete, gigantic inevitable famine stalks in the rear, and with one mighty blow levels the population with the food of the world.[1]

Who Had It Right, Osler or Malthus?
Death tolls and the causes of death in armed conflicts and famine are notori-ously difficult to measure or validate. When one is able to critically evaluate

the ultimate cause of most deaths due to war or to famine, either associated with armed conflict or not, it turns out that far more people are killed by the infectious diseases associated with the squalid living conditions, lack of safe drinking water and sanitation, and chronic malnutrition associated with armed conflict or poverty in general than have ever been killed by bullets, or directly by starvation per se (in fact, it was not until World War I that more people were killed by bullets than by disease).[2]

A well-documented example of this is offered by Florence Nightingale's experience during the Crimean War. During that conflict, Nightingale was one of the first in health care to use direct measurement and statistical analysis to demonstrate that ten times as many soldiers were dying from typhoid, typhus, cholera, and dysentery than from injuries incurred in battle. Appalled at the state of the sanitary conditions in which the wounded soldiers lived, she arranged for these conditions to be improved (she happened to be friends with the Secretary of War). Within six months of her arrival and the improvement in the sanitary conditions, mortality rates dropped from over 40 percent to 2 percent.[3] The generally agreed-upon death toll in the American Civil War (which had the highest number of American casualties of any war before or since) was approximately 620,000. Of these, 204,000 deaths are attributed to battle deaths, while 414,000 are considered the direct result of disease (25 percent of these felt to be due to typhoid fever).

As an example of causes of mortality in famines unassociated with armed conflict, the Great Irish Famine of the 1840s is estimated to have resulted in the death of 1,000,000 people, but actual death by starvation was uncommon—the majority of these deaths were ultimately due to infectious disease.[4] Even in populations not affected by conflict or chronic malnutrition, infectious disease has historically been responsible for the majority of deaths up to and including those in the twentieth century. It is estimated that smallpox alone accounted for 300–500 million deaths worldwide during the twentieth century, more than all of the wars of that century combined. While we are becoming increasingly proficient at killing each other directly through the use of sophisticated weaponry, and while chronic metabolic diseases such as coronary disease, diabetes, obesity, and hypertension are now leading causes of death worldwide—in large part due to unhealthy choices in nutrition and habits such as smoking—infectious diseases have been the major ultimate cause of death throughout the vast majority of human existence, and they continue to be the agent of death in essentially all of the premature, preventable deaths attributable to chronic undernutrition in the present day.

If we return to the quotes at the beginning of this chapter, we can begin to understand why Osler said what he did (fever being a cardinal manifestation of infection) and why Osler's statement was more accurate for the time than Malthus's. The lines from Revelation introduce the Four Horsemen of the Apocalypse, the agents of man's destruction as prophesized by Jesus and told by John. The white horse represents pestilence (a term used to describe highly contagious and virulent infectious diseases that cause illness and death in epidemic proportions); the red horse war; the black horse famine; and the fourth horse—the pale horse—death. While each of these bleak realities of the human condition carries its own terror, it has long been recognized that two of them, the twin fruits of war—famine and pestilence—are in fact of greatest significance in the production of human suffering and eventual death. Perhaps it is not coincidence that pestilence is riding the first horse.

Chronic Malnutrition and Susceptibility to Disease

Why are chronically undernourished people so vulnerable to infection, and why do they succumb to infections that would otherwise be at worst debilitating but survivable, and frequently nothing more than an inconvenience? In order to understand this, it will require us to review a brief primer in infectious disease and the immune system.

Virulence is a term used to describe the propensity for an organism to cause disease. It can be used to describe characteristics of contagion; ability to invade or destroy tissue; the likelihood of associated morbidity or mortality; or a combination of the above traits. The word itself comes from the Latin root for poison (Latin: *viru-*, also *veno-* as in venom). We may also recognize the use of this root in the word *virus*, used by Louis Pasteur for agents of disease (in this case rabies) that were "filterable," that is, not visible and not clearly demonstrable as particulate or living organisms with the technology available to him at the time, and therefore thought to represent some type of poison or "liquid infectious agent," as opposed to the living (depending on your definition) submicroscopic organisms they were later found to be.

Microorganisms that cause disease are termed *pathogens*. The virulence of any one pathogen is dependent on characteristics of both the organism and the host. The characteristics of the organism that determine its *pathogenicity* and degree of *virulence* are genetically determined gene products that increase the ability of the microorganism to cause disease. These gene products are generally specialized proteins that allow the pathogen to interact in very specific ways with a particular host. As examples, the proteins may act as *exotoxins* secreted by the bacteria into the external environment (as seen in staphylococcal food poisoning); specialized molecular receptors that allow the pathogen to adhere to target cells or *adhesins* (toxigenic *Escherichia coli*); proteins that allow the organism to invade healthy tissue or *invasins* (*Salmonella typhi*—the organism that causes typhoid fever); receptors that allow the organism to "hide" from the host's immune system by coating itself with host proteins (*Treponema pallidum*—the organism that causes syphilis); proteins that will destroy protective antibodies (*Hemophilus influenzae*—a common cause of severe bacterial pneumonia in infants and children); or even trick the host's body into stimulating production of immunosuppressive substances (*Mycobacterium tuberculosis*).[5] Of some interest is the fact that most human pathogens are specific only for human beings, an indication of the fact that they have evolved right along with us, many times having evolved from similar pathogens that infect our domesticated animals.[6]

Whereas some host characteristics may be genetically determined (a good example would be the resistance to falciparum malaria infection that benefits individuals with a single copy of the hemoglobin S gene—the gene responsible for sickle cell anemia in those who have two copies of it), most characteristics that determine a host's response to infection are determined by either environmental factors or factors that affect the state of the host's defenses. Environmental factors might include overcrowding, conditions that do not allow adequate hygiene, or poor sanitation. Situations such as this increase the probability that any one individual will encounter a pathogenic organism and, once encountered, increase the likelihood that the organism will gain entry to the host's body. Consider, for example, the lightning speed with which a common cold or case of infectious diarrhea can move through a class of kindergarten students (and their respective families). These environmental factors can cause quite serious illness in individuals, and in fact epidemics in situations in which the social infrastructure has either broken down or is nonexistent, such as in areas of armed conflict or poverty. These are the biological analogies of the "loud emergencies" discussed elsewhere in this book. The factors that affect the host's own defenses, however, are more insidious. These can be considered the biological equivalents of the "silent emergencies" that slowly debilitate individuals and populations, so that even the most innocent-seeming viral respiratory infection can quickly develop into progressive bacterial pneumonia and death.

Many if not most organisms exist in some sort of relationship with other organisms. These relationships are developed more by coevolutionary proximity and need. As a group these interspecific interactions are known as *symbiosis* and are categorized by the relative effect each organism has on the other. Relationships in which both organisms benefit belong to the category of *mutualism*. An example of this would be lichen—a very primitive member of the plant kingdom that is part fungus and part algae, neither of which would survive without the other in the harsh environments colonized by lichen. Relationships in which one organism benefits while the other is neither helped nor harmed, such as the relationship between the shark and the remora that hitches a ride (and may benefit from scraps of food), is termed *commensalism*. A relationship in which one of the organisms benefits but the other is harmed is considered *parasitism*. Infectious diseases, diseases caused by microbial organisms and that by definition are contagious to a greater or lesser degree, can be considered to be a form of microscopic parasitism. Just as organisms have evolved very effective, and at times remarkably sophisticated, means of defeating our defenses, invading our bodies, and causing disease, we have developed multiple means of defending ourselves. Our first line of defense is our physical barriers. Our skin and mucous membranes are extremely effective living barriers to attack and invasion by most organisms we encounter, as long as they are intact. When pathogenic organisms succeed in gaining entry, we have multiple mechanisms for recognizing them, neutralizing their molecular weapons, and killing and disposing of them with extreme prejudice. Our armamentarium includes various weapons such as humoral immunity, cellular immunity, chemical messengers known as cytokines, the complement system, and phagocytosis.

Humoral immunity, the part of the immune system that is based on soluble proteins circulating in the blood, is mediated by antibodies. These are highly sophisticated, complex proteins produced by specialized white blood cells called B-lymphocytes. When a B-lymphocyte encounters an antigen, usually a foreign protein, it is able to recognize it as such and produce an antibody that facilitates neutralization and destruction of that foreign protein. As it does so it forms a clone of identical B-lymphocytes that are not only programmed to generate the same antibodies but also have a memory that enable them to react immediately when exposed to an identical or nearly identical antigen again. As these antibodies are preformed and circulating in the blood, or can be prepared and released as soon as the antigen is encountered, this form of immunity is also called *immediate hypersensitivity*. Most forms of food allergies involve this part of the immune system.

Cellular immunity, as the name implies, involves more direct participation by a different type of white blood cell—the T-lymphocyte. T-lymphocytes are also able to recognize foreign antigens, and they also have a memory. Instead of producing and secreting antibodies, however, they can variably act to kill invading organisms, help other cells kill the organisms, or, along with other white blood cells called macrophages, secrete extremely potent cell-signaling chemicals that act as highly effective mediators of inflammation. These signaling proteins or peptides are called *cytokines* (Greek: *cyto*, cell; *kine*, motion).[7] Some cytokines that might sound familiar include the interferons and interleukins. Cellular immunity requires not just the activation of cells but also magnification of response by cellular division and building of active clones at the time of antigen exposure. As such, the response takes time and is also called *delayed hypersensitivity*. The blistering rash that occurs twenty-four to forty-eight hours after exposure to poison ivy is an example of a cellular-mediated immune response.

In addition to the humoral and cellular immunity systems, there is an additional humoral system of a group of proteins known as the complement system. These proteins, when activated by mediators of inflammation, adhere to the surface of invading bacteria, form complexes that disrupt the integrity of the cell wall and cell membrane of the organism, and in doing so overcome the bacteria's ability to maintain its osmotic balance with the environment. As fluids flow into the bacterial interior, the organism swells and bursts. Finally, as the invading organisms are disabled and killed, other specialized white blood cells seek out and engulf the remains, a process enhanced when the invading organisms are coated with antibodies and complement factors (a process known as *opsonization* (Greek: *opsonein*, to prepare food). This is called *phagocytosis* (Greek: *phago*, eat; *cyte*, cell).

This brief description of our innate defenses, as superficial as it is, still requires more explanation than the most basic details already mentioned as to how chronic malnutrition impairs these defenses. The answer to that complex question is: "in every way." Protein energy malnutrition (as we discussed in chapter 8) and multiple vitamin and mineral deficiencies cause breakdown and sloughing of the skin and weakening and atrophy of mucosal surfaces. Once these physical barriers are breached, even organisms that cannot usually gain access to our internal tissues are able to invade. When they do, they are opposed by a weakened internal defense system. Malnutrition leads to depletion and functional defects of T-lymphocytes and complement, depression of opsonic activity of the serum and phagocytosis, and to reduced activity of cytokines leading to inadequate inflammatory responses. All of these defects lead to a greater predisposition to infection, infections caused by organisms that would not be pathogenic in the intact host, and much more severe complications in otherwise minor infections. The medical profession is well aware that people who have suffered from debilitating, chronic diseases for many years—poorly controlled diabetes, untreated HIV infection and the resulting AIDS, chronic lung or liver disease—are at risk for this type of infection. People at risk for these *opportunistic infections* are considered *compromised hosts*. Chronically malnourished populations, especially children under five years of age, are the ultimate compromised hosts—made doubly vulnerable by the social inequities that allow them to live in poverty and the harsh biological consequences caused by the attendant lack of access to adequate infrastructure and nourishment.

Pestilence—the Diseases of Famine

As we noted in chapter 3, scientific and medical studies of chronic malnutrition, large-scale famine, and actual starvation have been restricted. Due to the ethical issues surrounding human experimentation and the limitations imposed by the very circumstances underlying the inadequate nutritional status and the associated illnesses, most studies have been observational (frequently at a distance) and generally retrospective.

Historically, the diseases linked to chronic malnutrition that have gotten the most attention have been those with the highest "profile": those most likely to cause widespread epidemics (especially if they might spread to previously unexposed populations); diseases that have been identified as responsible for high case fatality rates in vulnerable populations; or diseases that have been particularly "interesting" to the medical profession (that is by the nature of medicine directed much more to the treatment of disease than it is to its prevention). These "diseases of famine" include scarlet fever, diphtheria, dysentery, cholera, typhus, typhoid (enteric) fever, and tuberculosis.[8] In order for us to get an understanding of the different ways in which diseases spread, establish themselves in a host, and cause sickness, we will discuss four of them: dysentery, cholera, typhus, and typhoid fever.

Dysentery (Greek: sick bowel) is the term used to describe an infectious disorder of the large intestine (colon), characterized by inflammation, abdominal pain, and frequent stools containing blood, pus (fluid and cellular debris that are products of an inflammatory response), and mucus. Unlike diarrhea, the stool output associated with dysentery is not watery and may be quite limited in volume. The hallmark is the presence of blood and pus in the stool, as dysentery is caused by invasion and destruction of the tissue of the bowel.

The prototypical organism for invasive bacterial dysentery is *Shigella*. *Shigella* is an enteric bacterium, related to *Escherichia coli*, that is transmitted from person to person via fecal-oral spread or by contamination of the water supply. (The genus is named after the Japanese physician and bacteriologist Kiyoshi Shiga, who identified the organism as the causative agent of bacterial dysentery during an 1897 epidemic in which 90,000 cases were reported with a mortality rate of 30 percent.) To put this disease in perspective, *Shigella* is the most contagious of bacterial enteric infections and is reported to have been responsible for more casualties than battle-related injuries in wars as early as the Peloponnesian War of early 400 BCE through the Sino-Japanese War of the late nineteenth century (with infection rates still high but deaths relatively uncommon during the post-antibiotic era).[9] Ingested bacteria pass through the stomach and small intestine and invade the colonic epithelium, spreading from cell to cell and invading and destroying tissue. Its ability to do this is due to production of a variety of genetically coded virulence factors known as *shiga toxins*, cytotoxic proteins that damage and destroy cells by inhibiting protein synthesis at the ribosomal level.[10] Although these toxins are felt to have originated with *Shigella* species, the genes responsible for their production can unfortunately be passed to previously nonpathogenic strains of *E. coli* by the activity of bacteria-specific viruses called bacteriophages.[11]

Shigella infection is endemic (always present) in most of the world, with an estimated 120 million cases occurring annually, mostly in developing nations. Its ability to pass easily from person to person and to contaminate water supplies enables it to cause widespread epidemics in conditions associated with poor hygiene and inadequate infrastructure. Annual death rates have been reported to be as high as 1.2 million, with 60 percent of these occurring in children under the age of five years.[12] More recent reports have estimated the case rates to have decreased to about 90 million a year with fatalities much lower at slightly over 100,000. Although estimates of worldwide mortality rates from *Shigella* dysentery vary, the evidence that the disease is more severe, associated with more dangerous complications, and has a higher mortality in chronically malnourished individuals is not debated. In one study the incidence of death due to shigellosis in children under the age of five years in the United States was 27 in 100,000 (0.027 percent), whereas the mortality rate in rural Guatemalan Indian children was 10,000 in 100,000 (10 percent).[13]

Unlike bacterial dysentery, bacterial diarrhea is associated with multiple, watery stools frequently in large and sometimes voluminous quantities. The prototypical organism for noninvasive bacterial diarrhea is *Vibrio cholerae*. Also spread by fecal-oral contact or by contaminated water supplies, cholera is able to live in either a free-living or dormant state in aquatic environments, attached to algae or copepods (minuscule crustaceans). Because of this trait, cholera can remain endemic in all infected areas, and because it is highly contagious, it also has the biological ability to cause widespread epidemics and even more extensive pandemics.[14] Of some interest, the first successful "modern" epidemiologic study was performed by John Snow, a London physician, during the cholera outbreaks in London in the mid-nineteenth century. Snow plotted the known cases of cholera on a street map of the city and noted that the majority of cases were clustered around the Broad Street pump (which, unlike the other pumps, happened to get its water supply downstream of the sewage being dumped into the Thames). He was able—having overcome substantial resistance from a skeptical and corrupt Board of Public Health—to convince the local Board of Guardians to remove the handle of the Broad Street pump. Cases of cholera rapidly declined, and the outbreak was contained. This accomplishment is all the more impressive as it predated the recognition that microorganisms were at all related to disease, and the development of the germ theory of disease by Louis Pasteur and Robert Koch decades later (Robert Koch was awarded the Nobel Prize in Medicine in 1905 for his work demonstrating the causal relationship between microbes and disease).

The mechanism by which cholera causes disease is through the production of an exotoxin, a toxin that is secreted by the bacteria into its immediate environment. This exotoxin has an avid affinity for the cells lining the small intestine. Once attached to these cells, the toxin promotes intracellular production of the cell-signaling molecule cyclic adenosine monophosphate (CAMP). This in turn stimulates the cell to pump chloride ions (and accompanying sodium and water) into the lumen of the small bowel in copious amounts, overwhelming the ability of the large bowel to reabsorb the fluid and resulting in voluminous diarrhea. The toxin is so effective that, after an incubation period of 12–72 hours, the abrupt onset of diarrhea is so severe that the resulting dehydration can lead to shock and death in a matter of hours. Of course, the diarrhea is contaminated with millions of active cholera bacilli, likely to contaminate the water supply in areas with inadequate sanitation. Fatality rates are high, up to 10 percent of all cases, with higher fatality in young children (especially those who are malnourished). Fetal mortality rates in infected pregnant women can be as high as 50 percent.[15]

With proper treatment, mortality from cholera should be less than 1 percent, and the key to proper treatment is rehydration. (Antibiotics may shorten the length of illness, but without rehydration they will not significantly lower the mortality rate.) Of course, to adequately provide rehydration therapy, people must have access to water that is not contaminated by the bacteria.

A third type of bacterial enteric infection is caused by *Salmonella typhi* (and *paratyphi*), the causative organisms of typhoid fever. The genus *Salmonella* has many species, most of which can cause severe but self-limited disease in humans (the genus *Salmonella* itself was named after one of the first graduates of the School of Veterinary Medicine of Cornell University, Daniel E. Salmon, who along with Theobold Smith described the bacteria as the causative agent of swine cholera—Dr. Salmon was the administrative head of the USDA research effort, and the genus was named after him).[16]

The *Salmonella* species that causes the less severe, self-limited enteric infection, *S. enterica*, can be carried and transmitted by animals, either by contamination of food products such as poultry or eggs with fecal organisms, or directly through contact with animal carriers such as reptilian pets, especially turtles. The causative organisms of typhoid fever, on the other hand, are found only in humans and can only be spread by fecal-oral contact with an infected individual (including asymptomatic carriers) or ingestion of contaminated water. Typhoid fever (so-called as it was initially confused with typhus until they were clearly distinguished from each other in 1836) is endemic in many developing countries in Asia, Africa, Central and South America, and on the Indian subcontinent. It has been pointed out that these regions share certain traits, among them rapid population growth and urbanization with infrastructure for sanitation and safe water supply that have not kept up with the increasing demand.[17] Unlike shigellosis and cholera, typhoid fever is not mediated by a toxin. The ingested bacteria invade the mucosa of the small intestine, cause a primary bacteremia, and when they are ingested by phagocytic mononuclear cells (white blood cells), they are not killed but reproduce within the protective environment of these white cells. As the bacteria multiply, they destroy the cells they are in, cause a secondary bacteremia, and invade the gall bladder, lymphoid tissue in the lymph nodes, and intestine, from where they can be excreted back into the environment. The resulting disease may be relatively mild and pass unnoticed but is usually a prolonged (four to eight weeks) febrile illness that is extremely debilitating, with a high mortality rate of 10 percent to 30 percent in untreated cases (with higher mortality rates seen in compromised hosts). The possibility of a mild case of the disease explains the possibility of asymptomatic carriers. The first recognized instance of an asymptomatic carrier of typhoid fever (and a famous instance of prolonged involuntary quarantine of an otherwise healthy individual) is that of Mary Mallon, known better as Typhoid Mary, a young woman with no personal history of typhoid fever who, in her job as a family cook, was responsible for causing about fifty cases and an estimated three deaths from the disease.[18] This carrier state is caused by the tendency of the organisms to colonize in the gallbladder, from where they are constantly excreted with the bile into the small intestine and eventually into the environment.

The final disease historically associated with famine that we consider is typhus. Unlike the previous three, typhus is unique for three reasons.

○ It is not an enteric disease, that is, it is not a disease of the bowels.
○ It is transmitted by an arthropod vector (an insect that incubates and transmits the disease—in this case the human body louse).
○ It is a *zoonosis*.

This last term means that the causative organism can be found in other species and transmitted to humans (a reservoir in the wild has been identified in the Eastern flying squirrel in the United States). Although there are actually three specific types of the disease, caused by different microorganisms, the most common, and the one that concerns us, is most frequently transmitted not from flying squirrels but from human to human by the human body louse, *Pediculus humanus corporis*.

The causative organism belongs to a group of obligate intracellular bacteria (they can only survive inside a host cell) known as *Rickettsia*. Other rickettsial diseases include Rocky Mountain spotted fever, Q fever, and the closely related Cat Scratch fever. Independent early work on the organism that causes typhus was done by the scientists Howard Taylor Ricketts, Stanislau von Prowazek, and Charles-Jean-Henri Nicolle (among others). The agent is so contagious that many of the investigators, including Ricketts and von Prowazek, contracted typhus and died. Nicolle (the only survivor of the early workers) received the Nobel Prize in 1928 for demonstrating that the disease was transmitted through the body louse as a vector. As some consolation, the organism had been named *Rickettsia prowazekii*, after the two senior scientists who died researching the disease (the Nobel Prize is never awarded posthumously).

Throughout history typhus epidemics have been contemporaneous with war and the famine and squalid living conditions associated with it. It is estimated that 8 million Germans died of typhus during the Thirty Years War. Of the 600,000 soldiers in Napoleon's Grande Armée that invaded Russia in 1812, the vast majority, already weakened by lack of food due to the extended supply lines, died of typhus. During the period directly following World War I, 30 million cases of typhus were recorded in the Soviet Union from 1918 to 1922, with an estimated 3 million dead. During World War II, typhus was so prevalent that the German Army would test populations with a blood test called the Weil-Felix reaction that identifies individuals who are or have recently been infected with typhus so that they could avoid those areas. A group of Polish physicians, finding out about this practice, vaccinated groups of Polish citizens with a cross-reacting vaccine, successfully diverting the invading army.[19]

Typhus can present in two forms. Primary typhus is caused by the bite of the human body louse. As the louse feeds, it defecates, and there are large numbers of active rickettsial organisms in the feces. Scratching the louse bite rubs the infectious feces into the bite wound, allowing the organism to establish itself and multiply locally. Once established, it spreads through the bloodstream and invades the cellular lining of the small blood vessels, causing inflammation (microvasculitis) and tissue death. The organs most affected include the skin, heart, brain, muscles, and kidneys. Untreated the active disease lasts two weeks, followed by a prolonged period of convalescence. Mortality rates can be as high as 40 percent in vulnerable populations, such as the chronically malnourished or the senior population. Typhus can also present as a less acute illness in an individual who previously had the disease—recrudescent typhus or so-called Brill-Zinsser disease (named after the scientists who described it). Although the recrudescent form of the disease tends to be much milder, the danger lies in the fact that a person with the recrudescent form can transmit the organism to body lice that can then infect previously unexposed individuals, thereby kindling a typhus epidemic if the conditions are right. Treatment is actually quite simple. The organism is very sensitive to antibiotics, and a single dose can be curative. More important, however, are efforts directed toward prevention—adequate sanitation, facilities for bathing and cleaning clothes, and if necessary delousing of the population with malathion or DDT.

The Banality of Death

As we stated earlier, the diseases discussed above are a few of those historically associated with armed conflict and famine. In conventional times the additional epidemics of HIV/AIDS, multidrug-resistant tuberculosis (MDR-TB), and malaria have gotten a good deal of attention from the media and from celebrities interested in lending their names and faces to the advancement of important social causes. To extend the analogy made earlier in the chapter, these are the medical equivalents of the "loud emergencies." It happens that other major killers, the "silent emergencies," are much more ordinary and unexciting but no less deadly.

Hannah Arendt, a twentieth-century political theorist, coined the phrase, "the banality of evil" in describing Adolf Eichmann, the bureaucratic logistician of the Holocaust, during his trial in Israel in 1961. What she meant by this is best described in her own words: "The trouble with Eichmann was precisely that so many were like him, and that the many were neither perverted nor sadistic, that they were, and still are, terribly and terrifyingly normal. From the viewpoint of our legal institutions and of our moral standards of judgment, this normality was much more terrifying than all the atrocities put together."[20] Although Arendt disputed the application of her phrase to any other situation,[21] perhaps a similar statement can be made about the major killers of children under the age of five years living in resource-poor, poverty-stricken regions. These are not diseases that gain a lot of press coverage; nor are they diseases that would cause worrisome illness in children who have access to safe drinking water, adequate sanitation, and adequate nutrition. These silent medical emergencies are respiratory infections, diarrhea, and neonatal deaths due to severe perinatal infections and birth asphyxia. They are responsible for 10 million avoidable deaths annually in children under the age of five years.

How do these deaths occur? It is easy to think of this problem as a one-to-one, clear cause-and-effect relationship between a disease process and the individual child; that is, a young, vulnerable child gets pneumonia and dies because of it. This is not the case. These children are subjected to multiple episodes of diarrhea, respiratory infections (viral and bacterial), and perhaps a more severe episode of measles. One of the methods pediatricians use to monitor the health of children is by their position on a "growth curve"—a series of percentile curves based on normative values for height and weight for age and gender. Each time a child suffers another episode of infection, the lack of adequate nutrition or access to safe water or sanitation exacts a larger and larger toll; the child is never able to fully recover, and he or she relentlessly "falls off the growth curve." Ultimately a relatively "benign" infection tips these children beyond their bodies' capacity for recovery, and they die.

It is difficult to come by accurate, complete data on the details of the numbers of deaths, causes of preventable mortality, and factors that may be important predisposing, but not proximate, causes. An excellent series of five articles in *The Lancet*, one of the world's leading medical journals, sheds some light on this difficult problem.[22] A review of the available epidemiologic data from a number of sources led a group of international investigators to a number of interesting, and practical, observations. Using data from the year 2000 (the most complete, accurate available at the time of the study), they noted that 10.8 million children under the age of five years (considered to be the most vulnerable group in any population) die worldwide annually. Most of these deaths would be considered preventable, and almost all occur in resource-poor countries. Of some note, 50 percent of these deaths occur in only six countries; 90 percent occur in only forty-two countries. The proximate cause of deaths varies substantially by country rather than by geopolitical region—a critically important point when considering the design for workable interventions; that is, a program designed to address the larger picture in sub-Saharan Africa could well be ineffective when applied in Zimbabwe. As mentioned above, the investigators point out that the most common proximate causes of death are pneumonia and diarrhea; the presence of multiple concurrent illnesses plays an important role; and, central to the point of this chapter, malnutrition plays a major role in the deaths from infectious disease.

As of the year 2000, 41 percent of the preventable deaths in children under the age of five years occurred in sub-Saharan Africa, 34 percent in South Asia. Because of marked differences in the total populations of each country, the ranking by absolute total of deaths varies significantly from the ranking by mortality rate (deaths/1000 live births). So India leads the list of total number of deaths with 2.4 million, and Sierra Leone is number thirty-six on the list with 69,000 deaths, but Sierra Leone is number one in mortality rate at 316/1000 live births (almost one in three children under 5 years of age), whereas India is number fifty-four when ranked by mortality rate.

According to the statistical model used, lack of access to safe drinking water, water for hygiene, and lack of access to adequate sanitation facilities contribute to about 1.5 million deaths and 88 percent of the deaths from diarrhea; but the major underlying risk factor for death from these otherwise "minor" illnesses is clearly inadequate nutrition—either protein energy malnutrition or micronutrient deficiency. A review of ten community-based studies demonstrated that malnutrition increased the risk of death from diarrhea by 61 percent, from malaria by 57 percent, from measles by 45 percent, and from other infectious diseases by 53 percent. In total 53 percent of all the deaths were attributable to nutritional deficiency, with 20 percent to 24 percent of these deaths being attributable specifically to vitamin A deficiency.[23] In addition, the review goes on to note that there is a synergistic relationship between these infectious diseases and the degree of malnutrition, with those children who are mildly underweight facing a twofold increased risk of mortality, whereas children who are moderately or severely underweight face a fivefold to eightfold increased risk of dying.

As part of the report in *The Lancet*, profiles were developed defining the percentage of deaths from specific causes in different regions. In all such cases, pneumonia and diarrhea were prominent, major causes of preventable mortality. Nearly two-thirds of the deaths in the forty-two countries analyzed, and 57 percent of the deaths worldwide, occurred in only nineteen countries where pneumonia, diarrhea, and neonatal causes were predominant, with little mortality from malaria and AIDS—the diseases, along with multidrug-resistant tuberculosis, that would be considered the major threats today.

The second article in this series reports findings that are at the same time reassuring and yet disturbing. A review of available interventions that would be considered "feasible for delivery at high coverage in low-income settings" were classified as either level 1 (sufficient evidence of effect), level 2 (limited evidence of effect), or level 3 (inadequate evidence of effect). The investigators found that there is at least one level 1 intervention available for the prevention or treatment of each main cause of death in children under the age of five years except for birth asphyxia, for which there is a level 2 intervention.[24] They note that, should these interventions be made available globally, 63 percent of these childhood deaths could be prevented. The disturbing bit is that, at the time of this publication, global coverage was estimated to be less than 50 percent. So although we have the technological, and even the economic, wherewithal to prevent these deaths and meet the Millennium Development goal of reducing by two-thirds the number of childhood deaths by the year 2015, we have not yet developed either the political will or the healthcare systems that will enable this to happen.

11

The Biological Basis
for Political Behavior

Man is by nature a political animal.
—Aristotle (384–322 BCE)

We began this book with a description of an event that determined how we view and think about famine—the Ethiopian famine of 1973. In embarking on our journey to simultaneously understand the biology and the politics of starvation, we ended that prologue with the observation that the physical sciences tell us what is, whereas the social sciences strive to help us define the way things should be. In this chapter, we ask the following question. If, as Aristotle implies, political behavior is innately human, can we also say that it is biologically determined? That is, is there a stronger link between our biological "selves" and our social "selves" than we might presently believe? Is there a scientific explanation for the discrepancy between how we behave on a large scale and how we should behave? The answer to both questions, of course, is yes—but what is the scientific evidence with which we back up this unequivocal statement?

The study of the human mind is an extraordinarily complex subject involving multiple disciplines—neurobiology, neuroanatomy, neurophysiology, behavioral science, and psychology, among others. Although these disciplines overlap to some degree, they are considerably different in regard to the paradigms and tools of investigation used to define the workings of the human mind, and yet the findings of the scientific investigations in each of these fields are remarkable in their congruence, all pointing to the answer given above. We do not intend to present an exhaustive account of all the experimental evidence in each subject that has led to our final conclusion. Rather, we shall present representative arguments, borrowing from the literature in the neurosciences, behavioral sciences, and psychology that have informed our conclusions as to why we have been unable to transcend the behaviors that limit our ability to fulfill the basic needs of our fellow human beings.

If we are the good, decent, socially responsible people we all consider ourselves to be, or if we are created in the image of God, as some of us believe, we must reconcile our policies and performance on the one hand with our failure to reach this basic humanitarian goal on the other. In order to begin to understand the answer to this apparent paradox, we will need to understand the following four basic concepts.

- The evidence leading to our belief that at some level human behavior is genetically based and has evolved in much the same way as our physical attributes.
- The origin of intraspecific aggression; its function as a trait that confers "genetic fitness" and its relationship to the ability to form individual and group bonds.
- The curious but incontrovertible evidence that the linkage of the traits of aggression and bond formation leads to acceptable (unavoidable) aggressive behavior toward members of our own species, if they are seen (or can be portrayed) as "other."
- The evidence that cooperative behavior is also an evolutionary robust behavior that has evolved in tandem with aggressive behaviors because it is ultimately a successful behavioral strategy.

Genetic Basis of Human Behavior

First, we should address the question as to whether or not human behavior (what we call human nature) is in any manner genetically determined and, therefore, fixed in particular ways. In other words, are we *hard-wired* for certain behaviors: do we see the world in certain ways that are determined by our biology and evolutionary history? On reflection these are very sensitive questions. The potential answers involve not only consideration of scientific study and empirical evidence but millennia of strongly held human beliefs, core values, and moral structure. There are a number of moral arguments as to why this *should not* be true, or even suggested. If we are purely biological entities, and all of our structure and function, including our thoughts and behavior, are products of a Darwinian evolutionary process, does this mean that we are not divinely created; that we are not part of a greater process; that we are only meant to live and then die; that there is no such thing as free will or self-determinism?

The biologist E. O. Wilson makes it clear in his book *On Human Nature* that he believes all but the last point to be so (although he concedes that God may certainly have created matter—the protons, neutrons, electrons, and other atomic and subatomic particles that make up everything in our universe).[1] We suggest the following. The belief that we are biological organisms, products of a natural process of abiotic creation and subsequent evolution driven by mutation and natural selection and the belief that the universe and all that it contains (including us) were created by a Supreme Being, are in no way mutually exclusive. If God created matter, as Wilson allows, and we evolved from that matter in a process of a natural world created by God, then we are God's creation. In the same way, if we have certain behaviors that are directed by (and certainly constrained by) our biology, that in no way precludes our ability to exercise free will or the possibility that we have souls and spirituality. It is not our intent, nor do we feel it necessary, to defend or promote a philosophy of either biological or divine determinism, and our personal beliefs are frankly irrelevant to the discussion, as we are comfortable that the truth of one does not preclude the truth of the other. This particular difficulty is not one of exclusive truths but of exclusive ideologies—scientific as well as political belief systems.

Another concern, that a proof that human behavior is biologically determined would be used to justify the creation of oppressive, prescriptive societies based on racial or religious discrimination, is not a valid reason for ignoring scientific evidence, as the cognitive scientist Stephen Pinker points out. These societies have already developed and failed, and they will again—"the Nazi pseudoscience of racial superiority" to justify the horrific genocide of the Holocaust, "the Marxist pseudoscience based on the malleability of human nature" used as justification to force everyone into a communistic, one-size-fits-all society that would be more appropriate for ants than for people to name just two.[2] The German philosopher Georg Wilhelm Friedrich Hegel (1770–1831) pointed out that "What experience and history teach us is that people and governments have never learned anything from history, or acted on principles deduced from it." The one thing we should all have learned, however, is this— oppressive rulers clearly do not need a scientific basis from which to rationalize their appalling agendas—if the existing facts do not fit their political needs, those with a goal of forcefully imposing their will on others will not hesitate to suppress any inconvenient facts and create their own.

So we would ask that the thoughtful reader place ideological arguments aside for the time being and consider the body of facts that lead us to believe that our minds, in form and in function, much as our bodies, have been shaped by the evolutionary forces of mutation and natural selection. We can then individually decide if that makes us any less special, in the eyes of man or the eyes of God.

Sociobiology, Evolutionary Psychology, and Animal Behavior

Sociobiology, a subject area dealing with the concept that human behavior is a genetically determined trait, has been a controversial subject since the term was first used by John Paul Scott in 1946. The fact that human behaviors are, at least to some extent, determined by genetic elements molded by the same biological and evolutionary pressures that shaped our bodies has been recognized by psychologists and behavioralists for decades, but the concept did not receive much attention until E. O. Wilson's book *Sociobiology: The New Synthesis*[3] was published in 1975, at which time it ignited something of a firestorm of scientific debate and recrimination—ending in a frustrated colleague pouring a pitcher of ice water on Professor Wilson's head. Parenthetically, we believe it may have been Henry Kissinger, when asked why academic battles were so vicious, who answered, "Because the stakes are so small." There is even contentious debate on this point, however, and it may well be that the concept was first noted by Woodrow Wilson when he was the president of Princeton University.[4] The intensity of the discussion involving the part played by evolutionary pressures in forming human behavior has substantially diminished, in part due to the work of the anthropologist John Tooby and the psychologist Lena Cosmides in the field of evolutionary psychology,[5] which deals more with theories of evolution and less with biological determinism.

Stephen Pinker, the Harvard cognitive scientist, points out in *How the Mind Works*, that "the brain is an incredible organ" and asks the reader to consider "the complexity involved in the control needed to walk, pick up an object (both require motor coordination, sensation, proprioception), seeing, smelling," and so forth. (Proprioception is the ability to know exactly where any one part of your body is in relation to the other parts and the environment without looking.) Pinker goes on to point out that no one would claim that these functions are not biologically based, both evolutionarily and functionally, and asks why behavior should be any different: "The mind is a system of organs of computation (the brain) designed by natural selection to solve the kinds of problems our ancestors faced in their foraging ways of life, in particular, understanding and outmaneuvering objects, plants, and other people. . . . The mind is what the brain does."[6]

In *On Human Nature*, E. O. Wilson accepts as established fact that human behavior is in large part genetically determined, having evolved over millions of years through our prehominid ancestors, hundreds of thousands of years in our prehistoric hunter-gatherer ancestors, and only over 10,000 years during the development of civilization and culture. He bases this opinion on a number of demonstrated hard-wired behaviors such as the universality of incest taboos, socially appropriate behaviors in individuals born without the upper cerebral functions that would have allowed them to learn these behaviors, and remarkably similar if not identical behaviors in identical twins (who are genetically identical) who have been separated at birth.[7] An additional example he provides, which is our favorite in its obvious simplicity, is the smile. Recognition of facial expression is a critical part of human communication. Although certain behaviors may differ depending on cultural influence (as we will discuss below), the one that is acknowledged as universal and clearly innate is the smile. The smile is present in all cultures, all people, appears within weeks of birth, and is seen even in infants who are born blind and deaf. Thus, the fact that this behavior is a function clearly determined by inherited characteristics is hard to deny.

For the present time the controversy appears to have been settled. Our physical abilities are determined and constrained by our genetic complement; without the help of devices, we are unable to fly, we are unable to see through solid material, we are unable to breathe under water. We are, however, able to do all of those things thanks to our intellectual abilities and advances in technology; we fly with airplanes, see through solid material with X-rays, and can explore under water with scuba gear and submersible vehicles. By the same token it is generally accepted that human behavior is in large part genetically determined, present in the infant as potential and predisposition, and in many ways biologically constrained (we cannot read each others' minds, foresee the future, or project our thoughts); but our behavior is clearly substantially directed culturally and environmentally. Our intellect and our ability to advance social "technologies" as we have scientific ones should enable us to advance beyond our biological limitations socially as they have scientifically. Therefore, the answer to the question, is human behavior determined by nature or nurture, is a resounding "yes," both genetic predisposition and cultural and environmental determinants are at play here.

A great deal of work has been done in demonstrating that human intellectual and emotional responses have developed evolutionarily from the more basic responses of less highly evolved animals.[8] There is even recent work demonstrating the origin of laughter from similar responses in the various species of apes—gorillas, chimpanzees, and orangutans—in their provoking stimuli and meaning if not in their acoustic identity, that is, they are provoked by similar stimuli and communicate the same pleasure and desire to "play" but do not sound the same.[9]

If we accept the fact that human behavior is, to a greater or lesser extent, determined biologically, and that it evolved from similar behaviors in our less advanced ancestors, it will be helpful to further our understanding by considering animal behavior through the lens of behavioral science. Since the latter part of the nineteenth century, biologists have been fond of pointing out that *ontogeny recapitulates phylogeny*—a statement that has immediately caused millions of young minds to lose interest in the biological sciences. The statement is a general but fundamental truth of life, although the original theory used to demonstrate linear development of embryos from primitive organisms through progressively higher life forms has since been shown to be inaccurate if not actually fraudulent.[10] Ontogeny refers to the progressive growth and development of the individual: *ontos* from the Greek "to be," and *genesis*, of course, from the Greek "creation." To recapitulate is to restate. Phylogeny refers to the development of a species, from the Greek *phylon*—tribe or race, and again genesis or creation. So translated, the statement becomes "the maturational development of the individual restates the evolutionary development of the species." This theory illustrates the simple fact that all life has developed in progression: one molecule from the other, one cellular function from the other, one organism from the other[11]—and that one can see evidence of that progression in the stages of development of an individual both embryologically as well as in the process of individual maturation (although not necessarily in a strictly linear fashion). This is true on a physical level, and in the past two decades the science of evolutionary psychology has advanced to the point where this is known to be true of behavioral (mental) processes as well.[12] As a result, we can learn much about our behavioral characteristics by following the development of certain behavioral traits in other animals.

Throughout this book we have presented behaviors and failed policies that have frustrated our attempts to end world hunger. We produce enough food to reach this goal, and we certainly have the technologies and economic wherewithal to achieve this. Can we determine, in our discussion on the origin and function of some aspects of human behavior, an explanation for why those of us with excess resources (the "haves") are willing to tolerate a situation where others not only have little to no resources (the "have nots") but also have inadequate access to the basic necessities for survival? We as a species are highly intelligent, extraordinarily complex beings. In view of the fact that we evolved alongside other organisms, and that all living organisms shared common ancestors at one level or the other, it will be instructive for us to develop an understanding of animal behaviors at more basic, less complex levels before attempting to appreciate even isolated areas of human psychology. Very specifically, in focusing specifically on our seeming indifference to the suffering of others, we need to gain insight into the apparently polar opposite behaviors of aggression on the one hand and cooperation on the other.

Aggression and the Formation of Bonds

Perhaps the most basic, certainly the first, empirically based discussion on the evolution, specific elements, manifestations, and functionality of aggressive behavior was presented by Konrad Lorenz in his book *On Aggression*.[13] (Lorenz is credited as one of the founders of ethology, the scientific study of animal behavior, and shared the Nobel Prize in Physiology or Medicine in 1973 with his co-workers Niko Tinbergen and Karl von Frisch for this work.) Although some of the observations Lorenz made in regard to cause and effect and the genetic advantage conferred by certain behaviors on a species rather than on an individual (or on an individual gene) have undergone some criticism and reconsideration as our knowledge of evolutionary biology has advanced,[14] his experimental work and basic insights have made seminal contributions to our understanding of why we are the way we are. As such his insights are very useful as a foundation for understanding the biological basis of political (human) behavior. Very specifically his analysis of the evolution of intraspecific aggressive behavior on the one hand, the development of intraspecific bonding on the other, and their apparent mutual interdependence are very useful as illustrative examples for our analysis. From this perspective, it is not so much whether or not Lorenz got it exactly right in defining *how* these behaviors enhanced genetic fitness and therefore evolved preferentially as it is that he was correct in recognizing the fact that they did.

Lorenz begins his analysis of aggressive behaviors by asking the question: Why are coral reef fish so highly colored in such species-specific patterns (the scientific term for this is *aposematic*, or warning colors)? It turns out that the highly colored, patterned fish are those that are relatively sedentary and that are highly evolved to inhabit a very specific feeding niche in the reef. They tolerate individuals of other species because they do not compete for food or shelter with them, but they will relentlessly drive away members of their own species — the brilliant and starkly contrasting colors of their own species incite extreme aggressive behavior, much as the classic red flag does to a bull. The outcome of this behavior is that each species becomes evenly distributed throughout the environment, and from the perspective of "genetic fitness" (physical traits or behaviors that increase an individual's or species' chances of survival and reproduction), the species as a whole benefits by maximally exploiting the available environment with minimal intraspecific competition. Other families of organisms use different signaling mechanisms — territorial song in birds, scent marking in mammals — but the purpose and the outcome are the same. Lorenz goes on to elaborate on the three basic functions of aggressive behaviors that enhance genetic fitness and, therefore, reproductive and evolutionary success:

1 Creation of a balanced distribution of same-species individuals in the environment.
2 Selection of the strongest male for breeding by rival fights.
3 Defense of the young.

The obvious next question to answer is how do they ever get together to reproduce if they are so instinctively programmed toward this aggressive behavior (assuming, of course, that sexual dimorphism—visible differences between male and female—is not readily apparent to them). Untempered aggression is in fact potentially detrimental on several levels: it might decrease the likelihood that any two individuals will tolerate one another long enough to mate, and rival fights occurring as a result of a need to protect territory or a potential mate could also be dangerous for the aggressor and subsequently the species. If we think about this, at the very moment that the need for aggression is at its highest point so that the young, territory, and food sources may be protected, the parents also need to inhibit that aggression to avoid aiming it at the very object needing protection: the young or the other parent. As Lorenz points out, any measurable decrease in aggression at that time could lead to loss of territory or access to food sources and thereby decrease survival or reproductive success. The fact is, however, that animals are quite able to defend their territory, their mates, and their young and yet successfully reproduce and raise their young (without injuring them); and rival fights seldom if ever result in serious injury or death (not always true in some species).

How is this aggressive behavior modified so that successful reproduction and the raising of young are not jeopardized? Lorenz demonstrated, through empiric study of geese and other social animals, the development during individual maturation of very specific, ritualized behaviors leading to what he termed "redirection of the attack." What he meant by this was that otherwise aggressive behaviors would either be directed away from the "partner" in the mating pair (seen in many waterfowl as ritualized courtship) or, more ominously from the perspective of true hostility, toward another member of the same species but not the partner (this trait becomes very important when we consider ourselves). He went on to observe that these behaviors became increasingly complex in more "advanced" species, with threatening behavior becoming intermingled with protective behavior. This eventually becomes a symbolic ceremony leading to the creation of a pair bond—particularly strong in certain waterfowl species such as geese. Depending on the particular species, such bonding may include only two individuals of the same species or larger groups such as families or colonies. In addition to the three basic functions of aggressive behavior, there are also three basic functions of this pair-bonding behavior:

1 Fighting is suppressed within the group.
2 The group is held together by constant reiteration of the bonding behavior enactment.
3 The group is established as a separate, independent entity (against other groups).

Again, the latter point is very important in understanding certain aspects of human behavior.

The complexity of these behaviors increases measurably as one compares more primitive, less highly evolved genera of waterfowl to the more highly evolved geese (the phylogenetic development). The fascinating observation that Lorenz makes is that the same progression one sees as one follows the line of development among distantly related species of waterfowl can be witnessed in the development of progressive behaviors seen as an individual gosling matures (the ontogenetic development). Amusingly, as each behavior develops, the gosling at first may appear surprised or confused at his or her own somewhat inexplicable new behavior. The similarity between that and the baffling behaviors we encounter in human adolescents—sometimes carried well into early adulthood, and clearly motivated by drives other than conscious forethought—is too obvious to avoid mentioning.

As we develop our understanding of the importance of aggressive behaviors on the one hand and bond formation on the other, we should take a moment to ask: can we make the leap between development of behavior in geese (or lower primates) and behavior in humans? Humans are far more complex as individuals and as a species. Animals such as geese are truly hardwired in their behavior patterns. They are unable to modify their behavior to any real extent due to environmental pressures, and they have no culture and therefore no cultural contribution to their behaviors. Many mammals can learn to modify their behaviors through purposeful training—obvious examples would be dogs, cetaceans (porpoises, killer whales), and of course the higher apes, in whom there is ample evidence for the existence of culture, defined as a body of accumulated knowledge and behaviors transmitted horizontally (from one individual to another) as opposed to vertically (genetically).[15] Humans, however, have far more plasticity in their behavior patterns. The innate behaviors, that is, those that are genetically determined, formed by evolutionary pressure, and present in the infant as potential and predisposition are substantially altered, for better or worse, by environmental and cultural factors such as family dynamics, education, and societal expectations. Having said that, it is obvious that there are clear stages of development, physical, motor, social, and cognitive, that are recognizable as progressive, definable, and completely due to the biology, and not the sociology or culture, of the individual child.[16] A few examples of these behaviors would be imitative behavior around age one, defiant and ritualistic behavior around age two, the development of cooperative behaviors around ages three and four (or sometimes never). So it is fair to say that, although we differ in degree of complexity and plasticity from other animals, we share with them innate behaviors that are based in our biology and that are transmitted genetically.

Returning to the functions of aggressive behaviors on the one hand and pair-bonding behavior on the other, Lorenz described three forms of social order to demonstrate the phylogenetic development of the complex "human" behaviors of personal friendship and love, how they might manifest, and how they might enhance the genetic fitness of a species. He called them the anonymity of the flock, social organization without love, and the bond.

The Anonymity of the Flock

This describes an aggregation of anonymous members and would be considered by ethologists as the most primitive form of society. Examples would be a school of fish or a herd of ungulates such as horses, deer, or different species of cattle and bison. These types of animals depend on the concept of strength and safety in numbers. Depending on the species involved, they may actually attack a predator—a behavior known as mobbing, such as is seen when small birds might harass a cat or owl caught out in the daytime. Large groups of relatively vulnerable animals might also use their large numbers to maximize the probability that one member of the group will spot a stalking predator and notify the group at large through an alarm call, a behavior again seen in flocks of small birds. (This is a particularly interesting behavior as it raises a number of questions about altruistic behavior. If the bird that calls out the alarm is endangering itself by calling attention to itself while it increases the safety of the other members of the flock, what is the genetic advantage that would select for this behavior?)

Other more highly developed animals will engage in similar activity. For example, monkeys will follow a leopard through the jungle (from the safety of the treetops, as Lorenz points out) screaming at the tops of their lungs to alert all in the surrounding area that a leopard is passing through. The concept of safety in numbers is a particularly interesting one and does not have anything to do with members of the group banding together to fight off an intruder (although some species, such as water buffalo, musk ox, and other ungulates will do this). Lorenz theorizes that the safety factor has to do with the difficulty involved in focusing on catching one particular individual when it is surrounded by many more. Think of how difficult it is to catch one particular fish in an aquarium full of fish, or one particular bird in a cage full of birds. It is extremely difficult to focus on one individual target when it is surrounded by so many others. It is for this reason, among others, that predators do not try to attack the center of a herd (or school) but hunt around the edges. The other reason, of course, is that the predator is looking for the weakened or vulnerable prey more likely to fill its nutritional needs with the least expenditure of energy.

Clearly there are disadvantages to an anonymous existence in a large group.

There is obvious competition for food; concealment is out of the question; there is always the risk of diseases spreading through a large group and taking a significant toll. As one might expect, the animals that live in flocks, herds, or schools can be considered "grazers," depending on large quantities of readily available food sources—mostly herbivorous, although there are a number of examples of fish that live in large schools and are exclusively carnivorous. However, concealment tends not to be an issue for the safety in numbers reason given above, and generally widespread disease is not a problem in otherwise healthy (well-nourished) populations. In addition to the above there are two fundamental points to recognize here. Except during specific seasons (and only in certain herding species) associated with reproduction, animals that live together in these large groupings do not manifest two very specific animal behaviors: they do not demonstrate intraspecific aggression, and they do not form individual bonds. This is a crucial point. As we are about to see, *the behaviors associated with intraspecific aggression are linked to the ability to form group or individual bonds—the necessary behavioral elements of an "us versus them" paradigm.*

Social Organization without Love

These are complex aggregations of individuals of the same species that begin to approach the meaning of the word *society* in the sense we understand it. A particularly primitive form of this behavior is manifested by the night heron. These birds form colonies for the purpose of nesting and breeding. The nests are built exactly two neck-lengths apart (so they cannot quite reach each other, and thus their inhabitants avoid individual squabbles associated with the need to defend territory). The mates recognize and tolerate each other while on the nest, but once the birds leave the nest they do not recognize each other, and they act accordingly. The primitive "bond" these mating pairs develop is present only on the nest and nonexistent away from the breeding area.

Two other more complex social structures fitting this description, with which we are more familiar, are those established by rats and the social insects such as bees and ants. Rats will form highly structured colonies resembling in superficial ways communistic societies. Individuals are treated as "same" based on a specific smell associated with members of the colony. The young may be treated communally, fed, and protected by all (depending on population density).[17] Members of the colony greet others of the colony when encountered with minimal aggressive behavior except among territorial males and again depending on the density of the population. The signal for recognition, as noted, is a specific colony smell, generated by rats' tendency to urinate in the colony, on each other, and even on food sources they consider to be safe. These apparent individual bonds, however, are directed to the colony alone and not the individual. If one removes a rat from the colony and sequesters it long enough for it to lose the colony odor, then reintroduces it to the colony, the resulting behavior is gruesome. The previously isolated rat will approach its former colony mates in greeting, but the other rats will not recognize their former mate and perceive it instead as alien, and they will tear it to pieces if it is not removed.

Similar behavior is seen in the social insects—the hive members in a bee colony recognize each other by smell, are cooperative to the point of acting as if they are one extended individual as opposed to many separate individuals (which, in a way, they are, since all members of the hive except the queen and the few males are haploid, that is, have only one set of chromosomes and are genetically identical). Within the hive they demonstrate no intraspecific aggressive behavior whatsoever, but they will kill any bee of the same species not of their colony put into their hive (or a bee from their hive whose smell has been altered). These societies demonstrate an evolutionary midpoint of complex behaviors, with intraspecific aggression controlled by inhibitory behaviors signaled, in these cases, by odors and by social bonds directed toward the group, but not specific to the individual. Although very much an "us versus them" paradigm, this behavior is driven purely by sensory input and not an individual bond based on personal interaction, recognition of the individual, and memory.

The Bond

Lorenz describes these relationships, seen in as disparate species as certain fish such as the freshwater cichlids, advanced waterfowl such as geese, and of course human beings, as driven by more "sophisticated" behaviors with very complex interactions between the aggressive tendency on the one hand and inhibitory or appeasement behaviors on the other. He describes the development of the individual bond in geese, which are monogamous and mate for life, very explicitly, noting that the aggression is always there, but redirecting it seems to strengthen the bond—and the "us versus them" paradigm—"the ontogeny of a ritualized ceremony follows roughly the path of the phylogeny."[18] That is, in a young pair the male really does want to attack the female, but at the last minute he is inhibited and redirected by newly forming behaviors, while later in the more mature relationship the behavior becomes more "theatrical" and is performed for its own sake, not as redirected aggression but as specific bond-strengthening behavior. As Lorenz notes, one can trace the evolution of behavior from aggression through appeasement to love. Unlike aggression, love cannot be discharged to any and all but only to a specific individual (or group of individuals).[19] These bonds are no longer directed generally to a group of individuals identified by a colony stimulus such as smell, but to a specific individual very clearly identified, even after a long separation either by distance or time.

These behaviors are more easily dissected and interpreted in less complex animals such as geese, but analogous behaviors, sometimes quite primitive, can be readily observed in humans as well. As we begin to understand the fact that aggression on one hand and strong interpersonal bonds on the other are inextricably linked, and that this seeming paradox is strengthened, indeed appears to rely on an "us versus them" paradigm, we can begin to understand the attitudes and behaviors that can allow otherwise intelligent, well-meaning, kind human beings to let one group of humans (them) suffer from chronic malnutrition, disease, and preventable death as long as our group (we) are well fed and safe from harm. In addition it seems that aggression is a necessary component for the development of individual bonds, but it is not sufficient. In order to fully develop those bonds the aggression cannot just be inhibited; it must be discharged toward an "other"; that is, there must be an enemy!

A particularly disturbing example of this complex of behaviors—redirected aggression as a bond-strengthening behavior—in humans is presented by Lorenz as "militant enthusiasm"—a physical and mental response associated with specific physical sensations (a "chill" down the back and outside of the arms—caused by stimulation of the *erector pilae*, the muscles that would make the hair on your arms and back stand up—if you had hair there—but clearly seen in our closest relatives, the chimpanzees and other apes when they are defending their territory, and which makes them look larger and more threatening); a sense of fullness in the chest associated with a more upright, expansive posture; and a loss of rational thought. This is a predictable response that can be purposely produced with three elements, the effect of which is amplified when presented to a large group:

1 Your group is at risk/under attack.
2 There is a hated enemy.
3 There is an inspiring leader.

This response is well known to politicians, or would-be politicians, who once studied the science of rhetoric to understand the concepts and the nonverbal communications that could be used to move individuals and masses to accept them as leaders (and their ideology as valid).[20] The most obvious historical example of this in recent history is the successful use of these techniques by Adolf Hitler in subjugating an entire population of otherwise normal, intelligent people and leading them down a path of horrific behaviors that led to their near total destruction. Most of us have experienced this sensation at one point or another; when listening to a particularly rousing speech given by a politician we view as inspiring or listening to our national anthem at a particularly moving moment. Would we define this reaction as a political response or a biological one?

In understanding these concepts, we can begin to make analogies between these behaviors in animals that are clearly hard-wired and instinctively enacted and the cultural extension of similar predispositions in humans by the development of mores and norms. Lorenz asks us to consider the development of all forms of "good manners," that are essentially appeasement gestures (essentially representations of submissive signals) meant to inhibit aggression. To understand their importance, think of what happens when you choose to leave them out. Consider, if you will, what would happen if you walked into your home at the end of the day, headed to your room, and failed to greet or even acknowledge your mother or your significant other. Lorenz uses as other examples the fact that the physical signs of "polite listening" in one culture may seem obsequious to someone from another culture, whose gestures of politeness might be interpreted as coldly hostile by the other. Lorenz himself felt that he was perceived as being rude during a visit to America because he could not bring himself to smile quite as much as he felt was expected in American conversation.[21] So although the behavioral predisposition to inhibit or redirect aggressive behavior (which in fact appears to be the default behavior inasmuch as it needs to be inhibited at all) seems to be a ubiquitous human trait, the actual appeasement gestures, "good manners" in our everyday life, are established by cultural determinants.

The importance of this "us versus them" paradigm in human behavior is well recognized. E. O. Wilson noted our predilection as a species to dichotomize one another, separating individuals or groups into artificial categories—member or nonmember, friend or foe, us or them.[22] The developmental psychologist Erik Erikson describes this tendency of humans as inventing pseudospeciations—portraying other cultures as inferior subspecies (the basis of the concept of racial inferiority) not deserving of human rights ("life not deserving of living" in the parlance of the Nazis) and who can therefore be treated inhumanely (or killed).[23] This concept of pseudospeciation—denial of an individual's or group's humanity in order to deny them basic human rights—is well described in the treatise on racism by George Fredrickson.[24] He notes that in order to systematically oppress or exterminate another people, they must first be dehumanized, either by establishment of their biological inferiority or by a process of demonization. Either way, by establishing the "otherness" of the individual or group in a way that is seen as innate (an inherited, intrinsic characteristic), unchangeable (not related to a belief or cultural attribute), and unbridgeable (intolerable), one can create a situation in which it is not only acceptable to eradicate others but in some cases make their obliteration obligatory. This insight into the fundamental difference between races as a social/ethnic/cultural construct (situations in which the difference is a belief or behavior, are seen as changeable, and the "other" can be assimilated) and a biological construct (situations in which the difference is innate, cannot be changed, and therefore the "other" must be excluded or exterminated) is helpful in understanding the development of the vitriolic, murderous forms of racism that developed in the nineteenth and twentieth centuries, characterized by the slave racism mentality of the American South, the color-based racism of apartheid South Africa, and the metamorphosis from a religious to a race-based attempted genocide of European Jewry by the Nazis during World War II. Whether or not the concept of true "races" of *Homo sapiens* actually exists as a meaningful, scientifically based entity or not is a discussion beyond the scope of this chapter; however, advances in genetic research in the past three decades point to the incontrovertible fact that we are all descended from a common ancestor living in Africa as recently as 60,000 years ago, and we are genetically far more similar than we are different.[25] The issue of consequence here is not whether race is a valid concept or not in regard to the differentiation of human beings—some of us are taller than others, some of us are smarter; some of us have darker pigmentation, some of us have bigger noses. The issue of consequence is not race but racism—the hard-wired human behavior of differentiating "us" from "them." This is a very human trait; a very biological trait. And although it may have stood us in good stead during the hundreds of millennia we evolved as hunter-gatherers, it is a dangerous behavioral remnant of our ancestral past, and it is maladaptive if we are to become contributing citizens in a global society.

Cooperation

So, if we are in fact genetically programmed to view others in an adversarial way, how do we explain our ability to interact cooperatively within our groups? Why do our individual and group interactions not invariably deteriorate as each perceived enemy is confronted and overpowered into a "last man standing" scenario? Is there an additional set of genes that code for a propensity toward cooperation, and if so, what could be the genetic advantage that would cause these genes, or those individuals who carry them, to be selectively advantaged from an evolutionary perspective? In 1971 the evolutionary biologist and sociobiologist Robert Trivers presented the concept of *reciprocal altruism*, relying heavily on the earlier work of two of the great evolutionary biologists J. B. S. Haldane[26] and W. D. Hamilton[27] to explain these cooperative behaviors, including such diverse human behaviors as "friendship, dislike, moralistic aggression, gratitude, sympathy, trust, suspicion, trustworthiness, aspects of guilt, and some forms of dishonesty and hypocrisy," as "important adaptations to regulate the altruistic system."[28] Since then a large body of additional observational and experimental work has documented the existence and evolutionary advantage of these remarkably complex, interdependent behaviors.

As we might expect from the previous discussion, cooperative behaviors have developed evolutionarily in the same way as aggressive behaviors. The social insects cooperate to the point of behaving as if they are one single entity —and this makes perfect genetic sense as these individuals are essentially genetically identical. Many species of the dog family hunt cooperatively, and even some cats, specifically the African lion, hunt in groups and share their kills. We are not surprised to see groups of higher primates such as the gorillas and chimpanzees cooperating regularly, and there is even recent work that shows behaviors at the molecular level that can only be described as cooperative in such basic life forms as yeast.[29] Such "cooperative" molecular behavior has been recognized in advanced plant life such as trees for decades.[30] Darwinian theory would suggest that cooperative behavior would be quickly extinguished in any competitive environment by the natural selection of "selfish" behaviors that would advantage the aggressive individual and disadvantage cooperation. This assumption, however, turns out to be too simplistic and incorrect. We can turn to lessons learned in game theory, a type of applied mathematics used in a number of disciplines to model the potential for success of various strategies and used in studies by behavioral scientists to demonstrate that cooperative behavior is a very successful strategy for long-term survival in the game of life.

Winning strategies can be predicted by applying mathematical models to situations in which the success of one individual depends on the choices that others might make. This concept of cooperative versus noncooperative game theory received popular attention in the movie *A Beautiful Mind*, based on the life of John Forbes Nash, who shared the Nobel Prize in Economics in 1994 for his earlier work on noncooperative games.[31] One of the concepts developed by Nash is the Nash equilibrium, which basically states that, for any competitive process in which there are two or more "players," each player will develop his or her best strategy based on the decisions the others are making, and that those strategies will not change, that is, they achieve equilibrium. This is true even if the players could actually improve their own potential outcome if they chose to change their strategies in a cooperative mode.

John Maynard Smith, the British evolutionary biologist, applied the relatively young discipline of game theory to biological science in defining what he called the evolutionary stable strategy (ESS), originally proposed in 1973 and developed in his 1982 book *Evolution and the Theory of Games*.[32] ESS is defined as a strategy of behavior that, if adopted by the majority of an existing population, cannot be "invaded" by a new, initially uncommon behavior; the best strategy for any one individual will depend on the behavior of the population as a whole. Sir Richard Dawkins, in his book *The Selfish Gene*, gives a comprehensive explanation of how this might work.[33] He explains Maynard Smith's hypothetical model of a population made up of hawks (individuals that always attack and never relent) and doves (individuals that always run away and never confront). One might think that a population made up of a mixture of behavioral types such as these would quickly evolve into a purely hawk-dominated society, as hawks will always "win" over doves. It does not take much analysis, however, to show that this is not so. Although hawks may in fact initially begin to dominate, as the number of hawks increases and the number of doves decreases, it becomes more and more likely that one hawk will encounter another hawk, not a dove, and then the hawk behavior becomes more of a liability. It turns out that the ESS for this very simplistic model is not a pure population of hawks or doves, but a balanced polymorphism (a stable equilibrium of more than one form) in which the mathematical model shows that the population will stabilize at $7/12$ hawks and $5/12$ doves. This mathematical model or game can be made increasingly more complex, and the polymorphic ESS will change accordingly—the point being that the ESS (behavior) will evolve; much like the physical attributes of a species evolve as a result of the pressures of natural selection brought about by a changing environment.

Maynard Smith's concept of the evolutionary stable (behavioral) strategy represents the biological extension of the Nash equilibrium, and as such it allows us to consider behavioral strategies as they might affect the evolutionary success of a theoretical population. Dawkins goes on to describe the use of game theory as used by biologists and evolutionary psychologists in explaining how cooperative behavior is mathematically advantageous evolutionarily. The relationship between cooperation/noncooperation and "winning" versus "losing" can be clearly demonstrated by a game called "the Prisoner's Dilemma" and is used by Dawkins to explain the evolutionary advantage of cooperative behavior.[34]

The prisoner's dilemma, originally developed as a model of game theory at the Rand Corporation, can be simply stated as follows.

The police arrest two men for the same crime, but they have insufficient evidence to convict them. They separate the two men and offer them a deal. If one of them cooperates with the police and betrays the other, but the other individual remains loyal, the man who betrays his partner will go free but the other will get a ten-year sentence. If they both remain loyal and refuse to betray the other, they both get six months in jail for a lesser charge, and if they each betray the other, they both get five-year sentences.

ANALYSIS OF "PRISONER'S DILEMMA." Assuming that each individual will do what most benefits him individually, and that each man is unaware of the choice the other will make, the only rational choice for each to make, the choice that maximizes the individual's payoff with the least risk, is to betray the other man. If we think the choices through, regardless of what prisoner A does, prisoner B always does best if he defects. If prisoner A remains loyal, prisoner B gets six months in jail if he too remains loyal, but gets off with no jail time if he betrays prisoner A. If prisoner A betrays B, B gets ten years in jail if he remains loyal, but only five years if he also betrays. So B does not really have to worry about what A is going to do—he always betrays because that is always in his best interests. The same logic applies to prisoner A's choices, so the only rational choice for both is to always betray. Therefore, in game theory parlance, the option of silent loyalty is *strictly dominated* by the betrayal option, and this would be considered the "Nash equilibrium" of this construct (and also the ESS).

With some thoughtful consideration we can see that, despite the obvious logic that each of the players has no choice but to defect, they would in fact both be much better off in total if they both cooperated; that is they would each only get six months in jail—but they never will—hence the dilemma. For this reason, game theorists would call this inevitable equilibrium Pareto suboptimal (Pareto was an Italian economist best known for his 80/20 rule— for example 80 percent of an enterprise's business frequently can be attributed to 20 percent of its customers. His concepts and formulas are used in economics and game theory to explain or predict efficiency and distribution of, for example, resources or risk, and the term *Pareto optimal* does not necessarily imply a desired or equitable outcome but just the greatest gain.) This particular outcome is Pareto suboptimal because the logic leading to the inevitable Nash equilibrium does not lead to the optimal total outcome (which would be a total of only twelve months of jail time for the two prisoners combined—much less than either ten years for one of them or five years for each).

Only if each was assured of cooperative behavior on the part of the other would someone take the chance of remaining silent and not betraying the other, so that both would receive the lightest sentence (and by the way, we believe it safe to say that this would only occur if both prisoners were closely related—such as brothers, or father and son—a concept explored more fully in The Selfish Gene, and reliant on the fact that the more closely related two individuals are, the more genetically alike they are, and therefore the more "genetically fit" cooperative behavior would be).

And yet when a group of us are asked to play this game, a substantial percentage will at first cooperate. Either those people are not paying attention or they are somehow inclined to cooperate, and they expect others to as well. Why should they have this predisposition to cooperate? If there is only one round of the game, of course these people "lose," but *if the game is iterative*, they have the opportunity to retaliate and "punish" the other person for noncooperation. Game theorists can demonstrate that if the game is played a finite number of times, the dominant strategy will remain to betray.

The interesting outcome for the purposes of our discussion is seen when the game is infinitely iterative, that is, continues to be played either as a never-ending game or until a state of equilibrium is reached—or is finite but no one knows when it will end. In this model, the contestants have the opportunity to build trust, or mistrust, and to reciprocate loyalty or retaliate against betrayal. This is exactly what was done in an experiment run by the American political scientist Robert Axelrod, reported in his book *The Evolution of Cooperation* and used as example by Dawkins in *The Selfish Gene*.[35] Axelrod invited colleagues from around the world to enter a computer program in a tournament to play the prisoner's dilemma game, based on a few simple rules and either a "betray" or a "remain loyal" strategy. Fifteen individuals entered programs, varying in complexity, that for the purpose of this discussion can be defined as nasty (initiates betrayal with no provocation) or nice (always remains loyal until it is betrayed by another). The result of this tournament was surprising—the winning strategy, submitted by the Canadian psychologist Anatol Rapoport, was also the simplest and was called "Tit for Tat." This simple strategy always initially remained loyal, and continued to do so until it was betrayed. At that point it would immediately retaliate, and betray on the next round, but would go back to a loyalty strategy if the other contesting program reverted to loyalty. Depending on which program Tit for Tat was playing, it would gain more or less points; but in composite it gained more points than any other program and was the clearly dominant strategy. In fact, of the fifteen strategies submitted, the top eight were all "nice" strategies (always remained loyal initially), and the bottom seven were all "nasty." As Dawkins pointed out, this suggested that "nice guys finish first." Another program, Tit for Two Tats, which had not been submitted, actually did better than Tit for Tat. This program did not immediately retaliate but waited until it had been betrayed two times in a row. Again as Dawkins points out, this demonstrated two evolutionarily robust behaviors—niceness (cooperation) and forgiveness (understanding). Axelrod went on to hold a second tournament, and in this instance there were sixty-three entries. Once again Tit for Tat won (and all but one of the top fifteen strategies were nice, while all but one of the bottom fifteen were nasty).

The point made by Dawkins, and others, is that cooperative behavior is in fact a very strong and successful strategy, especially applied to a non-zero-sum game. (A zero-sum game is one in which, in order for me to win, you have to lose—like baseball, tennis, or poker. A non-zero-sum game is one in which both parties can benefit—like the prisoner's dilemma. The fact that the prisoner's dilemma is a non-zero-sum game is the reason that the Nash Equilibrium for the single game—both players betray—is Pareto suboptimal). This is also the reason why the saying "nice guys finish last," supposedly coined in the world of baseball (which is a zero-sum game) does not necessarily apply in life, which is not a zero-sum game. We can rephrase this in human terms to mean: *in order for me to have access to the basic necessities of life, it is not necessary for you to lose such access, and hopefully, life is an iterative game.*

Synopsis

We have reviewed a summary of the evidence and attendant reasoning supporting our belief that much of the potential and predisposition of human behavior are genetically determined and have been shaped by evolutionary forces in much the same way as our physical attributes. Among those behavioral traits is an innate tendency to aggression, tightly linked to the inevitable formation of strong personal bonds with specific individuals and groups of individuals. This behavioral dyad is initially formed, further strengthened, and in fact seemingly dependent on redirection of innate aggressive tendencies toward some "other," usually one that is despised, feared, or considered inferior in ways that enhance further polarization and encourage segregation and exclusion, if not actual extermination. Included in this group of fundamental behaviors is a basic predisposition to cooperate, tempered by judgment and experience.

The manifestations of these behaviors depend, of course, on the contextual situation in which they might occur. The longstanding rivalry between the New York Yankees and the Boston Red Sox is a well-known source of generally friendly teasing and banter between residents of New York and Boston. Residents of Boston from widely disparate backgrounds will band together as one to tease the individual foolish enough to enter Fenway Park wearing a Yankees baseball cap—but those same Bostonians will behave remarkably discourteously to one another while driving on the city's streets and highways, sometimes leading to serious altercations and even fatal attacks associated with so-called road rage. High school and college sports events are generally marked by good natured rivalries as opposed to true hostility, but it is not unheard of for things to get out of hand, as they did in a high school hockey practice leading to one father beating another father to death with his bare hands.

Although our general aggressive tendencies as individuals are almost always tempered by equally strong inhibitory behaviors, be they instinctual or culturally determined, this is not always the case when the "us versus them" paradigm is between sovereign nations. For an excellent scholarly review of the extent of our tendency to define the "otherness" of large populations in ways that characterize them tautologically as inferior, therefore justifying their subjugation and cultural and economic exploitation, the reader is referred to Edward W. Said's seminal work *Orientalism*.[36] Each of us, in even the most superficial study of world history is aware of this very human of behaviors, and of course we see evidence of it every day in our newspapers and on the evening news.

There are two important points for us to take away from this chapter. The first is that the importance of understanding this behavior lies not so much in how these traits might lead to progressive international misunderstanding and conflict—this is relatively easy to comprehend. More importantly, awareness of this biologically based "aggression-bond" dyad, linked to the behavioral manifestation of an "us versus them" paradigm helps us to understand why we are able to maintain indifference and inaction when "others" suffer chronically from the pain, disability, and premature death caused by inadequate access to even basic nutritional needs. This is in fact a very human attribute, one that is genetically determined, and one that for the vast majority of our species' existence was evolutionarily successful in that it enhanced our genetic fitness.

The second point is that we are not enslaved by our genetics, doomed to a constant reiteration of historical misjudgments and social inequities borne out of the misapprehension that we are somehow not all one people. Just as we have been capable of developing technologies that have enabled us to overcome the constraints imposed by the biological nature of our bodies, we have the capability to develop the "social" technologies that will enable us to overcome the behavioral constraints that are limiting our ability to take our next evolutionary step in becoming a global society.

As Hamlet exclaims,

What a piece of work is a man! how noble in reason! how infinite in faculties! in form and moving how express and admirable, in action how like an angel! in apprehension how like a god! the beauty of the world—the paragon of animals!
—William Shakespeare, *Hamlet* act 2, scene 2

Lessons from the Great Irish Famine [1845–1850]
Who Starves and Why?

Why did some Irish starve, and not others? We know that the failing structure of the Irish economy made the Irish peasant and laborers vulnerable to an environmental disaster like the potato blight. But Clarkson and Crawford at the Centre for Social Research in Belfast question the assumption that the Irish were "born" to famine. In the seventeenth and eighteenth centuries, along with early shifts in landholding patterns, Irish wage laborers were often paid in small holdings on which they grew potatoes. At the time the potato was supplemental to their diet. Clarkson and Crawford cite the Irish diet of the sixteenth and seventeenth centuries that included cereals and legumes, livestock meat, cheese, milk, and butter for the gentry, and meat scraps and offal for the poorer classes. Potatoes were an additional food.[1] By 1800, those Irish who were "very well off" continued consuming a diet that included stirabout,[2] potatoes, maslin bread,[3] milk products, meat, poultry, fish, and fruit.[4] Even wage laborers in the linen trade and weavers, for example, who lived plainly, sometimes consumed stirabout and meat, dairy products, perhaps some salted herring, along with occasional tea and oatbread in a diet to which potatoes were also added.[5]

During the first quarter of the nineteenth century, rising births, continuing emigration, the weakening of the Irish economy, land reallocations, and the increasing concentration of Ireland's productive land in the hands of a small, wealthy class, began displacing large numbers of Irish poor, intensifying their hardship and narrowing their diet. Between 1800 and the 1830s, the rising exportation of livestock, dairy products, and grains further reduced the diet of rural Irish laborers to one based primarily on potatoes. Unless fed by their employer, they ate little else. In effect, a "nutritional transition" was taking place, as the gap between the diets of the wealthy and the Irish peasant and labor classes widened. This is also an early example of our current "nutritional crisis." In Ireland, it was the landed wealthy who made the "transition" to a more diverse diet, much as rising incomes are shifting diets today in the "nutritional transition." The peasant diet narrowed into a "crisis." When The Poor Inquiry of 1835–1836 gathered information about diets from two-thirds of the 2500 parishes in Ireland, it "demonstrated that dependence on the potato by the poor was virtually complete."[6] They were in a "nutritional crisis" and one "ecological accident" away from tragedy.[7]

We discover similar patterns of diet change, single food crop dependencies, and wealth disparities as we examine modern developing states early in the twenty-first century. In sub-Saharan Africa today, for example, we find widespread dependence on a single food crop, maize (corn). This crop, like the potato, is easy to grow and requires little preparation before eating. Also like the potato, maize was an introduced crop brought to Africa from the Americas and moved inland with the slave trade. Maize was also a colonial crop, widely grown in "settler" (or agriculturally based) colonies. Maize adapted well to the sub-Saharan African climate of those colonies, especially in Kenya, Tanganyika/Tanzania, Nyasaland/Malawi, the Rhodesias/Zambia and Zimbabwe, Ghana, Nigeria, and parts of South Africa. Like the potato, maize became a "political" crop supporting a colonial economic system. White settlers in Southern Rhodesia/Zimbabwe, for example, produced large amounts of maize during the colonial period and exported it to the metropole, Great Britain, in a closed economic system that guaranteed an overseas market at a fixed price.

Maize transformed Africa, much as the potato did Ireland and Europe during the Industrial Revolution. Depending on the researcher, the introduction of maize into Africa during the nineteenth and early twentieth centuries created a "maize revolution," a "delayed green revolution," or a "failure" that caused "peasant impoverishment."[8] Today, maize is planted almost everywhere in modern Africa, even in city parks and along the edges of roadways. It is widely eaten—raw, cooked over an open fire, or pounded into flour. Maize is also fed to livestock, as was the potato in Ireland. Ground maize is served across sub-Saharan Africa as coarse grits, sometimes supplemented (as income allows) with greens or the occasional chicken. As one travels southward from Kenya to South Africa, only its food name changes, from *ugali* to *fufu* to *sadsa* to *pap*. But it is still maize.

In Africa, maize replaced a balanced, indigenous diet. In sub-Saharan Africa that diet included millet and sorghum, both of which are nutritious grains high in protein and total amino acids.[9] They are also more drought-resistant than maize but require longer and more physically arduous preparation to turn into flour. The adaptability of maize to the African climate, its easy preparation, and its ability to grow anywhere quickly established it as a staple food and bypassed the more durable indigenous crops.

Because it is a staple crop, maize is also a political food, as was the Irish potato of the nineteenth century. Maize shortages have caused riots in many African capitals, from Egypt to Malawi. Yellow maize, grown in the northern hemisphere and sent as emergency food aid south of the equator (where white maize is more common), has been returned by African states despite their starvation as unfit or a plot to sterilize the hungry. Genetically modified maize has also been rejected, until it was turned into flour. In general, African political leaders make certain that their urban dwellers have maize, sometimes to the detriment of starving rural people, to deter riots over food shortages, a lesson seen (if not learned) in England and Scotland at the time of the Great Irish Famine. As described earlier, rioters in England got food diverted to them, but not the Irish.

Maize and potatoes also share an environmental weakness. It is thought that the potato succumbed to a fungus encouraged by Ireland's damp weather. Maize is not drought resistant, and drought is a recurring environmental condition for much of sub-Saharan Africa. As we have seen in both regions, when an environmental catastrophe strikes these staple crops, starvation often results. Like the Irish, the Africans have also paid a high human price for their heavy dependency on a single food crop. (This is also true, nutritionally, for some Africans' dependency on root crops like cassava.) Blight and drought, dependency on a single staple food, agrarian economies held in balance by distant markets, disparities between large landholders and peasant laborers, are all preludes to catastrophe. Not surprising, many Irish in the Great Famine, and many Africans today, also share a final, predisposing characteristic: extreme poverty.

In 1808, Thomas Malthus began revising his theory of population and food production. Ireland at the time was experiencing a sequence of small famines, but mortality was far lower, in part because of interventions with emergency relief grains. Considering Ireland, Malthus thought about its poverty and wrote that the "wages of the labouring classes of [Irish] society" might stabilize its population growth, and thus prevent "a gigantic, inevitable famine" as the check on Irish population.

Malthus had it right. Wages would allow the Irish to purchase food and avoid possible starvation, if not outright poverty. But this is exactly what did *not* happen in Ireland during the Great Famine. Wages fell with the "Clearances," one of the defining events of the Famine. Landlords were obligated by tradition to feed their labor; people belonged to the estates. "Local property," Liz Young writes, "was held responsible for relieving local poverty."[10] Faced with this, landlords evicted tenant farmers; "one of the most ruthless illustrations of local social control and power. The power to grant charity was another."[11]

As we examine the conditions of today's "silent emergencies," we should remember that hunger, chronic malnutrition, and opportunistic diseases are not "inevitable" conditions of the poor. We have always had the means to alleviate poverty. Indeed, public interventions in earlier Irish famines from the

1740s onward had been essential to prevent the scale of poverty and mortality that occurred in 1845–1850. "However," Young continues," the obligations of the state and the private sector to the relief of poverty, then as now, were highly politicized."[12] In this, the Great Irish Famine, a distant mirror of today's food crises, carries yet another enduring lesson for modern Africa.

PART V

The Way Forward

[12] The Right to Food

Is There a Right to Food?

Following the first World Food Conference in 1974, as detailed in chapter 1, the international donor community established an increasingly accurate system of satellite observations of the world's arable land. Today we in the developed world *know* when and where food shortages, food insecurity, chronic hunger, starvation, and famine are taking place. We can go to "www.fao.org" or "www .usaid.gov" or "www.who.int," select a country, and get the latest famine early warning system (FEWS) or international health information. Our donor agencies also have the means to deliver emergency food relief quickly, even by air if they wish, and to assist with long-term development aid. The knowledge of hunger, starvation, and disease, and the means to respond to them, are easily at hand.

Further, our governments and international agencies have written and deployed the legal structures to move food from donor to recipient. They have also drafted and signed documents agreeing to the "moral right to food." We know, and we can respond. Yet food assistance is not always moved swiftly; neither is this "right" universally agreed to; nor does it always serve as the foundation for humanitarian responses to food needs. Jean Zeigler, UN Special Rapporteur on the Right to Food, points out that: "On the one hand, the UN agencies emphasize social justice and human rights. . . . On the other hand, the Bretton Woods institutions [World Bank and IMF], along with the government of the United States of America and the World Trade Organization, oppose in their practice the right to food—emphasizing liberalization, deregulation, privatization, and the compression of state domestic budgets—a model which in many cases produces greater inequalities."[1] These two positions—the humanitarian and the "secular" or "market"—delineate the struggle over "the right to food" that continues today, despite the fact that this right is defined as "fundamental" in two International Human Rights Covenants (discussed below).

What makes a claim to food a "right"? Xiaorong Li, writing in *World Hunger and Morality*, states: "The right to food should be understood as a need-based right. The right to food is a right of access to the means to procure adequate food. The right to food must be supported by social practices conducive to a stable social and economic order. Such an order is necessary to prevent deprivation and to insure that each person has the opportunity to secure adequate access to food. Governments are primarily responsible for instituting and maintaining this order and thus for protecting the right to food."[2] The right to food, Xiaorong Li concludes, "is thus a basic right."[3]

The right to food is well established in international law. It has its origins in the 1948 United Nations *Universal Declaration of Human Rights*. The *Declaration* is a commendable and broad-based statement of the "rights" that *should* be available to all human beings. Written just three years after the end of World War II, it calls for "recognition of the inherent dignity and of the equal and inalienable rights of all members of the human family" in a world where "disregard and contempt for human rights have resulted in barbarous acts which have outraged the conscience of mankind." It stakes out a wide tent of social justice and human rights. The *Declaration*'s articles declare "the right" to freedom of movement and speech and assembly; "the right" to employment and even "rest and leisure." Article 1, writes Asbjorn Eide of the Norwegian Institute of Human Rights, "lays the foundation of ethical behavior by stating that everyone is born free and equal in terms of dignity and rights and that everyone is endowed with reason and conscience and should act toward one another in a spirit of brotherhood." Ethical behavior, he believes, requires that people go beyond self-interest and care for one another.[4]

Article 25, which defines the core issue and framework of this book, also articulates the moral and human rights of ethical behavior. This includes a wide moral ground where "everyone" has "the right" to health and "well-being." That includes "food, clothing, housing and medical care and necessary social services," and "the right to security" when one is unemployed, sick, disabled, widowed, elderly or experiencing any "other lack of livelihood in circumstances beyond his control."[5]

The *Universal Declaration of Human Rights* was drafted, in part, to serve as a foundation for further legislation. It is often used as the fundamental instrument of a Human Rights Covenant. This has spawned a complex and extensive humanitarian legal structure that now includes the following:

1. *The International Covenant on Civil and Political Rights (ICCPR)* and *The International Covenant on Economic, Social and Cultural Rights (ICESCR)*. Both were based on the *Universal Declaration of Human Rights* and adopted in 1966; they even share similar phrasing. Article 11 of the *International Covenant on Economic, Social and Cultural Rights* recognizes the "right of everyone to an adequate standard of living for himself and his family, including adequate food, clothing and housing, and to the continuous improvement of living conditions."[6] Article 11 also proclaims the "fundamental right to be free from hunger," which is often argued as the "right not to starve."[7] Together they form a broadly applied

legislative instrument; for example, Article 11 has become "a guiding principle" for the UN Food and Agriculture Organization's (FAO) mission to provide "food security for all."

Two concepts included here are often debated. How is the term, "To be free from hunger" measured? Is it measured by the number of malnourished people, or only by those actually dying from starvation? Second, how is the "right to adequate food" to be achieved? A more complex standard, this calls not only for the elimination of malnutrition, but also for accessibility to food that is safe, varied, and adequate for a healthy life. Which standard—or both— should be met?

The *International Covenant on Economic, Social and Cultural Rights* also codifies "the right of everyone to the enjoyment of the highest attainable standard of physical and mental health." This has been incorporated as a guiding principle of the World Health Organization (WHO). The concept of "continuous improvement" in living conditions (Article 1) and the right "to health" and not merely "health care" (Article 2) form a nuanced difference. "The right to food," writes Onora O'Neill, "is viewed as a right to *adequate food*, not to the *best available food*; the right to health is viewed as a right to the *highest attainable standard . . . of health*, and not as a *right to adequate health*." (Italics in original text.) But, she asks, is the right to "the highest available standard" the right to a standard of health attainable only with local and affordable treatment "however meager that may be?" Or, she continues, "is it a right to the highest standard available globally—however expensive that may be? The first is disappointingly minimal, and the latter barely coherent (how can everyone have a right to the best?). And what is required of the farmer, the physician, and others who actually have to provide food and health care?"[8]

2. *The International Convention on the Rights of the Child.* Several "rights" and concepts in the *Universal Declaration of Human Rights* are found in the *Rights of the Child*. Article 25 of the *Declaration*, for example, sets out the right of care and assistance for mothers and children, "whether born in or out of wedlock." Article 26 protects "the kind of education" parents choose for their children. The rights of children are further defined in Article 27, which calls on countries and other interested parties to "recognize the right of every child to a standard of living adequate for the child's physical, mental, spiritual, moral and social development."[9] This includes clean drinking water and foods that help combat malnutrition and disease.

Other conventions and declarations bearing the imprint of the UN *Declaration of Human Rights* include the *African Charter on Human and Peoples' Rights* (also known as the *Banjul Charter*), the right to food found in the *Geneva Conventions of 1949* and their two Protocols of 1977,[10] the *Convention on the Elimination of All Forms of Discrimination Against Women*, and *UN Resolution 57 "The Right to Food,"* which states "food should not be used as an instrument of political or economic pressure."[11] The right to food has also been further affirmed by individual states and international conventions and conferences. This includes the *Universal Declaration on the Eradication of Hunger and Malnutrition* passed by the first World Food Conference in November 1974, and the 1984 UN General Assembly, which again asserted that "the right to food is a universal human right." The *Declaration* is also enshrined in some twenty individual state constitutions.[12] Notably absent are the constitutions of the Western European countries and of the United States, which are more broadly worded, thus allowing for greater interpretation and wider application. In some cases other documents adapted by these countries serve to establish the rights of their citizens, including the "right to food" and the "right to health."

Nongovernmental organizations (NGOs) often incorporate the right to food and adequate health as part of their mission statements. One of the most active agencies is UNICEF "which promotes breastfeeding as a chief right of the child and mother, and child nutrition as a right and indicator of development."[13] FAO, WFP, the Inter-American Commission on Human Rights, Oxfam International Global Exchange, Food First Information and Action Network, International Fund for Agricultural Development, WHO, International Labor Organization, UNICEF, and UNDP are among the international UN agencies and NGOs with right-to-food and/or health statements.

This human rights history reached a temporary, but important, culmination in 2000 with the *Millennium Declaration* and the Millennium Development Goals (MDGs), adopted by all members of the United Nations. In effect, and in practice, the *Millennium Declaration* is a "rights" document. As discussed in earlier chapters the first Millennium Goal proclaims "the eradication of extreme hunger and poverty." It calls for cutting by half before 2015 the number of people who suffer from chronic hunger and those living on US$1 a day or less.[14] "The MDGs represent virtually universal acceptance of the right to be free from hunger," writes Smita Narula, the New York University law professor, "which is the core minimum component of the right to food." The Millennium Goals and "rights" have been reconfirmed and readapted by the World Trade Organization's Doha Ministerial Declaration, the FAO's Guidelines, and other declarations, conventions, documents, and charters.[15] Thus we find constructed on the UN *Universal Declaration of Human Rights* an international legal and moral framework for defining and meeting a broad range of human rights issues. Despite this, however, the basic *Declaration* and these documents remain largely unfulfilled, "a promise diluted."[16]

Why? For one thing, the right to food is not universal law, or international legal obligation, or even a binding norm. The problem, Prof. Narula continues, comes from "weaknesses in implementation, enforcement, and a lack of universal ratification."[17] One example of this weakness rests with the United States, which has not ratified ICESCR, with its powerful Article 11 that articulates rights to "adequate food" and "freedom from hunger." Instead, the U.S. government at this writing has opposed "rights" legislation (other than nonbinding resolutions) and calls the right to food "overly burdensome and inconsistent with constitutional law."[18] Yet, the United States seeks to alleviate hunger at home through its federal food stamp programs, women and child nutrition projects, and supplemental feeding efforts. Overseas, as detailed earlier, the United States has supplied about 60 percent of all food aid each year between 1995 and 2003 and more than 48 percent of food contributions to WFP between 1995 and 2005. Most recently, in 2007, the United States shipped about 44 percent of all global food relief deliveries, more than 2.6 million tons; the next largest donor was the European Community with more than 12 percent and 756,000 tons.[19] Clearly, U.S. *actions* at home and abroad support the *Declaration*'s legislative intent and the humanitarian "right" to food.

This dichotomy is ironic. "Few human rights have been endorsed with such frequency, unanimity or urgency as the right to food," says Philip Ashton, also a law professor at New York University, "yet probably no other human right has been as comprehensively and systematically violated on such a wide scale in recent decades."[20] The issue, as Zeigler pointed out earlier, is divided between politically progressive advocates of social justice and human rights—the humanitarian—on the one hand, and a more normative path taken by legal, political, and financial experts—the "secular"—on the other. The former include health and nutrition advocates, NGOs (Oxfam, Save the Children), and citizens groups (Food First). The latter are more "market" driven and include the World Trade Organization, international financial institutions (including the World Bank and IMF), and the United States. The humanitarians "are not major players in the normative discourse of covenant making and interpretation that dominate the UN HRF [Human Right to Food] discourse that results in action."[21] Put another way, the humanitarians are currently not winning the struggle to feed the world's hungry or care for its diseased. The secular "market" proponents are.

If endorsement of the right to food and health is so universal, why has the international community not united around these "rights"? Prof. Ashton puts forward three reasons:

First, "moral and humanitarian considerations alone will not move governments or other relevant actors to respect the right to food." In this view,

"... food is first and foremost a commodity which is traded annually for billions of dollars and its status as a human right is very much secondary to this fact."

Second, the complexity of promoting the "right to food" and the "absence of a universal consensus" on either the causes of or solutions to the problem "make it virtually impossible to establish effective machinery for implementation of the right to food." The right is not enforceable.

Third, "civil and political rights are of prior importance" and "economic rights" like the right to food are "realized once freedom has been attained by the peoples of the world."[22]

We see more clearly, therefore, the rationale behind relief food being used as an instrument of foreign policy. On the one hand there is the moral argument that everyone has a "right" to food and health. On the other hand there is the more difficult action of obtaining and distributing that food to all who are hungry. Food is, in this view, an economic commodity; the Great Irish Famine illustrated this well. Moreover, a person's "right to food" has no power of enforcement. It is "moral persuasion" that causes donors to act. There may also be more powerful civil and political rights that complicate the equation. Should donors be obliged to feed people who are unfortunately starving under a dictator thus perhaps keeping him in power? Should they violate the sovereignty of a recognized nation to feed its starving citizens? Should donors withhold food from a starving country until other humanitarian conditions are met (such as democracy, child spacing, antiabortion policies, a halt to nuclear weapons development)?

American governments have opposed a formal recognition of the right to food for several reasons. As we discussed, the U.S. Constitution does not protect this "right." To some, the concept of "the right to food" is seen as the dogma of "un-American, socialist political systems"; to others, the obligations are "too expensive"; and, "culturally, it is not the American way, which is self-reliance." Advocates counter that the human right to food (HRF) is "not inconsistent with existing constitutional protection"; that Franklin Delano Roosevelt's concept of freedom from want, which was "a starting point for the HRF, is definitely an American political value enshrined in the U.S. political system"; that eliminating hunger is a significant "and overriding American value."[23]

Most U.S. administrations, with little variation between Republicans or Democrats, have taken the position of opposition to this "right." In June 2002, for example, during the first George W. Bush administration, the American delegation dug in their collective heels at the World Food Summit in Rome, Italy. The UN had called the conference to urge governments to fulfill their 1996 pledges to cut the number of the world's hungry people by half, from some 800 million to about 400 million, by 2015.[24] The United States stood alone among 182 nations in opposition to the "right to food" declaration. The U.S. delegation, headed by Ann Veneman, the secretary of agriculture at the time, announced that the United States would not sign a final summit declaration referring to food as a human right. In 1996, during the Clinton administration, the United States had also been the only nation that had refused to sign the final declaration of that World Food Summit because it also contained a reference to the right to food. According to U.S. negotiators at that conference, the 1996 declaration would have "made welfare reform illegal under international law."[25] Six years later, under a different president and party, Ms. Veneman, a Bush appointee, echoed that language when she voiced her administration's fears about creating "a welfare mentality." Instead, she offered, her administration preferred that the private sector respond to starvation, especially the biotechnology firms producing genetically modified grains.

The U.S. position, backing deregulation, privatization, budget-cutting, and free-market economics, echoes the views of the British Parliament in the mid-nineteenth century and the *laissez-faire* economics that had such dire effect in the Great Irish Famine. There is a fundamental moral inconsistency here, as there was in nineteenth-century Britain. On the one hand, as we discussed in chapter 7 and elsewhere, the United States is a generous donor and provides the largest amount of global food aid. The bulk of this is "emergency" food aid; total "program" relief aid responses have fallen by more than half since the 1990s, while "project" aid remains at steady, low levels. Basically, the United States acknowledges its moral and humanitarian "obligation" to feed those who urgently need emergency food. It is seen as our moral duty. On the other hand, the U.S. government retains—much as the British Parliament did during the Irish Famine—a long-standing aversion to anyone having a "right" or entitlement to food; these poor are historically viewed as freeloaders, lazy, unwilling to earn what they receive. This aversion emerges from Malthus's early writing, runs through British attitudes toward the Irish during the Great Famine (Elizabeth Smith states it clearly at the end of this chapter), and persists today. (This may also explain the persistence of the neo-Malthusian definition of famine to include numbers of deaths. As the number of deaths from starvation rises, it proves the presence of famine and dispels the lingering concerns about whether or not the recipients are deserving of "free food." If tens of thousands have starved, the doubts about "freeloaders" are dispelled.)

The United States in 2002 argued that the right to food meant "an opportunity to secure food and not a guaranteed entitlement."[26] Thus, the right to food was seen as subordinate to market forces: you may have a right to food, the United States argued, provided that you can pay for it. In the Great Irish Famine, *laissez-faire* proponents also argued that the market would resolve the famine:

"Left to the natural law of distribution, those who deserved more would obtain it."[27] The contemporary U.S. position held out a similar economic and political view: the right to food would be met by market forces, largely in the U.S. case with genetically modified (GM) grains from private-sector biotech firms. But although GM grains have been described as capable of "ending world hunger," their rejection has also been widespread, especially among some African states and in the EU. Here, "the right to food" meets free-market forces: those who produce and offer GM grains, and tout them as the solution to global hunger, remain unwilling to give them away to poor, seasonally hungry farmers in developing states. (Further discussion of GM foods is in chapter 13.)

"The fact is," writes Peter Rosset, co-director of Food First/The Institute for Food and Development Policy, "that the rather sad goal of the 1996 World Food Summit, which was to halve world hunger by the year 2015, is more out of reach than ever."[28] Between 1996 and 2000, the total reduction of hunger globally was just one-third of that needed to meet international goals, and 90 percent of the reduction took place in one country, China. "In fact, poverty and hunger have actually worsened in two-thirds of the developing nations and in most Northern countries as well," Russet continues. "In other words, we are moving in the wrong direction to end hunger."[29]

"Rights" and "Obligations"

Having examined the human *right* to food, we now ask: Do those donors or institutions that have surpluses of food incur or take on an *obligation* to feed those suffering from hunger? If people have a "right to food," do all people have equal rights to food? The answers to these questions are not as easy as they might seem. As we have detailed here, little progress appears to be occurring. In the 1980s, two decades of volatility in the world supply of cereals caused analysts to predict more catastrophic famines. The Green Revolution in Asia had failed; the bumper crops of the late 1970s proved short-term bounty. The 1960s and 1970s had "witnessed some of the worst starvation in the modern history of mankind." By 1980, wrote one observer at the time, "Mass hunger . . . is an everyday occurrence."[30] That year a World Bank report identified twenty-seven of the poorest countries of the world "where 258 million of the world's population barely survive amidst absolute poverty." The list of countries remains painfully familiar today—Uganda, Ethiopia, northeastern Brazil, Bangladesh, Kampuchea, Eritrea, and the Sahel regions of Africa—as does the number of people facing chronic hunger and malnutrition in 1980—800 million.[31]

"It is an intolerable situation," Willy Brandt wrote at the time. "The idea of a community of neighbors has little meaning if that situation is allowed to continue, if hunger is regarded as a marginal problem which humanity can live with."[32] Yet despite significant efforts by public and private relief agencies, the "intolerable situation" does indeed continue. Since the Brandt reports of the early 1980s the number of children, women, and men who are chronically hungry or malnourished has grown from between 700–800 million to more than 1 billion people. Global poverty has doubled to include more than 1.8 billion people. The debt of developing countries has increased from $700 billion to almost $3 trillion, thus locking in their poverty.

As we have learned here our advanced technology—FEWS, FAO crops reports, global communications—alerts us to their plight. Food crops are easily available to those in the wealthy developed states; famine ended there in the nineteenth century. Yet, equitable global food distribution and a systemic effort to alleviate poverty remain elusive. Even before the collapse of global economies in 2008–2009, the generosity of donors—"the donors' will to act"—was softening: By 2007, aid to developing states had fallen from 3.5 percent of GNP to 2.1 percent, using the international assistance standard.[33]

Are we then "a community of neighbors" looking out for one another? If so, do we have an obligation to help those less fortunate? Garrett Hardin offered several controversial responses to this question. One, his "Lifeboat Ethics," argues that the wealthy, responsible, developed nations do not incur obligations to respond to the needy. The right to food does not necessarily carry the obligation to act.

Hardin uses the metaphor of a lifeboat, with each lifeboat "full of comparatively rich people." In the surrounding ocean "outside each lifeboat swim the poor of the world." They wish to climb on board and share some of the advantages of the well-placed and fortunate. "What should the lifeboat passengers do?" Hardin asks.[34]

He considers the "reproductive differences" between wealthy and poor nations; those people in the lifeboats are doubling every eighty-seven years, but those swimming in the ocean are doubling every thirty-five years. As a result, in Hardin's argument, the poor are destroying the global commons. He describes world food reserves as "a commons in disguise. People will have more motivation to draw from it than to add to any common store. The less provident and the less able will multiply at the expense of the abler and more provident, bringing eventual ruin to all who share in the commons."[35] Hardin argues against providing any assistance to the starving; their condition is inevitable. He worried that the poor would swamp the lifeboats, drowning us all.

But the poor were and are largely created by actions of the wealthy who controlled and governed them as colonies and today, as mentioned earlier, continue to draw off natural resources and commodities from the developing world. As we discussed in several previous chapters, during the independence movements of the 1960s and 1970s Africans broke these colonial bonds only to exchange political freedom for a new economic colonialism. The wealthy states, or wealthy state actors like international financial institutions, still largely influence the economies of many developing countries through economic leverage such as debt and commodity extractions. How else can one explain today conditions in the oil-rich Niger delta of Nigeria, or in the Democratic Republic of the Congo? If Africans owned their valuable natural resources, would they be so poor?

Hardin's argument assumes that the rich are and will continue safeguarding the resources of the planet, much as they would the seaworthiness of their "lifeboats." But this is not the case. In general, citizens of the wealthy countries consume more resources and generate more waste than those of the poor. For example, one U.S. citizen annually eats more than three times the global average of meat per person (81.4 pounds); one African consumes less than half that amount and a South Asian just 13 pounds. The average European uses about 206 pounds of paper products per year; the average American, 726 pounds. And, states the American Association for the Advancement of Science, "The paper and board industry is the United States' third largest source of pollution, while its products make up 38 percent of municipal waste."[36] Further, we have detailed in chapter 9 the result of pollution from North America on the people of the African Sahel and the impacts of global climate change for the developing world. Who is really overgrazing the commons? Considering Hardin's "lifeboat ethics," let us reverse the story: if the poor were in the boats, and the wealthy in the water, would they actually benefit from lifting in the overconsuming rich to join them?

In fact, as this book details, those in the lifeboats have created—by colonialism and neocolonialism today—the circumstances that caused and continue to cause the conditions of those many poor in the water. Is there an *obligation* incurred by our status to lift them into the boats; that is, to feed them?

The ethicist and philosopher Peter Singer helps us answer that troubling question. We start with his thoughtful account of events in East Bengal that illustrates the entrenched priorities of the wealthy states that persist today. In November 1971, the people of East Bengal were suffering from prolonged civil war and intractable poverty. When a cyclone swept through their homes, 9 million Bengalis became, in Singer's account, "destitute refugees." The affluent nations could have sent assistance to reduce this suffering "to very small proportions," he writes. But few responded "in any significant way," and no government gave enough support that would have allowed these 9 million "to survive for more than a few days."

What were the priorities? The British government did donate £14,750,000 (about $35.5 million at the time),[37] but the same government, Singer points out, was spending perhaps as much as £440,000,000 (about $1 billion) on "non-recoverable development costs of the Anglo-French Concorde project," a luxury supersonic passenger airplane. "The implication is," Singer concludes, "that the British government values a supersonic transport more than thirty times as highly as it values the lives of the nine million refugees"[38] halfway around the world in East Bengal.

Could the donors not have known? Because of the size of the emergency, Singer argued, "neither individuals nor governments can claim to be unaware of what is happening."[39] Starvation and famine are not new, he later wrote, but what is new today is our ability to measure and watch food production everywhere in the world, and thereby to predict food shortages. What is also new—at least since the 1970s—is the ability of affluent nations to grow, harvest, and transport agricultural food to those in need. "These factors"—knowing, surplus food, and potential for global delivery—"impose obligations on individuals as well as nations to alleviate starvation," Singer wrote. "Thus, what one may do or refrain from doing has important consequences."[40]

There are further complexities. In the face of global climate change, and seeking to diminish carbon emissions from vehicles, some developed (and food-surplus) nations are converting corn to ethanol. The addiction to petroleum-based products among wealthy states (and China) is producing unintended (but well-known) consequences. The amount of corn being planted is increasing, but the use of corn for food is decreasing. Moreover the cost of corn in 2007–2008 doubled from a previously stable US$2 to US$4 a bushel. By 2010 it was falling back to its original level, but the price could rise again, and when that happens the add-on costs of meat, eggs, poultry, and milk will rise with it as they did in 2007.

The decision to shift corn to fuel was made for sound environmental reasons by developed states consuming large amounts of petroleum. But the real tension comes between the 800 million motorists who want to protect their mobility and the 2 billion people who are the world's hungriest and poorest. The U.S. Department of Agriculture reports that the consumption of grain globally increased by 20 million metric tons in 2006. Of that increase, 14 million tons went to fuel vehicles in the United States. That left only 6 million tons to meet rising demands for food assistance in the larger developing world. "In effect," writes Lester Brown, "supermarkets and service stations are now competing for the same resources."[41] We make individual choices daily in our purchases at those locations.

Can we identify moral principles that might serve as guidelines? How would those guidelines hold up when a recipient nation does not ask for food aid even in the face of widespread starvation of its own people, or when crops are deliberately destroyed and food shortages artificially created (Stalin in Ukraine, 1933; Mugabe in Zimbabwe, 2001–2007)? Some starvation continues for years, even decades (Ethiopia, 1973–1986; the Sudan, 1974–present; North Korea 1995–present). Can donors be asked to intervene continuously?

What are the *obligations* incurred from knowing about such tragedies and having the means to respond to them? Singer's analysis is informative. He forms his argument "with the assumption that suffering and death from lack of food, shelter and medical care are bad." We cannot discriminate against anyone on the basis that he/she, or the event (starvation), is physically far away; there is "no justification for discriminating on geographical grounds." Singer dismisses the fact, or the belief, that there may be "millions" of others in our position; they could act but do not. The view that "numbers lessen obligation" is an "absurdity," a position "that is an ideal excuse for inactivity." Therefore, Singer's central position is "if it is in our power to prevent something very bad from happening, without thereby sacrificing anything else morally significant, we ought, morally, to do it."[42]

Another wise voice joins this discussion. Onora O'Neill, a distinguished Cambridge University scholar and former principal (president) of Newnham College, places Immanuel Kant (1724–1804) at the center of her argument. Kant provides a set of "principles of obligation" often linked to human rights, O'Neill writes, and develops "a theory of human obligations" that gives it a wider scope.[43] The primary focus is "on action rather than either *results*, as in utilitarian thinking, or *entitlements*, as in theories that make human rights their fundamental category."[44] Singer argues that we have a "moral" obligation "to prevent something bad from happening." O'Neill suggests that we should act in ways that always treat humanity equally and fairly, "never simply as a means but always at the same time as an end." This includes a concern "for justice and benevolence."[45] John Rawls contributes his theory of "distributive justice," a set of normative principles that influence the allocation of resources such as food. Each human being, Rawls argues, has an equal claim to basic rights and liberties. Any social and economic inequities *must*, therefore, be rectified in order to achieve the greatest benefits for those suffering the greatest disadvantages.

Birth, privilege, and distance do not absolve us from obligation.[46] Neighbors who need food or other forms of assistance, O'Neill states, "are not entitled to justice at the expense of those who are far away." She writes: "Whether poverty and hunger are in the next street or far away, whether we articulate the task in utilitarian, in Kantian, or in other terms, the claims of justice and of beneficence for the two cases are similar. What may differ in the two cases are our opportunities for action." It may be easier to alleviate hunger and poverty nearby, rather than overseas. But act we must: "Since nobody can do everything, we not only *may* but *must* put our efforts where they will bear fruit."[47]

Singer, Rawls, and O'Neill agree that our actions cannot help those at hand if we create injustice or hunger for those at some distance.[48] Our obligations to help others and to end hunger and poverty include working with "agents and institutions across the world and across the generations of mankind to put an end to world hunger."[49] Nasir Islam summed this up well when he wrote: "The ethics of food aid must rest on the fundamental nature of human existence in society—the imperative of cooperation and interdependence."[50] Therefore, we must lift the world's poor into the lifeboat.

Should We Attach Conditions to Our Actions?

Given the moral obligation to act, is it immoral to attach conditions to such interventions? Between 2001 and 2009 roughly half the people of Zimbabwe faced severe food shortages generally caused by their own government. The WFP was, at various times, banished from the country by its autocratic president, Robert Mugabe, who allowed relief food aid to be distributed only to those who supported his government and political party, ZANU-PF. But these were the very agents that donors suspected of creating the starvation. Should WFP, in this case, donate food with "contingencies" attached to it regarding its distribution to *all* Zimbabwe's citizens whatever their politics? This sort of moral decision gets sticky. Donors might determine that they will deliver relief food only if certain services are provided or withheld (such as family planning practices) or conditions met (such as free elections or democracy). Should relief food be used to attain social, economic, or political justice in Zimbabwe, for example? Or is it always wrong to use food as a "tool" or "bargaining chip" because food is essential to human life and a "right"?

Advocates for "conditionalities" argue that food is the property of the country that produces it, much as oil belongs to the country under which it is found and drilled. It is theirs to use "as they see fit." Having surplus food and being a global food donor carries power with it: "To reject or ignore the possibilities of using food to enhance our own position in the world and to increase the world's peace and justice is to squander a valuable opportunity bequeathed to us."[51] Without conditions—at the least, an in-country donor presence and vigilant accountability—short- or long-term food aid "may serve only to prop up tyrannical regimes or stave off revolutionary reforms." Food given in this instance may work against the best interests and welfare of those who need it the most. It may perpetuate dependency, or postpone reform.[52]

Opponents of "conditionalities" argue that natural resources—oil, food-producing soil—are the arbitrary blessings of nature "to which their benefi- ciaries have no special moral entitlement." Moreover, as this chapter details, they advance the theory that food is a recognized and legislated "right." Food surpluses, given impartially as assistance by donor states, must be "weighed against the urgency of this universal human right."[53] Emergency and long-term food aid addresses such a basic human need that to use it for political, social, or economic preferences thus becomes inherently immoral. These preferences may be relevant, but only to the extent that they ensure that relief food is dis- tributed to those who are hungry and not withheld until certain "conditions" are met. No aid is apolitical; food sales, grants, concessions, food-for-work all carry economic, social, and political implications. But, we argue, it is immoral to block or control feeding those who are hungry.

There is also the question of moral legitimacy. We return to Singer and O'Neill. The shipping and distribution of both emergency and long-term food assistance must carry with them the moral power of preventing something bad—starvation, disease, death—from occurring. Tying food to conditions, however, strikes us as violating Singer's demand that this be done without "sacrificing anything of comparable moral importance."[54] Is not the promise of food or the threat of its withdrawal immoral when used to manipulate the behavior of starving individuals or nations?[55] Instead, as O'Neill writes, our obligations are to help others, and to end hunger and poverty by working with others around the world and across generations, "to put an end to world hunger."[56] Neither says anything about imposing conditions.

Thus, our "knowing" about chronic hunger, malnutrition, starvation, and famine globally, our continuing food surpluses, our technology and commu- nications and transportation abilities, directly inform and activate our moral responsibility. Stephen Devereux, reflecting Adam Hochschild's inquiry into the Belgian Congo, states that this responsibility in "its strongest form is the assertion that there comes a point where the suffering inflicted by design, neglect, or incapacity on citizens of a given country becomes so unjust that international responsibility overrides the sovereignty of the state involved and impels intervention."[57]

Is there a "right" to food? Yes. Is there an obligation to act (if we can) to prevent something bad from happening to another person? Yes, as long as it doesn't create a larger immoral action. "If people are hungry, it takes only the intervention of others who are aware of the situation to enable a person to have food," writes Nigel Dower. "The evil of hunger can be eliminated by the actions of others."[58]

Perhaps all of this moral philosophy and analysis comes clear in a single human observation. During the Great Irish Famine, the Scottish philanthropist,

Elizabeth Smith, echoing privileged women and men of her time, was torn between support for the anti-interventionist *laissez-faire* position and her own heart-felt humanitarian concern. She knew about the starving Irish, and she could certainly afford to help. But like many people then and now, Mrs. Smith felt that those who received free goods were those "who little deserve help and who would not be really benefitted by it."

But, she added, "when I see hungry children, I long to give them food."[59]

13   **Best Practices**

While researching this book we repeatedly encountered two fundamental realities: (1) the degree of human suffering from chronic hunger and disease is shameful, getting worse, and expanding to include more people; and (2) this suffering is avoidable. How might we reverse this trend? There are, in fact, some excellent ideas that may serve as models for addressing the problems detailed in this book. We call these "best practices." They are worth our consideration. We have placed them in four categories: food security, women and education, health care, and violence and conflict. This is not a comprehensive list, but it illustrates several things. First, it encourages us to do something about the problems set forth here. Second, it posits that some of the best models for addressing these problems are small in scale, comparatively inexpensive, and can be accomplished. Third, it shows that these models are successful because they are "targeted" and receive strong support, "inputs" (such as seeds, training, credit, and medicines), direct hands-on attention, and follow-up. And fourth, it reveals that the models employed come by working closely with the people in developing countries and are turned over to them.

Food Security and Smallholder Farming

Smallholder farmers produce much of the developing world's food.[1] They do this on small plots of land that produce enough for themselves, their families, and, when harvests allow, a little left over to sell or barter. Large numbers of Africa's people derive their livelihood from agriculture, which employs between 61 percent and 80 percent of the labor force, depending on the country; the majority of Africa's farmers are women. Agriculture contributes about 42 percent of the gross domestic product (GDP) of low-income African countries and 27 percent of the GDP of its middle-income countries; it accounts for between 40 percent and 60 percent of export earnings.[2] But most of the employment and production come from commercial farms growing commodity crops for export instead of food for internal consumption.

The challenge facing Africa's agriculture is formidable. According to a World Bank report, Africa's agriculture must over the next decades match the food demands of a growing population, maintain output per person, increase caloric intake, lower food imports and food aid needs, continue as Africa's principal employer, and compete on global markets to earn foreign exchange to fuel economic growth. "And it must do all that while reversing the degradation of natural resources that threatens long-term production," the World Bank states. *"This challenge requires a transformation of agriculture"*³ (italics added).

To do this, Africa's agriculture will have to continue commodity production and large-scale commercial farming, but it will also need to achieve and maintain food security and food self-sufficiency. Therefore, a paradigm shift is needed that would strengthen food security—that is, produce enough food to maintain health and productivity—and become self-sufficient in obtaining food. This will mean finding a better balance between smallholder and commercial farming. It will also mean addressing crop diversity and moving away from dependency on a single crop, such as maize, vulnerable to a "tragic environmental accident" similar to the potato blight. In addition increased regional food trade will need to become a central strategy by which food surpluses are moved as needed to nearby food-deficit countries. Food security and self-sufficiency also offer one way of addressing volatile world food trade markets. We have a possible "best practices" model in southern Africa currently in the productive farmlands of that region and within the 14-country Southern Africa Development Community.

The standard accepted wisdom that "large farms are more efficient than small-holder farms" ignores the potential in smallholder farming. It has led to land-ownership and agricultural policies in sub-Saharan Africa that have favored land alienation and expropriation in favor of large commercial farms and government-owned estates, and the production of commodity crops exported to earn foreign currency. Could resources of every kind—seeds, technology, credit, farm implements, and market access—be redirected to Africa's smallholders? What might be the outcome?

An excellent answer is found in an unlikely source: Zimbabwe. Using maize, Africa's staple food, as its principal crop, Zimbabwe actually produced two maize revolutions. How did they do it? The first began during the colonial period when the country was a British colony (Southern Rhodesia). White commercial farmers, each farming up to 1500–2000 hectares of land, were supported by large public investments in agricultural research, infrastructure (roads), subsidized loans and bank credits, favorable product prices, and a controlled colonial market linked to Great Britain. Regional cooperation with other nearby colonies like Nyasaland (Malawi) and Northern Rhodesia (Zambia), and even international sanctions following the Unilateral Declaration of Independence (UDI) in 1965, facilitated domestic agricultural research and the development and regional exchange of hybrid maize seed varieties. These farmers produced enough maize to feed the entire colony and export surpluses.

The first maize revolution jump-started the second. At independence in 1980 more than 4000 mostly large-scale, white commercial farmers cultivated half the country's arable land using mechanized farming and irrigation. On the other half of arable land about 700,000 African smallholder farmers tilled between 20 and 80 hectares each of rain-fed farmland. The principal legacy of commercial farmer to smallholder—from the first maize revolution to the second—came from gains in agricultural research made during the colonial period, especially new varieties of hybrid, drought-resistant maize that boosted the second maize revolution.

Within four years, Zimbabwe became a model of smallholder farming success. The new government under President Robert Mugabe—the only president the country has had to date—embraced the concept of food security. In 1980 Mugabe decided to increase the production of maize and, to a lesser extent, sorghum. He removed all racial and institutional barriers to credit, which gave the African smallholder farmer access to tools, seed, and fertilizers. Mugabe and his government expanded infrastructure deep into the rural areas; they built rail lines, roads, and market depots so farmers could haul harvests to market (and get paid) easily and quickly. Perhaps most important, Zimbabwe was at peace after more than a decade of brutal civil war. Land abandoned during the conflict—much of it in the fertile eastern highlands with its abundant rainfall—was brought back into cultivation.

Between 1980 and 1992, the proportion of maize produced by smallholders in Zimbabwe increased from less than 25 percent of national output to more than 70 percent.[4] These smallholders also doubled the country's production. Their surpluses enabled the country to export maize; as a symbol of its bounty, Zimbabwe was also the first and only sub-Saharan Africa country to send emergency food aid to Ethiopia during the 1983–1986 famine. By the late 1980s Zimbabwe was "awash with maize." During the next decade maize surpluses gave the country political stability and social and economic resilience; smallholders produced enough surplus grains for the country to overcome severe droughts in 1990–1993 by creating and then drawing down its food reserves (a good example of the "moral economy" concept working well). By 1997 Zimbabwe was being acclaimed in the *International Herald Tribune*'s financial pages as one of the "African lions," with a robust economy based on manufacturing, mining, tourism, and agriculture (maize, tobacco, and cotton).[5] As a result of the second maize revolution, Robert Mugabe received the Africa Prize for Leadership "for showing that smallholder farming was profitable and efficient."[6]

Zimbabwe's agricultural success of the 1980s and 1990s suggests that an African "green revolution" might be created using indigenous agriculture research and investments in smallholder farms in a country at peace. The International

Food Policy Research Institute (IFPRI) reported in 2002 that increasing production among Africa's smallholders could boost incomes and food security and lower food costs. An increase of 1 percent in agricultural GDP, for example, was shown to produce a 1.6 percent rise in per capita income among the poorest people in a developing state.[7] The result could also further reduce poverty. In a later report IFPRI added that "a one percent increase in food yields can help 6 million more people raise their incomes above US$1 per day. At this rate, a smallholder-led strategy might lead to large cuts in Africa's rural poverty within a couple of decades."[8] Because women are also the principal farmers in sub-Saharan Africa, there would be add-on benefits in family care and nutrition.

Maize is the logical African crop. It is the dominant staple food of sub-Saharan Africa, the equal to rice in Asia, and today plays a central role in African lives and diets. It is easy to cultivate, grows in both rural and urban areas, and transports easily. Maize is converted to flour with less effort (pounding in a mortar, for example) than sorghum or millet. Its principal drawback is nutritional: when eaten without protein additions (legumes, meat), maize is a poor food lacking in essential amino acids and micronutrients such as thiamine. It is also not resistant to drought. Although a dominant crop, with risks of blight mirroring those visited on the Irish potato crop, maize could (and perhaps should) be cultivated along with more hardy and drought-resistant foods like millet, sorghum and even cassava. Despite these drawbacks, as Derek Byerlee and Carl Eicher have proposed, maize produced by smallholder farmers offers "one of the few rays of hope for stepping up food production over the coming 10 to 20 years" in sub-Saharan Africa. Because it is an important food staple, "improvements in the performance of maize production will be crucial to solving Africa's food security problems and alleviating poverty."[9]

In chapter 6 we discussed the recovery of Malawi following its starvation, where smallholder farmers are again feeding the country and generating surplus maize. Elsewhere, intensive work with smallholder farmers in Kenya is also showing broad-reaching benefits. Sauri, a village of 5000 in western Kenya near Lake Victoria, is one of the UN's ten global Millennium Villages test cases challenged to cut poverty in half by 2015. Some 56 percent of Kenyans currently live below the UN's poverty line. Malaria kills one in five Kenyan children every year. Malnutrition is endemic.[10] In 2005 Sauri began receiving US$250,000 a year from the UN (to 2010) to support agriculture, health, and education. Much of the money went to farmers for crop improvements, and to health care, clinics, and school lunch programs. Sauri's example also adds a key element to food security and self-sufficiency: In addition to maize, beans, and groundnuts, its farmers planted leguminous plants and trees (nitrogen-fixing) to provide natural fertilizer for their depleted soils. They received inputs of other fertilizers and improved seeds and diversified their crops for local markets by adding sun-flowers, poultry, spices and vegetables. By 2007, three years after it had started, Sauri's farmers had tripled the district's food production.

There were further beneficial inputs: insecticide-treated bed nets were dis-tributed to all villagers, and the local health clinics received improved malaria diagnosis and treatment applications. As a result the prevalence of malaria dropped from 55 percent to 13 percent in two years. A new thirty-two-bed clinic was built, with additional village clinics refurbished, and seventy-four commu-nity health workers were trained. By 2008, all twenty-eight primary schools in the Sauri district provided lunch to 17,514 children; much of the food was locally grown. School enrollment increased 20 percent.

Today in western Kenya alone more than 55,000 people are benefiting from Sauri's example. The task now is to lift the Sauri model to the national level and make it self-sufficient and sustainable. There are some obstacles, such as increased teacher-student ratios (there are 55 children for each teacher), high costs of school-lunch preparation (for firewood and water), limited parental contributions during the drought months, and continuing household poverty. Also, "targeted funding" such as the Millennium Villages project almost always works in the short term. But not every village in every developing country can be targeted. What Sauri illustrates well is the effectiveness of the Zimbabwe model: smallholder farmers, a concentration of inputs, infrastructure, credits to smallholder farmers that boost food security, and diverse crops. Working together, they also create concomitant benefits to the community in terms of health care and education.[11] "The small-scale farmers and the poor rural land owners have been largely ignored," said Dr. Arthur G. O. Mutambara, a leader in Zimbabwe's opposition party. "When our poorest farmers finally prosper, all of Africa will benefit."[12]

Women and Education

The connections among increased food intake, the education of women and child spacing and reduced childhood malnutrition are increasingly well documented. Investments in a woman's education and health have been shown to improve her status in her community, extend the age at which she becomes pregnant with her first child, and reduce the incidence of malnutrition. A seminal IFPRI study states that "the countries with improved [child] nutritional status had larger increases in the enrollment of women in secondary school, in per capita food consumption, and in per capita incomes." The study links the importance of women's education to the reduction of malnutrition. The education of women and the subsequent improvement in their status within the community are estimated to make up almost 55 percent of the factors that assist in reducing childhood malnutrition. "The data do not establish strict causality," IFPRI warns, "but this analysis provided strong indications that women's schooling, women's status, per capita food intake and per capita incomes are important determinants of child malnutrition in Africa."[13]

Because Africa's farmers are predominately women, the education of women and girls matches well with increased food security and improved health care as "best practices." Educated mothers are 50 percent more likely to immunize their children. An extra year of girls' education can reduce infant mortality by as much as 10 percent; in Africa the children of mothers with even five years of primary education have a 40 percent better chance of living beyond five years of age. Studies by Goldman Sachs show that just a 1 percent increase in the education of girls in developing states also increases that country's economy as measured by its gross domestic product.[14]

It is also important to acknowledge that "the disproportionate impact of poverty on girls is not an accident, but the result of systematic discrimination."[15] Although women and girls account for about half the world's population, they are the majority of the poor and chronically hungry. ActionAid's report on women and the Millennium Development Goals states that "Ten million more girls than boys are out of primary school" and that girls make up two-thirds of the world's illiterate young people. In some countries girls have a 50 percent greater chance of dying before age five than boys; in Africa, 75 percent of all young people suffering from HIV/AIDS are girls or young women.[16]

Directing assistance toward girls and women, especially in regions like sub-Saharan Africa, should be a significant and obvious path toward decreasing child and maternal mortality, cutting the spread of HIV/AIDS, reducing childhood malnutrition, and boosting economic growth. With that in mind, in 1993 Ann Cotton of Cambridge, England, decided to address these issues. She created Camfed and sold baked goods to keep thirty-two girls in school in Zimbabwe.

Camfed initially focused on primary and secondary school girls in Nyaminyami, an area of subsistence farming and poor harvests, and in Chikomba, at the time a district of commercial farms where most Zimbabweans worked as paid farm laborers. In both areas families were poor, and young female school leavers had two choices: marry or leave to find work. Each carried risks: early pregnancy and childrearing or unemployment and the possible slide into prostitution. Camfed concentrated on keeping selected girls in school by funding their costs and providing close mentoring and support through the girls' families and teachers. When violence in Zimbabwe increased, further eroding options for postschool employment, Camfed focused on postschool career choices.

Camfed expanded its model to include four stages of support: primary education, secondary education, economic empowerment, and creating change.

This included continuing financial aid and local mentors, often teachers, to partner with girls throughout their education. Next, Cotton and Lucy Lake shifted Camfed beyond Zimbabwe into Zambia and more recently to Ghana and Tanzania. They expanded the model to include an alumnae support network for young women after their postsecondary education.

Each area offers something different in terms of the empowerment of girls. In northern Ghana, for example, Camfed works closely with primary schools allocating a "safety-net fund" to each school to pay costs (shoes or a school uniform, for example) that might cause a child to drop out. Teachers in the schools help Camfed to identify a child's needs and the urgency of response. In Zambia, Camfed's network supports promising young women and "guarantees" them four years of secondary education. Through its donors, Camfed pays for school uniforms, stationery, books, and fees; if a girl needs to attend boarding school, Camfed adds in soap, towels, pocket money, and a metal trunk to store her possessions. The selection of young girls, and their support, is tricky and carries the risks of identifying a needy girl to the exclusion of others and the possible stigma of favoritism or special status each designation might confer. To help a selected girl and her family adjust, Camfed also works closely with each girl and her teachers. So far, the program seems to work, and Camfed has seen 90 percent of its selected girls stay in school in the four countries.

In Tanzania, Camfed has more recently started microcredit training and peer support opportunities for young women no longer in school. Young Tanzanian women, many of them Camfed alumnae who themselves benefited from the Camfed program, run its "seed money program." They offer "non-repayable grants as the first experience of money ownership and control," guidance, and money management. Businesses operated by these Camfed alumnae identify a community need; for example, poultry raising, market gardening, tailoring, and trade in goods such as kitchen utensils.

Camfed's alumnae association, called Cama, now includes 9000 women. The women are "united by a shared background of rural poverty and transformation through education," says a Camfed publication. "The power for change is now in their hands." That empowerment addresses the issues faced by girls and young women in most developing states: choosing when and whom to marry; having and using their own money; participating in rural economies; becoming health educators concerned with nutrition, disease prevention (especially HIV/AIDS), child spacing, and nutrition. To date, Camfed has reached some 408,000 children, almost entirely girls, in its education programs. It has support from a range of donors for a budget of more than $16 million in 2008.

Camfed's weakness is that it is a "targeted" project with a small, narrowly focused, although well-financed, closely monitored, and maintainable program.

But it might work well in combination with the smallholder farming model. Investing in girls' education, as the IFPRI research shows, contributes directly to improving child and maternal health, boosting wages and income, and thus reducing poverty. It is also likely to increase farm production as well, given the fact that in Africa women are the principal farmers. The challenge is to sustain and gradually expand. Can the Camfed and the smallholder Millennium Villages farming models do it? Angeline Mugwendere, the first Chair of CAMA, answered that question this way: "If you think you're too small to be effective," she said, "you have never been in bed with a mosquito." [17]

Health Care

Health care, like food security and education, is a human right conferred by the UN *Universal Declaration of Human Rights*. We have detailed here some global health concerns, and some significant gains, according to World Health Organization (WHO) reports. Globally people are healthier and living longer than at the end of the twentieth century. Wider preventative measures, quicker interventions, and increasing primary care have greatly improved. This is perhaps best seen in child health care. If, for example, children in developing states were still dying at the 1978 rate, there would have been 16.2 million additional childhood deaths in 2006. Instead, there were 9.5 million deaths, still too many, but a difference of 6.7 million or the equivalent of 18,329 children's lives saved every day. This is the result of improved primary health systems and simple, basic gains in access to potable water, better sanitation, wider prenatal and postnatal care.

There are, however, sharp inequities that reflect deeper problems. Lack of access to a proper diet—part of the "nutritional crisis" detailed in this book—is a significant health problem that could be addressed through food security efforts. So, too, is the difference in life expectancy between rich and poor countries, which now exceeds forty years. The risk of dying prematurely is far greater in the developing world. Women in poor countries are 250 times more likely to die during pregnancy or childbirth than women in wealthy countries. In thirty-three of the world's poorest countries, more than half of all births annually occur *without any* medical assistance. [18]

As we have detailed throughout this book, the people—especially the women—of sub-Saharan Africa suffer disproportionately. In 2005, for example, of the 535,000 women who died worldwide during pregnancy or childbirth, 99 percent lived in developing countries. [19] African women accounted for more than half of those deaths. The possibility of a pregnant woman in Africa dying from complications during her pregnancy is 180 times greater than that of a European woman. [20] And more than 1 million people die annually from malaria, most of them African women and children.

There are other, systemic disproportions. Some wealthy nations spend as much as US$6000 per person annually on health care, whereas other countries are unable (or unwilling) to spend more than US$20 per person per year.[21] WHO reports that better health care is not always the result of higher health expenditures. Tajikistan and Sierra Leone spend about the same—less than $100 per person per year. But in Sierra Leone, life expectancy is less than thirty years, whereas in Tajikistan it is almost seventy.[22] WHO reports "the substantial progress in health care over recent decades has been deeply unequal . . . [with] considerable and often growing health inequalities *within* countries."[23] Access to and quality of health care vary enormously, not only from state to state but also just across a city. In Nairobi, Kenya, for example, the Emabakasi slum is one of the largest and poorest in the world, home to about a million people where more than one in every four children will die before age five. Across Nairobi, however, in a high-income district, the child mortality rate is one in almost sixty-seven.[24] "High maternal, infant and under-five mortality," UNICEF reports, "often indicates lack of access to basic services such as clean water and sanitation, immunization and proper nutrition."[25]

Best practices, therefore, are not necessarily the most expensive or complex. What works well in improving health care among developing states may simply be access to a health clinic or medical care and to low-cost preventive measures. For example insecticide-treated bed nets used in rural Africa cost about $10 a net but, as we just saw in the Sauri example, have "substantially reduced childhood mortality" in regions where malaria was "a major contributor to death."[26] Deworming children, a low-cost preventative care, is also shown to lower rates of childhood anemia and to increase a child's size. Moreover, "when younger children were dewormed, they attended school 15 more days a year."[27] In South Asia, researchers are trying to reduce newborn deaths by 20 percent simply by adding a vitamin A supplement to their diet. Iodine deficiency is "the single greatest cause of preventable mental retardation," and a factor in stillbirths, miscarriages, and learning disabilities. Consuming iodized salt can easily prevent these, but only thirty-four countries have universal iodized salt distribution.[28] Save the Children and Johns Hopkins University's Bloomberg School of Public Health have designed a simple "Better Beginning for Babies" kit for distribution by community health workers to more than 2 million new-born children in countries with high infant mortality rates. The kit contains soap, a clean razor blade (for cutting the umbilical cord), a clean cord tie, a sheet of plastic and educational materials on ways to improve new-born care. The cost to put the kit together and distribute it is about US$10 each.[29] Another "best practice" may be simply to improve health care records: in western Kenya, a WHO-sponsored program is integrating electronic health records with laboratory, drug procurement, and reporting systems. This effort has already "drastically reduced clerical labour and errors and improved follow-up primary care."[30]

Connecting these "best practices" carries even greater gains. A global assessment of Target 2 of Millennium Development Goal One, for example, indicates that food security and employment together with health care improvements and education could reduce the number of malnourished children globally by about 17 percent. These gains may also help close the health care gap between wealthy and poor countries and people. That, in fact, adds another benefit. As mentioned earlier in the book, there is a clear link between poverty—especially the lack of access to basic education, sanitation, health care, and food—and terrorism. It seems obvious that some of the people who have lost hope, who are without access to basic food, health care, and educational resources, carry out terrorist attacks. Closing the health care gap, therefore, may also be an important security "best practice." As Dr. Margaret Chan, director-general of WHO, puts it: "A world that is greatly out of balance in matters of health, is neither stable nor secure."[31]

Violence and Conflict Reduction

Food insecurity and health problems are often seen in countries also experiencing civil conflict and violence. The UN FAO has determined that almost 60 percent of the countries where more than half the people are malnourished have suffered from conflict. Conversely, only 8 percent of those countries with low levels of malnutrition have experienced conflict or violence.[32] Events in Zimbabwe since 1980 illustrate—as do other examples detailed in chapter 9—the benefits of ending conflict and violence. However, Africa still experiences the largest number of armed conflicts of any continent; one African in every five lives in a conflict zone. Violence has been the norm most recently in the Great Lakes region, Darfur, Somalia, and the Democratic Republic of the Congo. During the first decade of the twenty-first century alone, coups brought down governments in Guinea, Guinea-Bissau, Mauritania, and Madagascar.[33]

As chapter 9 also made clear, violence and conflict interfere with food security and economic progress. Studies have shown the obvious: the restoration of peace and security and the rule of law are linked directly to improvements in food production. Protracted violence and conflict undermine productive capacity and the ability to plant and harvest crops. Child mortality rates are directly proportional to the prevalence of food security; the greater the food *insecurity*, the greater the rate of child mortality.[34] Therefore, the reduction of conflict and violence helps in decreasing childhood mortality as well as increasing food security.

Some excellent first steps are already under way toward ending violence. African Union (AU) countries are making progress on the African Peace and Security Architecture (APSA), their initiative for joint peacekeeping action. The African Standby Force, composed of five brigades of peacekeeping troops and police from AU member states, had by 2010 several operational brigades in place ahead of schedule. This will allow Africans to monitor and enforce peacekeeping operations on their own continent. In addition, the Continental Early Warning System (CEWS), Africa's effort to create a collective security and early warning response to conflict and crises in their region, was approaching operational status by the end of that decade.

Although it is essential that Africans (and others) monitor and police their own conflicts, the reduction of violence and conflict is a global obligation. With that in mind, "best practices" models for conflict reduction and management are being deployed by The U.S. Institute of Peace (Washington, DC) and other agencies, including the United Nations. These models are based on incorporating conflict resolution skills training into international agency programs and on creating a global network of international "facilitators" to teach conflict-management skills to people in countries that have experienced violence and war. These now include Afghanistan, Pakistan, Iran, and the Middle East. In sub-Saharan Africa, conflict-management training is under way for civilian members of the Sierra Leone government, representatives of the North-South disputes in Sudan, and with Christians and Muslims in Nigeria. The U.S. Institute of Peace is also using South Africa's work in its Truth and Reconciliation Commission to develop model codes of justice.[35]

Why is this important? As WHO's Dr. Chan pointed out, global security will elude us as long as there are such wide gaps in health care, food security, peace, and stability. USIP's work in conflict resolution and management is essential to stability, which in turn allows work to progress on these other core problems and on the elimination of poverty.

Other Issues

"Land Grabbing"

"Land grabbing" is under way in sub-Saharan Africa and parts of Asia by food-importing countries with domestic land and water constraints. These include the oil-rich Gulf States, China, India, South Korea, and even Japan, which are acquiring farmland in developing countries. They are "land grabbing" largely because they cannot provide enough food for themselves and they have lost confidence in the global food markets to meet their domestic food demands. Governments or state companies have leased or bought more than 20 million hectares (50 million acres) in developing countries to grow food overseas for consumption back home.[36]

This might be seen as a beneficial investment that provides infusions of capital into developing countries, especially for the rural sector and the poor. Or, "land grabbing" might be challenged as promoting economic disparity between investors and local communities, displacing smallholder farmers, overusing soil and water resources to maximize production, and growing crops of value only for export to other markets. In addition "land grabbing" can be viewed as a global illustration of "the tragedy of the commons" now being played out over food: a distant "commons" (a poor country) is "over-grazed" by a foreign state or company that maximizes food production and exportation of resources. The "commons" bears the entire burden, while the "grazer" country suffers no environmental or resource liability or consequences but gains all of the benefits.

The expansion of food-growing opportunities is not new: Japan, for example, invested in farm land overseas more than a century ago and now holds overseas three times its own domestic food-producing land area. China has been active outside the mainland for 10 years, first in Cuba and Mexico and more recently in parts of sub-Saharan Africa.

To address this, IFPRI is promoting a code of conduct for foreign land acquisition that seeks greater sharing of the benefits, protects soil and water resources, and promotes environmental sustainability. The idea is not to halt the acquisition of land by foreign investors—but to control and monitor it. This model is worth further examination and bears watching.

Biofuels

Although the spike in food prices in 2007 caused by the biofuels controversy had quieted by 2009, the inherent conflict between alternative fuels and food production persists. This does not have to be the case. There are some models for shifting fuel sources from corn and other edible food crops to alternatives such as switchgrass or the jatropha tree. And although switchgrass and the jatropha lack the name recognition and lobbying power of corn-based ethanol, the energy industry is spending more research money to examine both as better biofuel sources. The product, cellulosic ethanol, may be years from commercial use, but proponents point out one major advantage: neither is a food source.

There are some good arguments for developing these two crops as fuel sources. Jatropha is easier to grow than corn. It is not a food source and thus untied to the food market. It is grown without carbon dioxide or sulfur emissions (from engines used for planting and fertilizing). It could be sown *along with* food crops. It already grows in India and Africa.

Some marginal farmers who diverted croplands to jatropha, however, have been hurt by low yields, land disputes, and weak or absent processing infrastructure—all of which can be corrected. So far, the plant seems to work well as a fuel: biodiesel made from jatropha has powered test airplane flights on Air New Zealand and Continental Airlines.

Regional Institutions

The support and expansion of regional institutions could also address issues of food security, education, and health care. For example the Southern Africa Development Community (SADC) consists of fifteen countries from South Africa to Tanzania and the Seychelles, an island-nation in the Indian Ocean. Similar regional entities exist in East Africa, Central Africa, and West Africa, and together they form an integral part of the African Union. Two of SADC's member states, South Africa and Zimbabwe, have been food-surplus producers and could, with support and inputs mentioned here, increase food security for the region. Efforts within SADC for regional cooperation and economic integration are also under way with the New Partnership for Africa's Development (NEPAD) agenda. These include a completed free trade and a common customs agreement, protocols concerning labor movement and water sharing, and plans for a common market by 2015, a common monetary union by 2016, and a single SADC currency by 2018—all of this reflecting their own model, the European Union. The blending of each SADC country's Poverty Reduction Strategy Program into a regional effort could construct a solid foundation for further regional cooperation.

Microfinance Institutions

Other more commonly mentioned "best practices" include the popular Grameen Bank microfinance loans, founded by Mohammad Yunus, for which he won the Nobel Prize in 2006. Largely unscathed by the global economic collapse, microfinance institutions based on this model continue to make loans of $100 or so for simple, local community-based projects, such as raising chickens, or buying a sewing machine to patch clothing. To date the Grameen Bank has dispersed some $8 billion in microloans to more than 8 million people with a 98 percent payback rate. Until recently, only wealthy investors could put money into the microfinance bank. Now smaller investors can contribute as well, through operations like Microplace.com (started by Tracey Pettengill Turner, a Dartmouth alumna). This appears to be an effective method of addressing poverty alleviation: it is bottom-up, small in scale, and works at the individual level, as do small-farm operations and Camfed mentioned here.

There are some cautions, however. On the whole, Africans have benefited the least from microfinance; 70 percent of the microfinance businesses are located in Asia, 20 percent in Latin America, and the rest are scattered about the developing world. Large, multinational financial institutions that are vulnerable to the perils of global market fluctuations have also taken up the industry. During the 2007–2009 recession, repayment of debt among the larger microfinance institutions became a problem worth watching.

The Internet

As we write, a new and potentially powerful expansion of the broadband Internet is under way in Africa. To date only 4 percent of all Africans have access to the Internet; they pay the most for it, about US$250–300 a month, and get the slowest connection service. Congo and Sudan, two of the largest African countries, have no public Internet at all. In West Africa, the SAT-3 undersea cable brings higher speeds and lower costs. SEACOM, the undersea cable connecting East Africa into high-speed internet, began in mid-2009. It is 75 percent owned by Africans and may reduce the cost of doing business within Africa and between Africa and the global economy. As we see it, the increasing use of the Internet inside Africa could also accelerate the distribution of food (through information sharing), thus assisting food security and health care.

Debt Relief

Relieving the burden of debt in the developing world should also be considered. Debt relief began in the late 1980s not long after developing countries ran up large levels of debt during the fuel spike and commodity collapse of the 1970s. In the 1990s, a campaign to relieve that debt focused on the IMF and World Bank and launched a scheme called the Heavily Indebted Poor Countries (HIPC) initiative to reduce the debt burden among developing states. At the time countries in sub-Saharan Africa were spending more on debt relief and interest payments than on education and health care combined. At this writing twenty-nine of the forty countries seeking debt relief under HIPC are in sub-Saharan Africa; some thirty-five countries (also many of them in Africa) have received full or partial relief from their debt. There are obvious benefits: in 2005, for example, Great Britain forgave Kenya its debt on the condition that it redirect the savings to eliminate school fees. When Kenya did so, more than a million "new" children—kept at home presumably because their parents could not pay the fees—showed up for school.

We cannot leave the topic of "best practices"—especially one so weighted toward food security—without addressing the discussion about genetically modified organisms.

Genetically Modified Organisms

Genetically modified organisms (GMO) or genetically engineered organisms (GEO) are food, plants, or even some animals whose basic genetic makeup has been altered. In terms of our topic, GMOs include genetic modifications to livestock and, most particularly, to foods such as maize and rice. Some believe GMO seeds will drive a new green revolution and see this as the solution to global hunger. Others believe genetic modification is further evidence of corporate greed. They view the attempt by a few multinational corporations like Monsanto, BSAF, Dow Chemical and DuPont, now litigating against one another for licensing rights, as proof of schemes to corner the global seed and food-production markets. In fact, acquisitions of smaller seed companies form a major undertaking by Monsanto, and the corporation has been identified by the American Antitrust Institute, an independent antitrust research resource, as creating "an impaired state of competition in transgenic seed."[37] The U.S. Justice Department was at this writing focusing an antitrust investigation on Monsanto for these and other actions aimed at cornering the genetic seed market. As evidence, the Department cited the sharp increase in grain prices: corn seed up 135 percent and soybean prices up 108 percent since 2001. By contrast, the Consumer Price Index rose 20 percent over that same period.[38]

Is GMO, therefore, a "best practice," the answer to global hunger? Monsanto's president dismisses "the Malthusian thing about running out of food." World hunger, he says, "is eminently solvable" with GMO seeds. Or, as opponents argue, is the genetic modification of food seeds, and the control of GMO seeds and other modified resources, a threat to biodiversity, human health, and basic farming practices?

We include this discussion here because it is relevant to emergency food aid and a part of the hunger-alleviation debate. By 2010, at least twenty-five nations were growing GMO crops on a cultivated area larger than Peru. GMO-seeded crops were worth more than US$130 billion.[39] GMO maize is widely used in the corn-soy blend that is basic to emergency food relief and supplementary feeding. Soy forms the basis of almost all short-term food aid, and the bulk of soybeans in international trade today are genetically modified.[40] In the United States, 90 percent of the soybeans and more than 80 percent of the maize are genetically modified.[41]

In seed form, GMO emergency relief food has been rejected by Zimbabwe and Zambia, among other states. During the drought of 2002–2003, Zambia's president refused GMO emergency maize relief food and declared, "I'd rather die than eat something toxic."[42] The solution at the time was to mill the emergency food maize into flour, thus keeping it out of the fields of the recipient state. India's government has heatedly debated the safety of genetically modified eggplants. Its farmers have protested that the seeds are expensive and must be purchased every year. The European Union still opposes imports of GM food; NGOs like Greenpeace cite environmental concerns and argue that GMO foods pose a health risk to humans. They claim that U.S. multinational corporations are exploiting emergency food shortages and poverty to introduce GMO crops into developing world diets and agriculture.[43] Yet Bill Gates and others promote GMO crops as necessary for increasing food production in the developing world.

We believe that GMOs should not be part of long-term solutions to developing state agriculture, especially a solution based on smallholder farmers; there are some problems with GM seed or food. One is the ability of small, impoverished countries to reject GMO offerings. The Cartagena Convention concerning biodiversity reserves the right for each country to decide whether or not to import GM seeds or food. This is the core of governance. A responsible and accountable government may carefully weigh its decision to admit or reject GM food aid, especially when its own citizens are facing food shortages or starvation. Also, the regulations under which GMO seeds and foods are allowed into a country place special agricultural and economic burdens on its farmers. Under Monsanto's terms of business, farmers must buy the corporation's fresh seeds every year; the farmer cannot stockpile seeds or try to replicate them, or even retrieve any for replanting from this year's gleanings. If a farmer breaks this license, Monsanto will deny the farmer access to its technology; in 2009 the corporation won a major legal battle with farmers in Canada who held on to their GMO seeds.

On the up side, Monsanto has "donated" its intellectual property, seed, and agricultural expertise for developing drought-tolerant genes to agencies like Water Efficient Maize for Africa (WEMA), "a public-private partnership" that has received grants from the Gates Foundation. The Millennium Villages project and five African countries are cooperating: Kenya, Mozambique, South Africa, Tanzania, and Uganda. The corporation says that the WEMA project will generate no royalties for Monsanto. It calls this cooperative effort "the democratization of technology." Perhaps so, but the corporation also sees the developing world as a significant growth region for its GMO products. For example, Monsanto already sells more GM cotton seeds to India than anywhere else. And of the 12 million farmers globally who plant at least a hectare with GM seed, 90 percent are smallholders in developing countries.[44]

This is creating what we see as unfortunate dependencies. The terms of agreement for GMO seeds lock developing-state agriculture into purchasing those seeds, and their supporting fertilizer and pesticides, from international corporations, in particular from Monsanto. These purchases, in turn, require foreign currency, which then forces that country and its farmers to produce crops (or other products) earning the foreign currency necessary for such purchases. This creates an economic loop inherently unfair to the developing state and its smallholder farmers: export commodities need to be produced to earn foreign currency to purchase GMO seeds, in an unbreakable cycle. If these commodities (such as tobacco, cotton, coffee, and tea) are grown, then finite arable land is withdrawn from food production. This is not a straight path to food security, food self-sufficiency, or poverty alleviation. Even if the GMO seeds are "donated," the farmer remains vulnerable to the whims (and shareholders) of Monsanto, or another corporate entity, which maintains licensing control of seeds, fertilizers, and pesticides essential to food production.

The result is agriculture unnecessarily dependent on untested technologies and international corporate beneficence. If the focus is truly on achieving food security and self-sufficiency, the greater benefit might come from helping indigenous farmers develop, maintain, and distribute their own hybrid seeds that are disease and drought resistant. They would own their own food seeds, and they would avoid the need for seed-licensing restrictions and foreign currency allocations. This is what farmers have done for millennia.

[14] **Prescription for Change**

As an end to our journey through the scientific and historical facts of hunger and starvation, let us consider where we have been, where we are going, what we can do, and what we *should* do.

From the biological perspective we have developed an understanding of the basics of nutrition as they relate to our health as individuals and as a species. Acquiring access to adequate nutrition is a primal driver of human behavior. Without sufficient nourishment, survival is not possible, so it is not hard to understand why our bodies have evolved so many redundant mechanisms, usually manifest as the sensation of hunger, to see to it that our nutritional status is maintained and defended above all else. It also follows that so much of our history is bound up in the acquisition and control of reliable, sustainable sources of food.

The details of how we internalize, incorporate, and use the energy and nutrients in our diets help us to understand the serious nature of events that follow inadequate access to nutrition, micronutrient as well as macronutrient deficiencies—not only the pain and suffering that accompany chronic hunger and malnutrition but also the preventable, usually minor illnesses to which the compromised host with malnutrition often succumbs. We have also discussed the body of evidence showing that our mental processes have been formed by the same evolutionary pressures as our physical processes. We have provided a brief description as to why the seemingly opposing behaviors of aggression and bond-forming behavior are successful evolutionary strategies. We have additionally discussed why these strategies would logically be linked to one another and how they would combine with the equally successful strategy of cooperation, explaining our predisposition to think in a dichotomous fashion, categorizing other humans either as "us" or as "them."

In parallel to our biological perspective, the political perspective reveals that a remarkably high percentage of the world's population goes to bed hungry every night. Many—between one and two billion people—are caught in a poverty trap without end. Their malnutrition is chronic, and their lives are reduced to obtaining food and staying alive. Their potential as human beings may never be fully realized.

There are differing theories as to the causes of widespread chronic malnutrition, starvation, and famine. Thomas Malthus's observation that our population grows at a rate that cannot be maintained by agricultural production remains a challenging and worrisome idea, which we should not and cannot ignore. Amartya Sen's presentation that starvation and famine are secondary to a loss of entitlement and that loss of access to food has been the primary cause of all famines in the modern era, is also compelling. Malthus's theory has been described as causation of famine through acts of God or food availability decline (FAD), basically a supply problem. Sen's theory has been categorized as causation through acts of man, or food entitlement decline (FED), a problem of demand.

The attentive reader will have observed that both of these explanations play a role, and in fact food availability and food accessibility are synergistic in producing and maintaining the degree of world hunger and malnutrition we see today. Our recent history has been replete with mechanisms to offer advanced warning of impending famine, and the policies of governments and efforts of a multitude of governmental and nongovernmental organizations have been dedicated to addressing the problem of world hunger.

With this in mind, can we begin to comprehend why we have failed to fulfill this basic need for adequate nutrition? And why we have done so universally, despite the fact that we have recognized this social gap, and our moral obligation to fill it, for more than sixty years? We now know when shortages will occur; satellites inform us every ten days about global agricultural production. We *know*. As our populations have grown, our ability to provide adequate food for them has grown accordingly; we practice irrigation, crop rotation, more advanced farming implements; we have highly effective fertilizers, hybrid seeds, and genetic modification to improve crop yields. Yet, none of these significant advances, nor market price incentives and agricultural subsidies, has solved the problem of world hunger.

There are, of course, some basic human problems. In chapter 1, we discussed the impending failure of the Millennium Development Goals to achieve its objectives by 2015. The basic *reasons* should concern us: (1) poor health care systems that prevent billions of people from receiving preventative and affordable care or proper medical attention when needed; (2) unremitting violence and conflict within states that disrupts agricultural development and harvests, economic planning, rule of law, and political stability; (3) the continuing global economic crisis that is widening the gap between wealthy and impoverished countries and peoples and diminishing the willingness and ability of donors to address and correct, or end, these inequalities. At the heart of this—for the Irish of the mid-nineteenth century and for the developing world today—is extreme poverty. As mentioned in chapter 1, the conditions of poverty and its attendant deprivations also lie at the heart of global terrorism. They engender resentment, hatred and eventually threats and actions endangering security. It is, we believe, the combination of population expansion and spreading poverty, the "wealth gap," and the "nutritional crisis" (among others), that are causing this global destabilization. We ignore these basic human problems at great peril. As the poet reminded us, "When you got nothing, you got nothing to lose."[1]

Can this be changed?

In chapter 5 we reviewed the metaphor of the "tragedy of the commons" and discussed it further in chapter 12. Although the core message of the un-sustainabilty of a commonly held resource is relevant to our discussion of agricultural resources in specific cases, and the world's resources in general, the more important point is that our failure to meet the expectations of Article 25 of the United Nations *Universal Declaration of Human Rights* is due to the fact that we have been attempting to address a moral problem with technological solutions.

We are biological entities, and as such we are constrained in our physical and mental abilities by our biological nature. As we evolved physically, however, we also evolved mentally to the point that we were able to do something that no other life-form before us has been able to do. We are capable of controlling and modifying our environments in a way, and to an extent, that is meant to ad-dress our needs as a species, as opposed to the other way around—the natural, Darwinian order of things. When we introduced the technology of agricul-ture—domestication of plants and animals, purposeful sowing, harvesting, and storage of crops, progressively improved methods for increasing reliability and amount of yield—we set the stage for a process of technological and social evolution that has exceeded our biological capacity to manage our resources morally. Although we can develop the technology to produce more food, we seem to be unable to develop the policies, or the political will, to apply that technology in a way that guarantees adequate nutrition for all. We seem to be able to live with the suffering of "others," even if we know that to be morally reprehensible, as long as the others are "other enough" that is, distant enough in appearance, cultural background, or just in space (far enough away)—that we can consider them to be "them," and not "us." We have also developed an understanding as to why that would be the natural response from an animal that evolved to live a hunter-gatherer lifestyle in an ancestral environment that existed prior to the advent of agriculture 10,000 years ago. Changing this will require altering fundamental human behavior. Not changing will mean accept-ing the unacceptable.

Feeding everyone should be an easy task. We grow plenty of food. We know when and where extreme hunger exists and crops will fail. We can communicate this globally and instantly. We have food surpluses, aid institutions, and advanced transportation systems. Why then, as Nigel Dower challenged us in our prologue, do we "not seem to be able to replicate the practices of past smaller societies of at least trying to ensure that everyone has enough of the one crucial thing it is in the power of others to provide—namely food"?[2]

Change of this magnitude will require a paradigm shift.

o We need to break the pattern, and acceptance, of a global "nutrition crisis." It forms the underlying problem of the silent emergency happening daily to those bottom 2 billion. This is the technological fix.

o We must focus on "food security" and "food self-sufficiency." René Dumont probably got it right. A country and its people who are self-sufficient in food— "food secure"—are far better able to recover from natural and man-made calamities. Smallholder farmers, as described in chapter 13, offer an excellent and inexpensive opportunity. Increased agricultural development and food security generally have the largest positive effects on economic growth and the alleviation of poverty.

o We must aggressively address the status and education of women. As chapter 13 also detailed, improving the status of a woman in her community, most quickly by continuing her education, offers documented paybacks in terms of food production, health care, and child nutrition.

o We must revisit the entire "moral economy" issue, first suggested at the World Food Conference in 1974. Stockpiling food reserves and goods, perhaps even medical supplies, and protecting them against theft and corruption strikes us as a good idea and is far less expensive than emergency food operations.

o We need to encourage "democracy," human rights, and term limitations for national leaders. Today, states with violence and conflict that are also suffering starvation are largely autocracies (and kleptocracies), where there is little or no peaceful election process and transition of leaders (North Korea, Zimbabwe, the DRC). Amartya Sen is probably correct that famines do not occur in democratic societies.

o With this in mind, we need to continue to build peace, and particularly a global enforcement to limit conventional weapons sales. The dumping of the AK-47 assault rifle, first by the old Soviet Union in 1991–1992 and then by the Chinese in the mid-1990s, has made this combat weapon available for everyone from game poachers to child soldiers. Tighter controls on conventional weapons *might* help to reduce violence in developing states. At any rate, it should be attempted.

o While we are at it, we should help developing states to shift governmental spending out of military budgets to agriculture, health care, and education.

Spending on rural roads, seeds, fertilizer, health clinics, and school buildings has significant positive effects on growth and poverty reduction.

o Regional cooperation is also an inexpensive and comparatively easy way to link countries together for sustainable development. The Southern Africa Development Community (SADC) and the Euro-regions in central Europe offer excellent models of transboundary cooperation based on sharing natural resource and cross-border economic exchanges and social benefits (such as tourism, health, and police security).

o We must further readdress the entire concept of "aid" and the neocolonial idea that "we" have the best answers for "them." Too often the aid projects of developed states define people in terms of what they lack, not what they can provide. This includes the support of smallholder farming, the construction of food reserves, and the end to the imposition of Western economic theories from "the haves" onto the impoverished "have nots"—some of the principal lessons of the Great Irish Famine and the African case studies today.

But there still remains the "moral" problem, "the right not to starve." Will poverty and disease persist because we *cannot* prevent them or because we *will not* prevent them?

To continue as we have, to maintain the status quo, honors hunger and poverty as acceptable conditions for the world's bottom 2 billion people. Echoing the words of James Grant in 1987, the time has surely come for the international community—all of us—to agree that it is intolerable for some 29,000 young children to die every day from preventable, poverty-related causes. "Can we really say that [this] is too difficult?" Grant challenged us. "We now have the knowledge. We now have the means. And if political and public opinion in the world were to burn with intolerance of readily preventable disease and malnutrition, then who would really deny that these evils could be brought to an end in our time?" [3]

We "have the knowledge." We know. All we need to do is work hard at telling the story, at speaking out, and taking action.

Or, we can remain silent. After all, "peasants always starve."

Notes

Prologue: "Peasants Always Starve"

1. Jack Shepherd, *The Politics of Starvation* (Washington, DC: The Carnegie Endowment, 1974), 1–2.

2. Nigel Dower, "Global Hunger: Moral Dilemmas," in Ben Mepham, ed., *Food Ethics* (London: Routledge, 1996), 1. Also Newsfeed@wfp.org, "1.02 billion people hungry," June 19, 2009.

3. "WFP and Millennium Villages Unite to Cut Hunger and Malnutrition," WFP/Millennium Villages News Release, September 28, 2009, 2.

4. http://www.millenniumcampaign.org/site/pp.asp?c=grKVL2NLE&b=185518.

5. Ibid.; http://www.alertnet.org/db/topics/HUNGER.htm.

6. World Health Organization, http://www.who.int/nutrition/challenges/en/index.html. See also WFP, "Weathering the Storm," WFP Fact Sheet, 2009, http://www.wfp.org/english/?n=999.

7. "Report: More Americans Going Hungry," *Washington Post*, November 16, 2009; also USDA, Economic Research Service, "Food Security in the United States," at http://www.ers.usda.gov/briefing/Foodsecurity.

8. http://www.alertnet.org/db/topics/HUNGER.htm from UNICEF and WFP sources.

9. Centre for Global Negotiations, "The Brandt Equation: 21st Century Blueprint for the New Global Economy," http://www.brandt21forum.info/.

10. "If the World Were Food, Nobody Would Go Hungry," *The Economist* 166, November 21, 2009, 61.

11. Jeffrey D. Sachs, "Commentary: 3 Billion Poor People Need World's Help," March 20, 2009, www.cnn.com.

12. "If the World Were Food, Nobody Would Go Hungry," *The Economist* 166, 21 November 2009, 61.

13. Josette Sheeran, "High Global Food Prices: The Challenges and Opportunities," in *Responding to the Global Food Crisis: Three Perspectives* (Washington, DC: International Food Policy Research Institute, 2008), 11.

14. WHO/UNICEF, "Progress on Sanitation and Drinking-water 2010 Update" (Geneva, Switzerland: World Health Organization, 2010), 6, 7; Fogarty Center for Advanced Study in the Health Sciences, "Strategic Plan: Fiscal Years 2000–2003" (Bethesda, MD: National Institutes of Health, n.d.), www.fic.nih.gov/about/plan/exec_summary.htm; UN-Habitat, *The State of the World's Cities 2010/2011* (London: UN-Habitat, 2010), http://www.unhabitat.org/pmss/listItemDetails.aspx?publicationID=2917.

15. "Economic Crisis is Devastating for the World's Hungry," Joint FAO/WFP news release, FAO/WP, October 14, 2009.

16. "Statement by WFP Executive Director Josette Sheeran on the world food summit and feeding the hungry billion," WFP Statement, November 17, 2009.

17. Dower, "Global Hunger: Moral Dilemmas," 9–10.

18. Ibid., 1.

19. Cormac Ó Gráda. *The Great Irish Famine* (Cambridge: University of Cambridge Press, 1997), 41. The Dutch Winter Famine of 1944 is considered an "artificial famine" created by the Nazi siege of sections of the Netherlands.

20. Albert L. Lehninger, *Bioenergetics: The Molecular Basis of Biological Energy Transformations*, 2nd ed. (Reading, MA: Addison-Wesley, 1971).

21. *Universal Declaration of Human Rights*, 7.

22. Thomas Pogge, "Unjust Social Rules: Killing and Causing Pain," 35th Annual Francis W. Gramlich Memorial Lecture, Dartmouth College, April 3, 2009.

I. The Silent Emergency

1. Mehari Gebre-Medhin and Bo Vahlquist, "Famine in Ethiopia—A Brief Review," *The American Journal of Nutrition* 29 (September 1976): 1016–20.

2. U.S. Congress, Committee on Foreign Affairs, U.S. House of Representatives, *Feeding the World's Population: Developments in the Decade Following the World Food Conference of 1974* (Washington, DC: U.S. Government Printing Office, 1984), 9.

3. Ibid., 20.

4. Ibid., 8.

5. Ibid., 9.

6. Ibid., 17.

7. Ellen Messer and Marc J. Cohen, "The Human Right to Food as a US Nutrition Concern," IFPRI Discussion Paper 00731 (Washington, DC: International Food Policy Research Institute, 2007), 11.

8. Ibid., 11–12.

9. "Food as a Human Right," Interview with Asbjorn Eide, in *News & Views* (Washington, DC: International Food Policy Research Institute, April 2001), 4.

10. Smita Narula, "The Right to Food: Holding Global Actors Accountable Under International Law," Center for Human Rights and Global Justice Working Paper Number 7 (New York: New York University School of Law, 2006), 64.

11. "Food as a Human Right," 5.

12. *Universal Declaration of Human Rights*, Article 25 (Lake Success, NY: General Assembly, United Nations, December 10, 1948), 1.

13. Ibid., 7.

14. Ibid., 3.

15. Thomas Pogge, "Unjust Social Rules: Killing and Causing Pain," 35th Annual Francis W. Gramlich Memorial Lecture, Dartmouth College, April 3, 2009.

16. http://www.wfp.org/aboutwfp/introduction/hunger_what. asp?section=1&sub_section=1.

17. "Flash Points Loom in War on Hunger," *New York Times*, November 18, 2002, 27.

18. Tracey Wilkinson, "UN Says 1 Billion Face Hunger," *Los Angeles Times*, June 4, 2008, A1.

19. Josette Sheeran, "High Global Food Prices: The Challenges and Opportunities," in *Responding to the Global Food Crisis: Three Perspectives* (Washington, DC: International Food Policy Research Institute, 2008), 11.

20. Joachim von Braun, "Responding to the World Food Crisis: Getting on the Right Track," in *Responding to the Global Food Crisis: Three Perspectives* (Washington, DC: International Food Policy Research Institute, 2008), 1.

21. "If the World Were Food, Nobody Would Go Hungry," *The Economist*, November 21, 2009, 61.

22. Sheeran, "High Global Food Prices," 11.

23. Mark W. Rosegrant, *Biofuels and Grain Prices: Impacts and Policy Responses*, (Washington, DC: International Food Policy Research Institute, May 7, 2008).

24. "Man-Made Hunger," *New York Times*, editorial, July 6, 2008, 9.

25. WFP News Release, "WFP says High Food Prices a Silent Tsunami, Affecting Every Continent," April 22, 2008.

26. Sheeran, "High Global Food Prices," 11.

27. Ibid.

28. "Economic Crisis is Devastating for the World's Hungry," Joint FAO/WFP news release, FAO/WFP, October 14, 2009, 2.

29. UNICEF, "A World Fit for Children, Statistical Review," *Progress for Children*, no. 6 September 2007, 2. Available at http://www.unicef.org/search/search.php?q=global +childhood+deaths+topics%3A%22Statistics%22+millenniumdevelopmentgoals%3A %22MDG+4%3A+Child+Mortality%22&Go_x=142&Go_y=13.

30. James Grant, United National Children's Fund, *The State of the World's Children, 1987* (Oxford: Oxford University Press, 1987), 5, 7.

31. UNICEF, *Progress for Children*, 2.

32. Global Hunger Index, "The Challenge of Hunger 2008" (Bonn: International Food Policy Research Institute, October 2008), 11.

33. Goal 1: Eradicate extreme poverty and hunger; Goal 2: Achieve universal primary education; Goal 3: Promote gender equality and empower women; Goal 4: Reduce child mortality; Goal 5: Improve maternal health; Goal 6: Combat HIV/AIDS, malaria and other diseases; Goal 7: Ensure environmental sust inability; Goal 8: Develop a global partnership for development (United Nations, *The Millennium Development Goals Report*, 2007).

34. UNICEF, "A World Fit for Children," 2, 4.

35. Ibid., 18.

36. Ibid., 36.

37. WHO, available at http://www.who.int/mdg/publications/en/.

38. Angel Gurría, OECD Secretary-General, "Innovative Financing Perspectives in the New Global Economic Outlook," speech, Paris, May 28, 2009.

39. We use the term *Africa* to refer to sub-Saharan Africa, that is, Africa south of the Sahara Desert.

40. The United States gets 16 percent of its oil and *all* of its strategic minerals such as platinum, cobalt, bauxite, and manganese from sub-Saharan Africa. See, for example, Michael Klare, *Resource Wars: The New Landscape of Global Conflict* (New York: Henry Holt and Company, 2001), 220.

41. UN Development Programme, "Human Development Index," in *Human Development Report 2007/2008* (New York: United Nations, 2008), 231–232.

42. Ibid.

43. "Trends and Current Status of Malnutrition in the World," *Hunger Notes*, available at http://www.worldhunger.org/africa.htm.

44. http://www.un.org/News/Press/docs//2009/dsgsm465.doc.htm.

45. "Human Development Index," 229–354.

46. World Health Organization, 2008. "The Global Burden of Disease: 2004 Update."

"Leading causes of death," 11. HIV/AIDS statistics are notoriously suspect. They initially were projections from tests randomly given to pregnant women seeking help in clinics.

47. PRIO, Centre for the Study of Civil War, "Data on Armed Conflict," Conflict Site Dataset 2006.

48. UNHCR, "Population Levels and Trends," in *UNHCR Statistical Yearbook 2007*, Chapter II, 25, 29–30; available at http://www.unhcr.org/4981b19d2.html.

49. UNICEF, "Global child deaths have reached a record low," *The Medical News*, September 13, 2007, available at http://www.news-medical.net/news/29841.aspx.

50. Philip Gourevitch, "The Life After," *The New Yorker*, May 4, 2009, 37, 38, 39.

51. White House, text of President Barack Obama's speech in Accra, Ghana, July 11, 2009.

52. Grant, *The State of the World's Children, 1987*.

53. Ibid., 1, 5.

54. UNICEF, "A World Fit for Children," 120–125.

55. Grant, *The State of the World's Children, 1987*, 1, 7.

56. Ibid., 7.

57. Raffi Khatchadourian, "The Kill Company," *The New Yorker*, July 6, 2009, 44.

2. The Framework of Understanding

1. Michael Watts, *Silent Violence: Food, Famine and Peasantry in Northern Nigeria* (Berkeley: University of California Press, 1983), 3.

2. M. K. Bennett, "Famine," in D. L. Sills, ed., *International Encyclopedia of the Social Sciences*, vol. E (New York: Macmillan and Free Press, 1968), 322.

3. Carl C. Mabbs-Zeno, *Long-Term Impacts of Famine: Enduring Disasters and Opportunities for Progress* (Washington, DC: U.S. Department of Agriculture, Economic Research Service, International Economics Division, 1987), 12.

4. John Field, *The Challenge of Famine* (Boston: Kumarian Press, 1993), 4.

5. N. S. Scrimshaw, "The Phenomena of Famine," *Annual Review of Nutrition* (1987), 2.

6. Jim Wurst, "Africa: Region Faces 'Unprecedented Crisis' WFP Tells Security Council," *UN Wire*, December 4, 2002, 1.

7. UNICEF, "A World Fit for Children, Statistical Review," *Progress for Children*, no. 6 (September 2007), 30.

8. Andrew Tomkins, "Comparison of Nutrient Composition of Refugee Populations and Pet Foods," *The Lancet* 320 (August 8, 1992), 367–68.

9. See, for example, J. Appleton, et al., "Nutrition of Refugees and Displaced Populations," in *The Fourth Report on the World Nutrition Situation, Nutrition Throughout the Lifecycle*, ed. Administrative Committee on Co-ordination, Subcommittee on Nutrition (Washington, DC: International Food Policy Research Institute, 2000); and Mike Toole, "Protecting the Health of Conflict-Affected Populations, Lessons Learned: 1976–2001," paper presented at the Global Health Council's annual conference (Melbourne: Centre for International Health), 2002.

10. *WFP News*, "Drought and Lack of Food Aid Threaten Millions of Ethiopians," November 12, 2002.

11. UNfoundation.org, "North Korea: WFP Calls for $201 Million to Feed 6.4 Million Next Year," December 3, 2002.

12. Wurst, "Africa: Region Faces 'Unprecedented Crisis.'"

13. Amartya Sen, *Poverty and Famines: An Essay on Entitlement and Deprivation* (Oxford: Clarendon Press, 1982), 1. Italics in text.

14. Stephen Devereux, *Theories of Famine* (New York: Harvester/Wheatsheaf, 1993).

15. Ibid., 21.

16. Ibid., 26.

17. Ibid., 26.

18. Ibid., 183.

19. Ibid., 27.

20. Ibid., 22.

21. Ibid., 22.

22. Ibid., 22.

23. ICIHI, 1985, 63; quoted in Devereux, *Theories of Famine*, 27–28.

24. Sen, *Poverty and Famines*, 459; quoted in Devereux, *Theories of Famine*, 28.

25. Devereux, *Theories of Famine*, 68.

26. Sen, *Poverty and Famines*, 454; quoted in Devereux, *Theories of Famine*, 72.

27. Devereux, *Theories of Famine*, 77.

28. Ibid.

29. Alex de Waal, "War in Sudan: an analysis of conflict," London: Peace in Sudan Group, 1990; see also Devereux, *Theories of Famine*, 77.

30. Amartya Sen, "The causes of famine: A reply," *Food Policy* 11 (May 1986), 9–10; Devereux, *Theories of Famine*, 78.

31. Devereux, *Theories of Famine*, 81.

32. Ibid., 81, 82.

Lessons: The Causes of Starvation

1. Cormac Ó Gráda, *The Great Irish Famine* (Cambridge: Cambridge University Press, 1995), 68.

2. N. S. Scrimshaw, "The Phenomena of Famine," *Annual Review of Nutrition*, (1987), 2.

3. The Dutch Winter Famine of 1944 killed an estimated 18,000 people. It is considered an "artificial famine" caused by the Nazi siege of parts of the Netherlands. It continued to be of significant medical interest long afterwards, however, because of the availability of medical records and survivors. Studies of them have contributed greatly to the understanding of the long-term effects of starvation on those who survive.

4. Richard B. Stott, *Workers in the Metropolis: Class, Ethnicity and Youth in Antebellum New York City* (Ithaca, NY: Cornell University Press, 1989), Table 9, 73.

5. R. Dudley Edwards and T. Desmond Williams, "Foreword," in *The Great Famine: Studies in Irish History, 1845–1852* (Dublin: The Lilliput Press, 1994), edited by R. Dudley Edwards and T. Desmond Williams, xiv.

6. Celticfestvancouver.com; "Calgary Tower Gets Full Green Bulb Treatment," *Calgary Herald*, http://www.calgaryherald.com/news/Calgary+Tower+gets+full+green+bulb+treatment/1378992/story.html.

7. Ó Gráda, *The Great Irish Famine*, 1–2.

8. Ibid., 3.

9. In 1997, the British Prime Minister Tony Blair apologized publicly to the Irish people for the failure of past British administrations to respond fully to the calamity of the Great Irish Famine.

10. Liz Young, "Spaces for Famine: a Comparative Geographical Analysis of Famine in Ireland and the Highlands in the 1840s," *Transactions of the Institute of British Geographers*, 21, no. 4 (December 1996), 666–80.

11. Edwards and Williams, *The Great Famine*, viii.

12. Ibid., x.

13. Ibid., 5, 26.

14. Mary E. Daly, *The Population of Ireland* (Dublin: Dundalgan Press, 1987), 8.

15. Irish emigration to the United States, available at http://www.irishinnyc.freeservers .com/custom3.html.

16. Ó Gráda, *The Great Irish Famine*, 7, 8.

17. John O'Beirne Ranelagh, *A Short History of Ireland*, (Cambridge: Cambridge University Press, 1994), 114.

18. Ó Gráda, *The Great Irish Famine*, 8.

19. The name comes from a current description of South Africa's poor, who are compressed across the bottom of their poverty and unemployment statistics.

20. Ó Gráda, *The Great Irish Famine*, 30–31.

21. Ibid., 23.

22. See, for example, Joel Mokyr and Cormac Ó Gráda, "Emigration and Poverty in Prefamine Ireland," *Explorations in Economic History* 19, no. 3 (July 1982).

23. Edwards and Williams, *The Great Famine*, 89.

24. Ibid., xi.

25. Ranelagh, *A Short History of Ireland*, 112.

26. Ó Gráda, *The Great Irish Famine*, 33.

27. Cecil Woodham-Smith, *The Great Hunger: Ireland 1845–1849* (London: Penguin Books, 1991), 50–51.

28. Ó Gráda, *The Great Irish Famine*, 32.

29. Ibid., 34.

30. Ibid.

31. Ranelagh, *A Short History of Ireland*, 114.

32. *The Economist*, January 2, 1847, 3b; and January 30, 1847, 4a.

33. Ó Gráda, *The Great Irish Famine*, 34.

34. Ibid., 45.

35. Ibid., 23.

36. Woodham-Smith, *The Great Hunger: Ireland 1845–1849*, 75.

37. Cormac Ó Gráda, *Ireland Before and After the Famine* (Manchester: Manchester University Press, 1993), 68.

38. Christine Kinealy, *This Great Calamity: The Irish Famine 1845–1852* (Boulder, CO: Roberts Rinehart, 1995), 160, 162

39. Ranelagh, *A Short History of Ireland*, 115.

40. Ibid., 115.

41. Stephen Devereux, *Theories of Famine* (New York: Harvester/Wheatsheaf, 1993), 71.

42. Young, "Spaces for Famine," 675.

43. Joseph McPartlin, "Diet, Politics, and Disaster: The Great Irish Famine," *Proceedings of the Nutrition Society* 56 (1997), 222.

44. Young, "Spaces for Famine," 672.

45. Data available at http://www.assumption.edu/ahc/Irish/TideofEmigration.html.

3. The Basics of Nutrition

1. P. Bellwood, *First Farmers: The Origins of Agricultural Societies* (Cambridge, MA: Blackwell Publishing, 2004).

2. G. Lechler, "Prehistoric Diet," *Michigan History Magazine* 27 (1943): 537–38.

3. C. C. Furnas and S. M. Furnas, *Man, Bread and Destiny* (New York: Reynal & Hitchcock, 1937), xix.

4. Available at http://www.biblegateway.com/.

5. University of Minnesota Laboratory of Physiological Hygiene and A. B. Keys, *The Biology of Human Starvation*. (Minneapolis: University of Minnesota Press, 1950).

6. Ibid.

7. Special to the *New York Times*, "Levanzin's New Charges: Fasting Professor Says He Was Nearly Killed by Sulphuric Acid," May 21, 1912; available online at http://query.nytimes.com/mem/archive-free/pdf?_r=1&res=9802E0DA153CE633A25751C2A9639C946396D6CF.

8. F. G. Benedict, W. R. Miles, P. Roth, and H. M. Smith, *Human Vitality and Efficiency under Prolonged Restricted Diet* (Washington, DC: Carnegie Institution of Washington, 1919).

9. *Leaves of Grass*, "Song of Myself," verse 31.

10. On acceptance of the Nobel Prize in Physics, December 8, 1983.

11. T. R. Gregory and R. DeSalle, "Comparative Genomics in Prokaryotes," in T. R. Gregory, ed., *The Evolution of the Genome* (Elsevier: San Diego, 2005), 585–675.

12. Available from: http://genomics.energy.gov/.

13. E. V. Koonin, A. R. Mushegian, M. Y. Galperin, and D. R. Walker, "Comparison of Archaeal and Bacterial Genomes: Computer Analysis of Protein Sequences Predicts Novel Functions and Suggests a Chimeric Origin for the Archaea," *Molecular Microbiology* 25, no. 4 (1997): 619–37.

14. A. L. Lehninger, D. L. Nelson, and M. M. Cox, eds. *Lehninger Principles of Biochemistry*. 4th ed. (New York: W. H. Freeman, 2005).

15. V. L. Mcguire, *Water-Level Changes in the High Plains Aquifer, Predevelopment to 2005 and 2003 to 2005*. Available at http://pubs.usgu.gov/sir/2006/5324/. Accessed March 22, 2007.

16. J. Bartam, Kristen Lewis, Roberto Lenton, and Albert Wright, "Millenium Development Project Focusing on Improved Water and Sanitation for Health, *The Lancet* 365, no. 9461 (2005): 810–12.

17. World Health Organization. *Global Health: Today's Challenges*. Available at http://www.who.int/whr/2003/chapter1/en/index2.html. Accessed June 20, 2008.

18. R. Lenton, Albert Wright, and Kristen Lewis. *UN Millennium Project Task Force on Water and Sanitation: Health, Dignity, and Development: What Will It Take?* [cited 2009 June 19]; Available at http://www.unmillenniumproject.org/documents/WaterComplete-lowres.pdf. Accessed June 19, 2009.

19. Ibid.

20. Charles Darwin, The Descent of Man (London: John Murray, 1871).

21. Lehninger, Nelson, and Cox, *Lehninger Principles of Biochemistry*.

4. The Anatomy and Physiology of Nutrition

The first chapter epigraph is from L. H. Sullivan and D. D. Walker, *The Autobiography of an Idea* (New York: Press of the American Institute of Architects, 1924).

1. H. Gray and P. L. Williams, *Gray's Anatomy*, 37th ed. (Edinburgh: C. Livingstone, 1989).

2. A. C. Guyton and J. E. Hall, *Textbook of Medical Physiology*, 11th ed. (Philadelphia: Elsevier Saunders, 1989), xxxv.

3. M. E. Shils and M. Shike, *Modern Nutrition in Health and Disease*, 10th ed. (Philadelphia: Lippincott Williams & Wilkins 2006), xxv.

4. P. S. Holzman, "Seymour S. Kety," *Nature Medicine* 6 (2000), 727.

5. G. F. Cahill Jr., "Starvation in Man," *New England Journal of Medicine* 282, no. 12 (1970): 668–75.

6. G. F. Cahill Jr., "Editorial: Nitrogen Versatility in Bats, Bears and Man," *New England Journal of Medicine* 290, no. 12 (1974): 686–87.

7. O. E. Owen et al., "Brain Metabolism during Fasting," *Journal of Clinical Investigation* 46, no. 10 (1967): 1589–95.

8. G. F. Cahill Jr., "Fuel Metabolism in Starvation," *Annual Review of Nutrition* 26 (2006): 1–22.

5. Agriculture

1. Jared M. Diamond, *Guns, Germs, and Steel: The Fates of Human Societies* (New York: W. W. Norton & Co., 1997).

2. R. Pumpelly and O. S. Rice, *Travels and Adventures of Raphael Pumpelly, Mining Engineer, Geologist, Archaeologist and Explorer* (New York: Henry Holt and Co., 1920).

3. Vere Gordon Childe, *Man Makes Himself*, 4th ed. (London: Collins, 1966), xvii.

4. A. B. Gebauer, T. D. Price, and Society for American Anthropology, *Transitions to Agriculture in Prehistory. Monographs in World Archaeology* (Madison, WI: Prehistory Press, 1992), vii.

5. C. O. Sauer, *Agricultural Origins and Dispersals* (New York: American Geographical Society, 1952), v; S. R. Binford, L. R. Binford, and American Anthropological Association, *New Perspectives in Archeology* (Chicago: Aldine, 1968), x.

6. D. Rindos, *The Origins of Agriculture: An Evolutionary Perspective* (Orlando, FL: Academic Press, 1984), xvii.

7. S. Wells, *The Journey of Man: A Genetic Odyssey* (New York: Random House, 2002), xvi.

8. Adam Smith, *An Inquiry into the Nature and Causes of the Wealth of Nations* (Dublin: Whitestone, Chamberlaine, W. Watson, Potts, S. Watson [and 15 others], 1776).

9. C. J. Wheelan, *Naked Economics: Undressing the Dismal Science* (New York: Norton, 2002), xxii.

10. M. Pollan, *The Omnivore's Dilemma: A Natural History of Four Meals* (New York: Penguin Press, 2006).

11. Childe, *Man Makes Himself*, xvii.

12. R. E. Leakey and R. Lewin, *Origins: What New Discoveries Reveal about the Emergence of Our Species and Its Possible Future* (London: Macdonald and Jane's, 1977).

13. D. L. Clarke, I. Hodder, G. L. Isaac, and N. Hammond, *Pattern of the Past: Studies in Honour of David Clarke* (Cambridge: Cambridge University Press, 1981), ix.

14. A. M. Watson, "The Arab Agricultural Revolution and Its Diffusion 700–1100," *Journal of Economic History* 34, no. 1 (1974): 8–35; A. M. Watson, "A Medieval Green Revolution: New Crops and Farming Techniques in the Early Islamic World," in *The Islamic Middle East, 700–1900: Studies in Economic and Social History* (Princeton: Darwin Press, 1981).

15. P. Steinhart, "The Second Green Revolution," *New York Times Magazine*, October 25, 1981, 46–53.

16. Genesis 39:2.

17. Genesis 41:14.

18. Genesis 41:1–54.

19. Genesis 47: 13–20.

20. W. F. Lloyd, "Two Lectures on the Checks to Population," in *Michaelmas Term* (S. Collingwood: University of Oxford, 1832), 75.

21. G. Hardin, "The Tragedy of the Commons. The Population Problem Has No Technical Solution; It Requires a Fundamental Extension in Morality," *Science* 162 (1968): 243–48.

22. R. DeYoung, "Tragedy of the Commons," in *Encyclopedia of Environmental Science*, R. W. F. D. E. Alexander, ed. (Hingham: Kluwer Academic Publishers, 1999).

23. W. Maathai, *The Green Belt Movement: Sharing the Approach and the Experience*, rev. ed. (New York: Lantern Books, 2003), x; W. Maathai, *Unbowed: A Memoir* (New York: Anchor Books, 2007), xvii; http://nobelprize.org/nobel_prizes/peace/laureates/2004/press.html.

Lessons: Nutrition

1. See, for example, Cormac Ó Gráda, *The Great Irish Famine* (Cambridge: Cambridge University Press, 1995), 5–8.

2. Liz Young, "Spaces for Famine: A Comparative Geographical Analysis of Famine in Ireland and the Highlands in the 1840s," *Transactions of the Institute of British Geographers* 12, no. 4 (December 1996): 676,

3. See, for example, L. A. Clarkson and E. Margaret Crawford, *Feast and Famine: Food and Nutrition in Ireland 1500–1920* (Oxford: Oxford University Press, 2001); and Cormac Ó Gráda, *Ireland: A New Economic History 1780–1939* (Oxford: Clarendon Press, 1994).

4. Joseph McPartlin, "Diet, Politics, and Disaster: The Great Irish Famine," *Proceedings of the Nutrition Society* 56 (1997): 212.

5. Both by Arthur Young in 1778 traveling around Ireland and during World War I by British nutritionists. See Ó Gráda, *The Great Irish Famine*, 54, 55.

6. Ó Gráda, *The Great Irish Famine*, 15–17.

7. Cormac Ó Gráda, "Poverty, Population, and Agriculture, 1801–1845," in *A New History of Ireland*, ed. W. E. Vaughan (Oxford: Clarendon Press, 1989), 122.

8. Young, "Spaces for Famine," 674.

9. Mary E. Daly, *The Famine in Ireland* (Dublin: Dundalgan Press, 1986), 17.

10. McPartlin, "Diet, Politics, and Disaster," 214.

11. Clarkson and Crawford, *Feast and Famine*, 121.

12. McPartlin, "Diet, Politics, and Disaster," 214; and, Ó Gráda, *The Great Irish Famine*, 18, 19.

13. McPartlin, "Diet, Politics, and Disaster," 216.

14. Ibid., 211–212.

15. Ó Gráda, *The Great Irish Famine*, 68.

16. E. Margaret Crawford. "Scurvy in Ireland during the Great Famine," *Social History of Medicine* 1, no. 3 (1988): 290.

17. "The Potato: Spud We Like," *The Economist* (March 1, 2008): 18.

18. Ibid.

19. McPartlin, "Diet, Politics, and Disaster," 216, 217.

20. John O'Beirne Ranelagh, *A Short History of Ireland* (Cambridge: Cambridge University Press, 1994), 115.

21. Mary E. Daly, *The Population of Ireland* (Dublin: Dundalgan Press, 1987), 113.

22. McPartlin, "Diet, Politics, and Disaster," 222.

23. Ó Gráda, *The Great Irish Famine*, 37, 38.

24. Ibid., 55.

25. McPartlin, "Diet, Politics, and Disaster," 217.

26. Ibid.; see also Mary A. Moloney, "The Famine Soup-Kitchens," available at http://www.limerick.com/lifestyle/soupkitchen.html.

27. Moloney, "The Famine Soup-Kitchens," 38.

28. http://www.theshipslist.com/1847/index.htm.

29. In 1992, almost 150 years after the Great Irish Famine and the Choctaw gift, eight Irish descendents of survivors of the Famine made the 500-mile walk from Broken Bow, Oklahoma, to Nanih Waiya, Mississippi—the "Trail of Tears"—in appreciation for that gift. The Irish and the Native Americans were seeking to raise $71,000—one hundred times the original amount—for famine relief in Somalia. See Mike Ward, "Irish Repay Choctaw Famine Gift: March Traces Trail of Tears in Trek for Somalian Relief," *American-Statesman Capitol* (1992), at http://www.uwm.edu/~michael/choctaw/retrace.html.

30. Piers Brendon, *The Decline and Fall of the British Empire, 1781–1997* (New York: Vintage Books, 2010), 123.

31. McPartlin, "Diet, Politics, and Disaster," 218.

32. Ó Gráda, *The Great Irish Famine*, 39.

33. Ibid., 42.

34. Thomas Gallagher, *Paddy's Lament: Ireland 1846–1847, Prelude to Hatred* (New York: Harcourt Brace & Co., 1982), 104

35. Cathal Poirteir, *Famine Echoes* (Dublin: Gill and MacMillan, Ltd, 1995), 11.

36. Cecil Woodham-Smith, *The Great Hunger, Ireland 1845–9* (London: Hamish Hamilton, 1962), 141.

37. Ibid., 159.

38. Ibid., 163.

39. Available at http://www.wesleyjohnston.com/users/ireland/past/famine/ summer_1847.html.

40. Ranelagh, *A Short History of Ireland*, 114.

41. http://www.theshipslist.com/1847/index.htm; see also W. A. Carrothers, *Emigration from the British Isles* (London: Frank Cass & Co., 1965), 305.

42. McPartlin, "Diet, Politics, and Disaster," 219; and, Poirteir, *Famine Echoes*, 182.

43. McPartlin, "Diet, Politics, and Disaster," 219.

44. Sam Porter, "Confronting Famine: The Case of the Irish Great Hunger," *Nursing Inquiry* 5 (1998): 115.

45. The Irish Brigade was composed of the 63rd New York Infantry, the 69th Infantry Regiment, the 88th New York Infantry, the 116th Pennsylvania Infantry, and the 28th Massachusetts Infantry. The Brigade fought at the First Battle of Bull Run, the Battle of Gettysburg, the Seven Days Battles, the Second Battle of Bull Run, the Battle of Antietam, and the Battle of Fredericksburg, among others. The Brigade took such high casualties (1,344 killed at the Battle of Fredericksburg; 60 percent at Antietam alone) that it was disbanded and reformed as the Second Irish Brigade in 1864. The 69th Infantry Regiment fought in World War I, and as part of the 27th New York Division in the Pacific in World War II. From 2004 to 2005, the 1st Battalion, 69th Infantry, fought in and around Baghdad, Iraq. See, for example, http://88ny.net/Battles.htm.

46. Brendon, *The Decline and Fall of the British Empire, 1781–1997*, 124.

6. Responses on the Ground

1. World Food Programme Report, August 16, 2005, at http://www.wfp.org/news/ news-release/wfp-increases-mali-appeal-help-175000-children-under-five.

2. By "artificial famines" we mean deliberate acts of starvation by one group of people against another. These include Stalin's starvation of the Ukrainians, 1933; the Nazi starvation

of the Dutch in the winter of 1944–1945; Robert Mugabe's actions against selected millions of Zimbabweans, 2000–2008; and the political and economic choices of North Korea's leaders to feed its army instead of its people, 1995–2008.

3. "The essential element is a relatively *sudden collapse* in the level of food *consumption* by *large numbers of people*. Starvation refers to people going without sufficient food, and during famines people do so on such a large scale that mortality is high. . . . [F]amine is not just the result of an extreme and protracted shortage of food, but also an *economic and social phenomenon* that can occur *when food supplies are adequate to prevent it*." Nevin S. Scrimshaw, "The Phenomenon of Famine," *Annual Review of Nutrition* 7 (1987): 2.

4. Scrimshaw, "The Phenomenon of Famine," 1.

5. John Osgood Field, ed., "What Is Famine," in *The Challenge of Famine* (Sterling, VA: Kumarian Press, 1993), 4.

6. Jack Shepherd, *The Politics of Starvation* (Washington, DC: The Carnegie Endowment for International Peace, 1974), 14.

7. Ibid., 19.

8. Perhaps as many as a million evicted Irish peasants went searching for food. See Cormac Ó Gráda, *The Great Irish Famine* (Cambridge: Cambridge University Press, 1995), 32–56.

9. Ó Gráda, *The Great Irish Famine*, 43.

10. Alexander de Waal, *Famine that Kills* (Oxford: Clarendon Press, 1989).

11. Ibid., 6.

12. Ibid., 6.

13. Ibid., 9.

14. Ibid., 76.

15. Ibid., 77.

16. Jenny Edkins, "Legality with a Vengeance: Famines and Humanitarian Relief in 'Complex Emergencies,'" *Millennium Journal of International Studies* 25, No. 3 (1996): 553.

17. Jeevan Vasagar, "Plenty of Food—Yet the Poor Are Starving," *The Guardian*, August 1, 2005. Available at http://www.msf.org/msfinternational/invoke.cfm?objectid =713F2725-E018-0C72-09A8820B841B1066&component=toolkit.article&method=full_html.

18. See Mike Davis, *Late Victorian Holocausts: El Niño Famines and the Making of the Third World* (London: Verso, 2001), 280–285; and, Michael Watts and Hans Bohle, "Hunger, Famine, and the Space of Vulnerability," *Geojournal* 30 (1993): 117–25.

19. Davis, *Late Victorian Holocausts*, 281.

20. Robert Stock, *Africa South of the Sahara* (New York: The Guilford Press, 2004), 232.

21. The idea has also been part of U.S. agricultural policy, but in a somewhat different form. During the Great Depression, Henry Wallace, the secretary of agriculture, created the "Ever-Normal Granary" concept in which the government guaranteed a pricing "floor" at which it bought crops from U.S. farmers and stored them. The crops could be sold, distributed, or even "sold back" to the farmer who could then put them on the market when prices rose. In the 1933 Agricultural Adjustment Act, the Roosevelt administration put some of Wallace's idea into law and created the Community Credit Corporation, still operating today, as accountants for the "Ever-Normal Granary." This included U.S. staples such as wheat and corn. See, for example, Henry A. Wallace, *Democracy Reborn* (New York: Da Capo Press, 1973); and John C. Culver and John Hyde, *American Dreamer: A Life of Henry A. Wallace* (New York: W. W. Norton, 2000).

22. Stock, *Africa South of the Sahara*, 232–233. See also Michael Watts and H. Boyle,

"Hunger, Famine, and the Space of Vulnerability," *Geojournal* 30 (1993), 117–125; and Sheldon Gellar, "The Colonial Era," in *Africa*, edited by Phyllis M. Martin and Patrick O'Meara, 3rd ed. (Bloomington: Indiana University Press, 1995), 135–155.

23. Richard Peet, *Modern Geographical Thought* (London: Blackwell Publishing, 1998), 96.

24. Liz Young, "Spaces for Famine: A Comparative Geographical Analysis of Famine in Ireland and the Highlands in the 1840s," *Transactions of the Institute of British Geographers* 21, no. 4 (December 1996): 671.

25. Barry Bearak, "Why People Still Starve," *New York Times*, July 13, 2003, 33.

26. "Death by Starvation in Malawi: The Link between Macro-economic and Structural Policies and the Agricultural Disaster in Malawi," An ActionAid Policy Brief, June 13, 2002, 1.

27. Stephen Devereux, "State of Disaster: Causes, Consequences and Policy Lessons," an ActionAid Report, June 2002, available at http://www.ids.ac.uk/go/idsproject/food-supply-crisis-and-food-security-in-malawi. "Nyasaland" was the colonial name for Malawi.

28. Raphael Tenthai, "Malawi Declares Famine Emergency," BBC News, February 27, 2002.

29. Devereux, "State of Disaster."

30. ActionAid, "Death by Starvation in Malawi," 1.

31. Tenthai, BBC News, February 27, 2002.

32. Bearak, "Why People Still Starve," 34.

33. Ibid.

34. Stephen Devereux, "The Malawi Famine of 2002: Causes, Consequences, and Policy Lessons," Lilongwe, Malawi, May 30, 2002; published online February 2, 2009, at http://www3.interscience.wiley.com/journal/121648427/issue.

35. BBC News, "Country Profile: Malawi," available online at http://www.fco.gov.uk/en/travel-and-living-abroad/travel-advice-by-country/country-profile/sub-saharan-africa/malawi/?profile=all.

36. Smita Narula, "The Right to Food: Holding Global Actors Accountable under International Law," Center for Human Rights and Global Justice Working Paper Number 7 (New York: New York University School of Law, 2006), 15–16.

37. Ibid., 16.

38. See, for example, impacts of ESAPs on Bangladesh, Ecuador, Hungary, Mexico, and the Philippines: Yassaman Saadatmand and Michael Toma, "IMF-inducted Structural Adjustment Programs and Women in Ecuador," available online at http://www.entrepreneur.com/tradejournals/article/180564341.html; *The Sapri Report: The Policy Roots of Economic Crisis, Poverty and Inequality*, prepared by the Structural Adjustment Participatory Review International Network (Washington, DC: SAPRIN), April 2002, http://www.saprin.org/global_rpt.htm; John W. Peabody, "Economic Reform and Health Sector Policy: Lessons from Structural Adjustment Programs," Division of General Internal Medicine, West Los Angeles Veteran's Affairs Medical Center, Los Angeles, California, February 24, 1999; William Easterly, "What Did Structural Adjustment Adjust? The Association of Policies and Growth with Repeated IMF and World Bank Adjustment Loans," *Journal of Development Economics* 76, no. 1 (February 2005): 1–22; Marc Lindenberg and Shantayanan Devarajan, "Prescribing Strong Economic Medicine: Revisiting the Myths about Structural Adjustment, Democracy," *Comparative Politics* 25, no. 2 (January 1993): 169–182; John W. Mellor, "Food Policy, Food Aid and Structural Adjustment Programmes," *Food Policy* 13, no. 1 (February 1988): 10–17; Padma Gotur, "Bangladesh: Economic Reform Measures and the Poor," in *Social Safety Nets: Issues and Recent Experiences*, edited by Ke-young Chu and Sanjeev Gupta (Washington, DC: International Monetary Fund, 1998), 117–129; "Trade Liberalization

Policies and Their Impact on the Manufacturing Sector," in *The Policy Roots of Economic Crisis and Poverty: A Multi-Country Participatory Assessment of Structural Adjustment*, prepared by the Structural Adjustment Participatory Review International Network (SAPRIN), April 2002; "Structural Adjustment Programs at the Root of the Global Social Crisis: Case Studies from Latin America," prepared by The Development GAP for the Social Summit in Copenhagen, 1995, available online at http://www.rrojasdatabank.info/stradj1.htm; Judith Adler Hellman, "Structural Adjustment in Mexico and the Dog That Didn't Bark," CERLAC Working Paper Series, April 1997.

39. http://www.globalissues.org/article/10/food-aid-as-dumping. See also Global Policy Forum, at http://globalpolicy.org/component/content/article/209-bwi-wto/43084.html; State of the World's Children, Table 2, 122.

40. Stock, *Africa South of the Sahara*, 143.

41. Narula, "The Right to Food," 16, 17.

42. House of Commons, International Development Committee, "The Humanitarian Crisis in Southern Africa," Third Report of Session 200–2003, *Volume I: Report and Proceedings of the Committee*, HC 116–1, March 4, 2003, 33.

43. Ibid., 34.

44. Mark W. Rosegrant, Sarah A. Cline, Weibo Li, Timothy B. Sulser, and Rowena Valmonte-Santos, "Looking Ahead: Long-Term Prospects for Africa's Agricultural Development and Food Security," IFPRI 2020 Discussion Paper 41 (Washington, DC: IFPRI, August 2005). See also Narula, "The Right to Food," footnote, 17.

45. John Iliffe, *Africans: The History of a Continent* (Cambridge: Cambridge University Press, 1995), 246.

46. Jesse Jackson, *Los Angeles Times*, September 29, 1998; at Africa Action, http://www.africaaction.org/docs99/dbt9903b.htm.

47. As did other African states, including Ethiopia and Mali.

48. ActionAid, "Death by Starvation in Malawi," 5.

49. Ibid., 4.

50. Ibid., 5.

51. Ibid., 2.

52. "Malawi Leader Blames IMF for Food Crisis," Reuters, June 6, 2002.

53. "Interview—IMF Denies Advising Malawi to Sell Food," Reuters, May 28, 2002.

54. ActionAid, "Death by Starvation in Malawi," 6.

55. Ibid., 3.

56. Raphael Tenthani, "Malawi Donors Suspend Aid," BBC News, November 19, 2001.

57. Bearak, "Why People Still Starve," 33.

58. "Evaluation of the 2006/2007 Agricultural Input Subsidy Programme, Malawi," Final Report, March 2008, School of Oriental and American Studies (SOAS), London, ii, iii.

59. Ibid., iii.

60. "Malawi: Can It Feed Itself?" *The Economist*, May 3, 2008, 57.

61. Bearak, "Why People Still Starve," 60.

62. Mali ranks 174/177 and Niger 173/177. UNDP, "The Human Development Index," available at http://hdrstats.undp.org/2008/countries/country_fact_sheets/cty_fs_NER.html. The Index measures life expectancy, education, "a decent standard of living," and serves as "a broadened prism for viewing human progress and the complex relationship between income and well-being."

63. WFP Newsfeed, August 9, 2005, available at www.wfp.org.

64. Ibid., August 5, 2005.

65. Duval Smith, "IMF and EU Are Blamed for Starvation in Niger" (*Independent*, August 1, 2005), 23; and Craig Timberg, "The Rise of a Market Mentality Means Many Go Hungry in Niger," *Washington Post*, August 11, 2005, A17.

66. Narula, "The Right to Food," 19.

67. Vasagar, "Plenty of Food."

68. "Embassy: Ongoing Coup Attempt Taking Place in Niger," February 15, 2010, available at http://www.cnn.com/2010/WORLD/africa/02/18/niger.coup/index.html?hpt=T2.

69. Ibid.

70. Médecins Sans Frontières, available at http://www.msf.org/msfinternational/invoke.cfm?objectid=C26C30E1-E018-0C72-094D3663807A34F5&component=toolkit.article&method=full_html, June 28, 2005.

71. Narula, "The Right to Food," 19; see also Smith, "IMF and EU Are Blamed," 23; and Timberg, "The Rise of a Market Mentality," A17.

72. Vasagar, "Plenty of Food."

73. Narula, "The Right to Food," 19; also Vasagar, "Plenty of Food."

74. "Acute malnutrition," also sometimes called "global acute malnutrition," includes severe and moderate malnutrition that occurs when a person's weight-to-waist ratio falls below 70 percent of the norm.

75. WFP Report, August 16, 2005, at www.wfp.org. A "ton" is 2000 pounds whereas a "metric ton" is 2,205 pounds, or roughly 1.1 tons. It is often abbreviated as "MT."

76. Jeevan Vasagar, "Don't Blame the Locusts," *The Guardian*, August 12, 2005. See also Narula, "The Right to Food," 19.

77. WFP Newsfeed August 5, 2005, available at www.wfp.org.

7. Responses: Government and International

1. U.S. Congress, "Feeding the World's Population: Developments in the Decade Following the World Food Conference of 1974," Committee on Foreign Affairs, U.S. House of Representatives (Washington, DC: U.S. Government Printing Office, 1984), 26.

2. Food and Agriculture Organization of the United Nations, "GIEWS: The Global Information and Early Warning System on Food and Agriculture" (March 2010), 4, 6–9, 10, 17, 22, 23. See www.fao.org/giews or http://www.fao.org/giews/english/about.htm.

3. Ibid., 2 ("Foreword" by Jacques Diouf).

4. Sophia Murphy and Kathy McAfee, "U.S. Food Aid: Time to Get It Right," (Minneapolis: Institute for Agriculture and Trade Policy, 2005), 4.

5. Ibid., 9.

6. Ibid., 10.

7. Ibid., 8.

8. INTERFAIS, Food Aid Monitor, June 2008, 17, 18. Available at http://one.wfp.org/interfais/index2.htm.

9. WFP News Release, "China Emerges as World's Third Largest Food Aid Donor," July 20, 2006.

10. WFP News Release, August 9, 2005; Murphy and McAfee, "U.S. Food Aid: Time to Get It Right," 11.

11. INTERFAIS, Food Aid Monitor, 20.

12. WFP Newsfeed, August 9, 2005.

13. See, for example, the endnote at "WFP Scales Up Emergency Distributions Under Operation Lifeline Gaza," WFP News Release, January 22, 2009.

14. UN Office for the Coordination of Humanitarian Affairs, "Southern Africa: Lessons learnt in early warning," January 8, 2003.

15. WFP News Release, July 20, 2006.

16. The Bill Emerson Humanitarian Trust is a food reserve for Public Law (PL) 480 administered by USDA. It is allowed to hold up to 4 million MT of corn, rice, sorghum, and wheat "to meet unanticipated emergency needs that cannot otherwise be met under Title II of PL 480." See http://www.fas.usda.gov/excredits/FoodAid/emersontrust.asp.

17. Title I, administered by the USDA, provides for program aid through concessional sales of agricultural commodities to developing nations. Title II, administered by USAID, sends emergency aid, usually donations of food, for humanitarian purposes either by direct feeding or purchase of agricultural products locally. Title III (USAID), food for development, is a government-to-government grant to least-developed states for long-term food and nutrition programs. Title IV is no longer funded. Title V (USAID) offers short-term technical assistance by U.S. farmers, who volunteer to work with farmers in developing states to improve their food production and marketing.

18. http://www.fas.usda.gov, 1.

19. http://www.fas.usda.gov, 2.

20. http://www.fas.usda.gov, 3.

21. Murphy and McAfee, "U.S. Food Aid: Time to Get It Right," 3, 4.

22. See, for example, Christopher B. Barnett and Daniel G. Maxwell, *Food Aid after Fifty Years* (London: Routledge, 2005), the basic primer; and Carol Lancaster, *Foreign Aid: Diplomacy, Development, Domestic Politics* (Chicago: University of Chicago Press, 2007); Brester Kneen, "The Invisible Giant: Cargill and Its Transnational Strategies," in Nora Haenn and Richard R. Wilk, eds. *The Environment in Anthropology: A Reader in Ecology, Culture, and Sustainable Living* (New York: New York University Press, 2006).

23. Murphy and McAfee, "U.S. Food Aid: Time to Get It Right," 1.

24. For a discussion about relief camps, see Peter Salama, Paul Spiegel, Leisel Talley, and Ronald Waldman, "Lessons Learned from Complex Emergencies over the Past Decade," *The Lancet* 364 (November 13, 2004), available at www.thelancet.com.

25. U.S. Congress, "Feeding the World's Population," 9.

26. Dean Baquet and Diana B. Henriques, "Abuses Plague Programs to Help Exports of Agricultural Products," *New York Times*, October 10, 1993. To see some of those donations in the House Agriculture and House Resources Committees, explore http://www.opensecrets.org/cmteprofiles/overview.php?cmteid=H02&cmte=HAGR&congno=111&chamber=H. For donations to members of the Senate Agriculture, Nutrition and Forestry Committee, and the Energy and Natural Resources Committee, see http://www.opensecrets.org/cmteprofiles/overview.php?cmteid=S02&cmte=SAGR&congno=111&chamber=S.

27. Peter M. Rosset, *Food Is Different: Why We Must Get the WTO out of Agriculture* (New York: Zed Books, 2006), 46; Brester Kneen, "The Invisible Giant," 444.

28. Timothy Egan, "Big Farms Reap Two Harvests with Subsidies a Bumper Crop," *New York Times*, December 26, 2004.

29. "Uncle Sam's Teat: Can America's Farmers Be Weaned from Their Government Money?" *The Economist*, September 7, 2006.

30. Michael Pollan, "When a Crop Becomes King," *New York Times*, July 19, 2002, A21.

31. Another problem with corn, as we have discussed elsewhere in this book, is its

nutritional deficit unless eaten with other foods. Although a staple crop in sub-Saharan Africa, for example, it has replaced millet and sorghum, which are highly nutritious and drought-resistant indigenous grains.

32. Harry S Truman, *Memoirs: Years of Decisions* (New York: Doubleday, 1955), 236.

33. Frances Moore Lappé, Rachel Schurman, and Kevin Danaher, *Betraying the National Interest* (New York: Grove Press, 1987), 12.

34. By contrast, as starvation was again rising across sub-Saharan Africa during the 1980s, Egypt received 1.7 million metric tons (MT) of U.S. food aid, while the top six sub-Saharan states needing emergency food relief received a total of 519,300 MT. See U.S. Department of State, Agency for International Development, *Congressional Presentation, Fiscal Year 1982, Main Volume, Amended Version* (Washington, DC: U.S. Government Printing Office, 1981), 115.

35. Ibid.; see also *Main Volume, Fiscal Years 1982–1985*.

36. Mengistu reportedly arrested Emperor Haile Selassie and put him in a cell directly beneath his palace office, where he allegedly denied him food and water and watched him starve to death.

37. Mengistu was taken in by Robert Mugabe and as of this writing was living in Harare, Zimbabwe in great comfort.

38. Independent Commission on International Humanitarian Issues (ICIHI), *Famine: A Man-Made Disaster? A Report for the Independent Commission on International Humanitarian Issues* (London and Sydney: Pan Books, 1985), 69.

39. "Food and Agriculture Organization (FAO): Special Meeting Discusses Drought," *Africa Research Bulletin*, September 15–October 14, 1980, 5695.

40. Frits N. Eisenloeffel, *Famine in Eritrea* (Utrecht, The Netherlands: Stichting Oecumenische Hulp [Dutch Interchurch Aid] Publications, 1983), 11–13, 15–16, 34–42.

41. Jack Shepherd, *The Politics of Starvation* (Washington, DC: The Carnegie Endowment for International Peace, 1974), 2–3.

42. Ibid., xii, xiii.

43. U.S. House of Representatives, House Select Committee on Hunger, "Situation Report #7," June 27, 1985, 2, 3, 5.

44. "Lives: WFP Hunger Facts for Africa," WFPNews, July 1, 2005; "WFP Chief Urges WTO to Support Food Aid in Doha Round," NewsFeed, May 9, 2005.

45. "Grim Christmas Awaits Millions of Desperately Hungry Southern Africans," WFP Press Release, December 22, 2004.

46. Jim Wurst, "Africa: Region Faces 'Unprecedented Crisis,' WFP Tells Security Council," *Unfoundation.org*, December 4, 2002.

47. Ramola Talwar Badam, "Amnesty Blasts North Korea on Food Report," January 21, 2004, available at http://news.yahoo.com.

48. UN Wire, "Donor Shortfall Forces WFP to Cut North Korean's Food Aid," January 20, 2004, available at www.unwire.org.

49. WFP Newsfeed, 30 June 2008, at www.wfp.org. See also, "US Announces N Korea Food Aid Package," *Financial Times*, May 16, 2008, at www.ft.com/cms/s/034bbd44-468a-11dd-876a-0000779fd2ac,d . . .

50. WFP News, "Horn of Africa Facing Another Year of Hunger as Millions Battle for Survival," June 9, 2009.

51. Timothy M. Shaw, "Towards a Political Economy of the African Crisis: Diplomacy, Debates and Dialectics," in Michael H. Glantz, ed. *Drought and Hunger in Africa* (Cambridge: Cambridge University Press, 1987), 129.

8. Responses to Malnutrition

1. K. Markandaya, *Nectar in a Sieve: A Novel* (London: Putnam, 1954), 91.

2. A. Maslow, "Theory of Human Motivation," *Psychological Review* 50 (1943): 370–96.

3. Oskar Minkowski and Joseph von Mering, "Diabetes mellitus nach Pankreasextirpation," *Centralblatt für klinische Medicin* 10, no. 23 (1889): 393–94.

4. F. G. Banting and C. H. Best, *The Internal Secretion of the Pancreas* (Toronto: The University Library, 1922).

5. G. Whitlock et al., "Body Mass Index and Cause-Specific Mortality in 900,000 Adults: Collaborative Analysis of 57 Prospective Studies," *The Lancet* 373, no. 9669 (2009): 1083–96; T. Pischon et al., "General and Abdominal Adiposity and Risk of Death in Europe," *New England Journal of Medicine* 359, no. 20 (2008): 2105–20; J. Manson et al., "Body Weight and Mortality among Women," *New England Journal of Medicine* 333, no. 11 (1995): 677–85.

6. University of Minnesota Laboratory of Physiological Hygiene and A. B. Keys, *The Biology of Human Starvation* (Minneapolis: University of Minnesota Press, 1950); A. L. Lehninger, D. L. Nelson, and M. M. Cox, *Lehninger Principles of Biochemistry*, 4th ed. (New York: W. H. Freeman, 2005); M. E. Shils and M. Shike, *Modern Nutrition in Health and Disease*, 10th ed. (Philadelphia: Lippincott Williams & Wilkins, 2006), xxv.

7. M. Gilbert, *The Holocaust: A History of the Jews of Europe during the Second World War* (New York: Holt, Rinehart, and Winston, 1986).

8. C. D. Williams, "Kwashiorkor: A Nutritional Disease of Children Associated with a Maize Diet," *The Lancet* 229 (1935): 1151–52.

9. Lehninger et al., *Lehninger Principles of Biochemistry*; Shils and Shike, *Modern Nutrition in Health and Disease*; Thomas M. Devlin, *Textbook of Biochemistry*, 6th ed. (New York: Wiley-Liss, 2006); M. Ezzati, A.D. Lopez, A. Rodgers, and C.J.L. Murray, *Comparative Quantification of Health Risks: Global and Regional Burden of Diseases Attributable to Selected Major Risk Factors*, 3 vols. (Geneva: World Health Organization, 2004).

10. A. Sommer, "Vitamin A Deficiency and Childhood Mortality," *The Lancet* 339 (1992): 864.

11. Ibid.

12. Bellagio Child Survival Study Group, "How Many Child Deaths Can We Prevent This Year?" *The Lancet* 362 (2005): 65–71.

13. "Iodine Deficiency—Way to Go Yet," *The Lancet* 372 (2008): 88.

14. Ezzati et al., *Comparative Quantification of Health Risks*.

15. Shils and Shike, *Modern Nutrition in Health and Disease*.

16. Ezzati et al., *Comparative Quantification of Health Risks*.

17. R. M. Stoltzfus, L. Mullany, and R.E. Black, "Iron Deficiency Anaemia," in Ezzati, et al., *Comparative Quantification of Health Risks*, vol. 1, 163–209.

Lessons: Nineteenth-century Ireland and Modern Africa

1. Cormac Ó Gráda, *The Great Irish Famine* (Cambridge: University of Cambridge Press, 1995), 68.

2. "Households Below Average Income, Department for Work and Pensions (DWP); Labour Force Survey, Office of National Statistics (ONS); at http://www.statistics.gov.uk/CCI/nugget.asp?ID=1815&Pos=1&ColRank=1&Rank=374

3. The National Center on Family Homelessness, "America's Youngest Outcasts: Report Card on Child Homelessness," 2009; available at www.homelesschildrenamerica.org.

4. Amy Goldstein, "Report: More Americans Going Hungry," *The Washington Post*, November 16, 2009.

5. U.S. Department of Agriculture, "Food Security in the United States," Economic Research Service, 2007; http://www.ers.usda.gov/Briefing/FoodSecurity/stats_graphs.htm.

6. W. E. B. Du Bois, *The Suppression of the African Slave Trade to the United States of America, 1638–1870* (New York: Longmans, Green, and Co., 1896), 1.

7. For example, see Joseph J. Williams, *Whence the "Black Irish" of Jamaica?* (New York: Dial Press, 1932); "Barbadosed: Africans and Irish in Barbadoes," Gilder Lehrman Center for the Study of Slavery, Resistance, and Abolition, Yale University, at http://www.yale.edu/glc/tangledroots/Barbadosed.htm ; and Valerie Robinson, "Barbados's Memorial to Irish Slaves Reignites Cromwell Row," *Irish News*, May 4, 2009.

8. Williams, *Whence the "Black Irish" of Jamaica*, 5; quoted in W. E. B. Du Bois, *Black Folk, Then and Now: An Essay in the History and Sociology of the Negro Race* (New York: Henry Holt and Co., 1939), 152

9. "Barbadosed: Africans and Irish in Barbadoes," Gilder Lehrman Center for the Study of Slavery, Resistance, and Abolition. See also Valerie Robinson, "Barbados's memorial to Irish slaves reignites Cromwell Row."

10. "Barbadosed: Africans and Irish in Barbadoes," Gilder Lehr Lehrman Center for the Study of Slavery, Resistance, and Abolition, 10–11.

11. Ibid. See also Don Jordan and Michael Walsh, *White Cargo: The Forgotten History of Britain's White Slaves in America* (New York: NYU Press, 2008), 191–192.

12. Joseph McPartlin, "Diet, Politics and Disaster: The Great Irish Famine," *Proceedings of the Nutrition Society* (1997), 56, 211.

13. Adam Hochschild, *King Leopold's Ghost* (New York: Houghton Mifflin, 1999), 6.

14. Gerald of Wales, *The History and Topography of Ireland by Giraldus Cambrensis*, translated with an introduction by J. J. O'Meara (Dolmen Press, 1982; Penguin Classics, 1982), chapter 1, "Irish People's Character and Customs, 1183–1185."

15. Gerald of Wales, chapter 5, "The Irish Form of Christianity."

16. Jan Nederveen Pieterse, "White Negroes," in Gail Dines and Jean M. Humez, eds., *Gender, Race and Class in Media*, 2nd ed. (Thousand Oaks, California: 2002), 112.

17. See, for example, David Quammen, "Megatransect" *National Geographic*, October 2000, 2–29; "Green Abyss: Megatransect Part 2," *National Geographic*, March 2001, 2–37; and, "End of the Line: Megatransect Part 3," *National Geographic*, August 2001, 74–103. Also at, http://ngm.nationalgeographic.com/static-legacy/ngm/0010. The series traces the fifteenth-month journey across northern Congo to the coast of Gabon, and is informative for its portrayals of J. Michael Fay, a white conservationist, his African porters and guides, the African people encountered, and the imagined and obsessive fears of the Central African rainforest.

18. Pieterse, "White Negroes," 112.

19. Piers Brendon, *The Decline and Fall of the British Empire, 1781–1997* (New York: Vintage Books, 2010), 120.

20. Ned Lebow, "British Historians and Irish History," *Eire-Ireland*, vol. III, no. 4 (Winter 1973), 11.

21. L. P. Curtis, Jr., *Anglo-Saxons and Celts: A Study of Anti-Irish Prejudice in Victorian England* (Bridgeport, CT: Conference on British Studies at the University of Bridgeport, 1968), 84.

22. Ó Gráda, 1995, 62.

23. British colonies in sub-Saharan Africa (directly, or as the result of various negotiated

agreements) included Botswana, Cameroon (Germany), Eritrea (Italy), The Gambia, Ghana, Kenya, Lesotho, Malawi, Mauritius, Nigeria, Sierra Leone, Somalia (Italy), South Africa, Sudan (Egypt), Swaziland, Tanzania, Togo (Germany), Uganda, Zambia, and Zimbabwe.

24. Helen Litton, *The Irish Famine: An Illustrated History* (Dublin: Wolfhound Press, 1994), 98.

25. Cathal Poirteir, *Famine Echoes*, (Dublin: Gill and MacMillan, 1995), 235

26. Ó Gráda, 1995, 20.

27. Ó Gráda, 1995, 50.

28. Hochschild, 305.

29. http://www.uwm.edu/~michael/choctaw/robinson.html

30. The American Society of Friends, or Quakers. See Christine Kinealy, "Emancipation, Famine & Religion: Ireland under the Union," Multitext Project in Irish History, University College Cork, Ireland.

31. In 1992, almost 150 years after the Great Irish Famine and the Choctaw gift, eight Irish descendents of survivors of the Famine made the 500-mile walk from Broken Bow, Oklahoma, to Nanih Waiya, Mississippi—the "Trail of Tears"—in appreciation for that gift. The Irish and the Native Americans were seeking to raise $71,000—1,000 times the original amount—for famine relief in Somalia. See Mike Ward, "Irish Repay Choctaw Famine Gift: March Traces Trail of Tears in Trek for Somalian Relief," *American-Statesman Capitol*, 1992, at http://www.uwm.edu/~michael/choctaw/retrace.html

32. "President of Ireland Mary Robinson Addresses the Choctaw People," Bishinik, The Official Publication of the Choctaw Nation of Oklahoma, June, 1995, at http://www.uwm .edu/~michael/choctaw/robinson.html.

33. Edward T. O'Donnell, "154 Years Ago: The Choctaw Send Aid," *Hibernian Chronicle*, 2001 Irish Echo Newspaper Corp., at: http://www.uwm.edu/~michael/choctaw/hiberian.html.

9. Why Do Some People Starve?

1. See, for example, Paul Collier, "Economic Causes of Civil Conflict and Their Implications for Policy," World Bank, June 15, 2000.

2. Mike Davis, *Late Victorian Holocausts: El Niño Famines and the Making of the Third World* (London: Verso, 2002).

3. L. Brown, *Who Will Feed China? Wake-up Call for a Small Planet* (London: Earthscan, 1995).

4. René Dumont, *False Start in Africa* (New York: Praeger, 1966); and René Dumont, *The Hungry Future* (New York: Praeger, 1969).

5. Ellen Messer, Marc J. Cohen, and Jashinta D'Costa, "Food from Peace: Breaking the Links between Conflict and Hunger," IFPRI Discussion Paper 24 (Washington, DC: IFPRI, 1998), 1.

6. Robert Stock, *Africa South of the Sahara* (New York: The Guilford Press, 2004), 237.

7. Paul Collier, "Economic Causes of Civil Conflict and Their Implications for Policy," The World Bank, June 15, 2000, 5–6.

8. Messer et al., "Food from Peace," 6.

9. Ibid., 3.

10. Ibid., 5, 9.

11. Ellen Messer and Marc J. Cohen, "Africa: Breaking the Links Between Conflict and Hunger in Africa," 2020 Africa Conference Brief 10 (Washington, DC: IFPRI, 2004), 2–3.

12. Stephen Devereux, *Theories of Famine* (New York: Harvester/Wheatsheaf, 1993), 148.

13. Messer et al., "Food from Peace," 3, 5, 6.

14. World Health Organization, "Emergencies Cited as Major Threat to Human Health in Africa, as Wars Cost Region $15 Billion per Year," World Health Organization, Regional Office for Africa, Brazzaville, Congo, March 13, 2003.

15. "Ethiopia: Food Supply Problems," *Africa Research Bulletin*, October 15–November 14, 1978, 4880–4881.

16. Devereux, *Theories of Famine*, 149.

17. "Horn of Africa: Threat of Famine," *Africa Research Bulletin*, February 15–March 14, 1978, 4880.

18. James Shambaugh, Judy Oglethorpe, and Rebecca Ham (with contributions from Sylvia Tognetti), *The Trampled Grass: Mitigating the Impacts of Armed Conflict on the Environment* (Washington, DC: Biodiversity Support Program, 2001), 4.

19. Michael Klare, *Resource Wars: The New Landscape of Global Conflict* (New York: Henry Holt and Co., 2001), 25.

20. Collier, "Economic Causes of Civil Conflict," 5. Collier defines a civil war as "an internal conflict with more than 1,000 battle-related deaths." During the period studied there were 73 civil wars in 161 countries.

21. Collier, "Economic Causes of Civil Conflict," 6.

22. Lisa Ling, "World's Most Valuable Resource, a Curse for Most Nigerians," available at http://www.cnn.com/2008/WORLD/africa/12/11/pip.nigeria.oil/index.html.

23. Convention on International Trade in Endangered Species, an international legal instrument protecting the globes endangered species.

24. Adam Hochschild, *King Leopold's Ghost* (New York: Houghton Mifflin, 1999), 42.

25. Ibid., 161.

26. Quoted in Hochschild, *King Leopold's Ghost*, 161.

27. Ibid., 165.

28. Ibid., 3, 4, 233.

29. "Report of the Panel of Experts on the Illegal Exploitation of Natural Resources and Other Forms of Wealth of the Democratic Republic of the Congo," available at http://www.un.org/News/dh/latest/drcongo.htm, April 12, 2001.

30. Ibid., 8. This is, of course, a violation of the Convention on International Trade in Endangered Species (CITES), a globally recognized international law that protects a long list of plant and animal species, including elephants and rhinos.

31. This rare ore contains *tantalum*, with the same word root as "tantalizing."

32. "Report of the Panel of Experts," 11.

33. Ibid., 16.

34. In June 2000, the UN Security Council asked the Secretary General to appoint a formal Panel of Experts to investigate the exploitation of the natural resources of the DRC. Four significant reports were issued between January 2001 and October 2002. They are available at http://www.natural-resources.org/minerals/africa/docs.htm.

35. Several NGOs, most importantly Global Witness and Human Rights Watch, have reports on resource extractions in the DRC. These are available at http://www.globalpolicy.org/security-council/dark-side-of-natural-resources/minerals-in-conflict.html. See especially, "Digging in Corruption: Fraud, Abuse and Exploitation in Katanga's Copper and Cobalt Mines" (Washington, DC: Global Witness, July 2006).

36. "WFP extends food aid to crisis-hit Zimbabwe," Reuters, November 19, 2008.

37. E-mail to authors from MP Trudy Stevenson, Harare, Zimbabwe, May 6, 2009.

38. http://www.globalissues.org/article/87/the-democratic-republic-of-congo; and "Mutual Convenience," in "A Ravenous Dragon: A Special Report on China's Quest for Resources," *The Economist*, March 15, 2008, 12, 13.

39. WFPNews, "WFP Starts Air Drops in Congo in Bid to Beat the Rains," May 20, 2009.

40. Ellen Messer and Marc J. Cohen, "Breaking the Links between Conflict and Hunger in Africa," 20/20 Africa Conference Brief, October, 2004, 2.

41. Messer et al., "Food from Peace," 1.

42. World Health Organization, "Emergencies Cited as Major Threat to Human Health in Africa."

43. Jim Wurst, "AFRICA: Region Faces 'Unprecedented Crisis,' WFP Tells Security Council," UNfoundation.org, December 4, 2002.

44. Davis, *Late Victorian Holocausts*, 6, 7.

45. Ibid., 8.

46. Ibid., 9.

47. WFP, "Emergency Situation Report," April 4, 2008.

48. WFP, "WFP helps Mozambique Flood Victims," February 20, 2007.

49. Famine Early Warning System Network, "FEWS Mozambique Food Security Update May 2009," May 31, 2009. Also struck by repeated cyclones were Angola, Lesotho, Madagascar, Malawi, Namibia, Swaziland, Zambia, and Zimbabwe.

50. See the Earth Observatory site at http://earthobservatory.nasa.gov/NaturalHazards/view.php?id=18226&oldid=14211.

51. Davis, *Late Victorian Holocausts*, 280.

52. Ibid., 310.

53. Hurricane Katrina killed more than 1600 people, displaced about 1 million, destroyed 200,000 homes, and created some 90,000 internally displaced refugees. More than 60,000 people were stranded without food or water inside New Orleans, many of them unable to leave because they were too poor and had neither cars nor bus fares. The U.S. government delayed and then botched relief responses. Emergency food aid came from overseas but was slow in arriving. Ceci Connolly writes that more than 400,000 emergency relief packaged meals, worth $5.3 million, were donated by Great Britain and flown into Little Rock Air Force Base but sat in a warehouse in Arkansas while U.S. officials dithered about whether or not to distribute the aid ("Katrina Food Aid Blocked by US," *Washington Post*, October 14, 2005, A1). Greece also sent emergency food aid.

54. "Human Impact Report: Climate Change—The Anatomy of a Silent Crisis," Global Humanitarian Forum, May 29, 2009.

55. "AFRICA: Failed Harvests Fulfill Predictions on Climate Change," UNfoundation.org, January 7, 2003.

56. "Development in the Balance: How Will the World Cope with Climate Change?" at www.brookings.edu/events/2008/0801_development.aspx.

57. Robert O'Neill, "Global Warning," *John F. Kennedy School of Government Bulletin*, Winter 2008, 17.

58. "Human Impact Report," 2.

59. "Climate Change and the Poor: Adapt or Die," *The Economist*, September 13, 2008, 67.

60. "Human Impact Report," 3.

61. Joseph M. Prospero and Ruby T. Nees, "Dust Concentration in the Atmosphere of the Equatorial North Atlantic: Possible Relationship to the Sahelian Drought," *Science* 196, no. 4295 (1977): 1196–1198.

62. Leon D. Rotstayn and Ulrike Lohmann, "Tropical Rainfall Trends and the Indirect Aerosol Effect," *Journal of Climate* 15, no. 15 (August 2002): 2103–16.

63. Ibid., 2110, 2113–2114.

64. "Drought: Air Pollution Link Found," CSIROnline, June 13, 2002, available at http://www.csiro.au/files/mediaRelease/mr2002/SahelDrought.htm.

65. Surabi Menon, James Hansen, Larissa Nazarenko, and Yunfeng Luo, "Climate Effects of Black Carbon Aerosols in China and India," *Science* 297, no. 5590 (2002): 2250–53.

66. Keith Wiebe, Nicole Ballenger, and Per Pinstrup-Andersen, eds. *Who Will Be Fed in the 21st Century?* (Washington, DC: IFPRI, 2001), 1. Some 265 million Africans are malnourished. See WFP Newsfeed, Joint WFP/FAO/IFAD Report, "1.02 Billion People Hungry," June 19, 2009.

67. Per Pinstrup-Andersen, Rajul Pandya-Lorch, and Mark W. Rosegrant, *World Food Prospects: Critical Issues for the Early Twenty-first Century* (Washington, DC: IFPRI, October 2001), 4.

68. Per Pinstrup-Andersen and Rajul Pandya-Lorch, "Meeting Food Needs in the 21st Century: How Much and Who will be at Risk?" in Keith Wiebe, Nicole Ballenger, Per Pinstrup-Andersen, eds. *Who Will Be Fed in the 21st Century?* (Washington, DC: IFPRI, 2001), 4.

69. Pinstrup-Andersen et al., *World Food Prospects*, 9.

70. Ibid. We should add that on average a person in the developing world will "in 2020 consume less than half the amount of cereals consumed by a developed-country person and slightly more than one-third of the meat products," 9.

71. Wiebe et al., *Who Will Be Fed in the 21st Century*, 9.

72. See, for example, Keith Bradsher, "China Fills Its Pantry with Global Commodities," *New York Times*, June 11, 2009, B1.

73. Sarah Schafer and Anne Underwood, "Building in Green," *Newsweek*, September 26–October 3, 2005, 30.

74. See, for example, Ansley J. Coale, *Rapid Population Change in China, 1952–1982* (Washington, DC: National Academy Press, 1984); and IIASA, Chart, "Population growth, crude birth and death rates, 1949–1996," Data—Population Growth, at http://www.iiasa.ac.at/Research/LUC/ChinaFood/data/pop/pop_10.htm. Yang Jisheng, a Chinese journalist, spent ten years investigating the famine and estimated the 36 million *premature* deaths. The IIASA chart suggests possibly 40 million.

75. Albert Ravenholt, "China Symposium," Institute of Current World Affairs, December 4–5, 1998, Washington, DC, 31.

76. WFP News Release, "As Last Food Aid Arrives, China Progresses from Recipient to Donor," April 7, 2005.

77. "Mutual Convenience," in "A Ravenous Dragon: A Special Report on China's Quest for Resources," *The Economist*, March 15, 2008, 18.

78. Ibid.

79. Gerhard K. Heilig, "Can China Feed Itself?" IIASA Land Use Project, July 2002, available at http://www.iiasa.ac.at/Research/LUC/ChinaFood/faq/faq_12.htm.

80. Ravenholt, "China Symposium," 32.

81. Richard McGregor and Mure Dickie, "China Aims to Lift Living Standard in Rural Areas," *Financial Times*, March 6, 2006, 3.

82. Ravenholt, "China Symposium," 31–32.

83. Bradsher, "China Fills Its Pantry."

84. Lester R. Brown, "China Replacing the United States as World's Leading Consumer," Earth Policy Institute, February 16, 2005, 3.

85. Ibid., 9–10.

86. Ibid., 10.

87. http://www.vegsource.com/how_to_win.htm, and http://earthsave.org.

88. WFP, April 7, 2005; Denis D. Gray, "Ravenous China Farming the World," Associated Press, May 5, 2008.

89. Ravenholt, "China Symposium," 32.

90. Lester Brown, *Who Will Feed China: Wake-up Call for a Small Planet* (London: Earthscan Publications, 1995), 18.

91. Ibid., 30.

92. Ibid., 32.

93. Vince Morkri, UN Wire, March 11, 2004. See also Lester Brown, statement, "China's Shrinking Grain Harvest," Earth Policy Institute, March 10, 2004.

94. Lester Brown, statement, "China's Shrinking Grain Harvest," Earth Policy Institute, March 10, 2004, 1–2.

95. Ibid., 2.

96. Ibid., 3.

97. "Major Foreign Holders of Treasury Securities," http://www.treas.gov/tic/mfh.txt.

98. Clifton B. Luttrell, "The Russian Wheat Deal—Hindsight vs. Foresight," Federal Reserve Bank of St. Louis, October 1973, 2.

99. David Walker, "The Great Grain Give Away," September 25, 2002, available at www.openi.co.uk.

100. Luttrell, "The Russian Wheat Deal," 2.

101. Ibid., 2.

102. Ibid., 2.

103. Ibid., 2–3.

104. Ibid., 4.

105. Ibid., 9.

106. Ibid., 6.

107. Ibid., 7.

108. The Comptroller General of the United States, Report to the Congress, "Russian Wheat Sales and Weaknesses in Agriculture's Management of Wheat Export Subsidy Program" (July 1973), 2, 25; see also Martha Hamilton, *The Great American Grain Robbery and Other Stories* (Washington, DC: Agribusiness Accountability Project, 1972).

109. U.S. Congress, report prepared for the Committee on Foreign Affairs, U.S. House of Representatives, by the Foreign Affairs and National Defense Division, Congressional Research Service, The Library of Congress, "Feeding the World's Population Developments in the Decade Following the World Food Conference of 1974" (Washington, DC: U.S. Government Printing Office, October 1984), 4.

110. Ibid., 7.

111. Ibid., 7.

112. Luttrell, "The Russian Wheat Deal," 4–5.

113. Hal Sheets and Roger Morris, *Disaster in the Desert* (Washington, DC: Carnegie Endowment for International Peace, 1974). Stephen S. Rosenfeld also stated in *Foreign Policy* that because of the Russian purchases in 1972–1973, the United States could respond "only

stingily to emergency appeals from West Africa and Bangladesh." Stephen S. Rosenfeld, "The Politics of Food," *Foreign Policy* (Spring 1974), 28.

10. Why Do Some People Die?

1. Thomas Robert Malthus, *Essay on the Principle of Population*, 1798; quoted in C. Ó Gráda, *The Great Irish Famine* (Cambridge: Cambridge University Press, 1995).

2. "Medicine: War and Pestilence," *Time*, April 29, 1940, available at http://www.time.com/time/magazine/article/0,9171,794989,00.html.

3. B. Cohen, "Florence Nightingale," *Scientific American* 250 (1984): 128–137.

4. C. Ó Gráda and J. Mokyr, "Famine Disease and Famine Mortality: Lessons from Ireland, 1845–1850," presentation at Les Treilles, France, 25–30 May 1999; available at http://faculty.wcas.northwestern.edu/~jmokyr/mogbeag.pdf.

5. D. Relman and S. Falkow, "A Molecular Perspective of Microbial Pathogenicity," in *Principles and Practice of Infectious Disease*, ed. G. Mandell, R. Douglas, and J. Bennett (London: Churchill Livingston, 2000), 3–12.

6. J. M. Diamond, *Guns, Germs, and Steel: The Fates of Human Societies* (New York: W. W. Norton & Co., 1997).

7. J. Hardman, L. Limbird, P. Molinoff, R. Ruddon, and A. Gilman, eds., *Goodman and Gilman's The Pharmacological Basis of Therapeutics*, 9th ed. (New York: McGraw-Hill, 1996), 618–619.

8. Minnesota University Laboratory of Physiological Hygiene and A. B. Keys, *The Biology of Human Starvation* (Minneapolis: University of Minnesota Press, 1950).

9. W. Davison, "A Bacteriological and Clinical Consideration of Bacillary Dysentery in Adults and Children," *Medicine* 1, no. 3 (November 1922), 389.

10. K. Sandvig, K. and B. van Deurs, "Entry of Ricin and Shiga Toxin into Cells: Molecular Mechanisms and Medical Perspectives," *EMBO Journal* 19, no. 22 (2000): 5943–50.

11. M. Bielaszewska et al., "Shiga Toxin Gene Loss and Transfer in Vitro and in Vivo during Enterohemorrhagic *Escherichia coli O26* Infection in Humans," *Applied Environmental Microbiology* 73 (2007): 3144–50.

12. S. Niyogi, "Shigellosis," *Journal of Microbiology* 43, no. 2: 133–43.

13. L. Mata, E. Gangarosa, and A. Caceres, "Epidemic Shiga Bacillus Dysentery in Central America—I. Etiologic Investigations in Guatemala," *Journal of Infectious Disease* 122 (1970): 170–180; E. Gangarosa, D. Perera, and L. Mata, "Epidemic Shiga Bacillus Dysentery in Central America—II. Epidemiologic Studies in 1969," *Journal of Infectious Disease* 122 (1970): 181–190.

14. R. Glass and R. Black, "The Epidemiology of Cholera," in *Cholera*, ed. D. Barua and William B. Greenough III (New York: Plenum Press, 1992).

15. C. Seas and E. Gotuzzo, "*Vibrio cholera*," in Mandell, Douglas, and Bennett, *Principles and Practice of Infectious Diseases*.

16. FDA, *FDA/CFSAN—Food Safety A to Z Reference Guide—Salmonella* (College Park, MD: FDA—Center for Food Safety and Applied Nutrition, 2008), accessed February 14, 2009, available at http://www.cfsan.fda.gov/~dms/a2z-s.html; R. Guerrant and T. Steiner, "Principles and Syndromes of Enteric Infections," in Mandell, Douglas, and Bennett, *Principles and Practice of Infectious Diseases*, 1215–27.

17. Mandell, Douglas, and Bennett, *Principles and Practice of Infectious Disease*.

18. G. Soper, "The Work of a Chronic Typhoid Germ Distributor," *JAMA* C48 (1907): 2019–22.

19. Mandell, Douglas, and Bennett, *Principles and Practice of Infectious Diseases.*

20. Hannah Arendt, *Eichmann in Jerusalem; A Report on the Banality of Evil* (New York: Viking Press, 1963).

21. U. Baer, *The De-demonization of Evil* (2001). Available at http://www.cabinetmagazine .org/issues/5/dedemonization.php. Accessed June 26, 2009.

22. R. Black, S. Morris, and J. Bryce, "Child Survival I: Where and Why Are 10 Million Children Dying Every Year," *The Lancet* 361 (2003): 2226–34; G. Jones, R. W. Steketee, R. E. Black, Z. A. Bhutta, and S. S. Morris, and Bellagio Child Survival Study Group, "Child Survival II: How Many Child Deaths Can We Prevent this Year?" *The Lancet* 362 (2003): 65–71; J. Bryce, S. el Arifeen, G. Pariyo, C.F. Lanata, D. Gwatkin, J.P. Habicht, and the Multi-Country Evaluation of IMCI Study Group, "Child Survival III: Can Public Health Deliver?" *The Lancet* 362 (2003): 159–64; C. G. Victoria, A. Wagstaff, J. A. Schellenberg, D. Gwatkin, M. Claeson, J. P. Habicht, "Child Survival IV: Applying an Equity Lens to Child Health and Mortality: More of the Same Is Not Enough," *The Lancet* 362 (2003): 233–41; The Bellagio Study Group on Child Survival, "Child Survival V: Knowledge into Action for Child Survival," *The Lancet* 362 (2003): 323–27.

23. S. Fishman, L. E. Caulfield, M. de Onis, M. Blossner, A. A. Hyder, L. Mullany, and R. E. Black, "Childhood and Maternal Underweight," in *Comparative Quantification of Health Risks: Global and Regional Burden of Disease Attributable to Selected Major Risk Factors*, vol. 1, ed. M. Ezzati, A. Lopez, A. Rodgers, and C. Murray (Geneva: World Health Organization, 2003), 39–162.

24. Jones et al., "Child Survival II."

II. The Biological Basis for Political Behavior

1. E. O. Wilson, *On Human Nature* (Cambridge, MA: Harvard University Press, 1978), xii.

2. S. Pinker, "My Genome, My Self," *New York Times Magazine*, January 7, 2009.

3. E. O. Wilson, *Sociobiology: The New Synthesis* (Cambridge, MA: Belknap Press, 1975), ix.

4. R. Keyes, *The Quote Verifier: Who Said What, Where, and When* (New York: St. Martin's Press, 2006), xxi.

5. J. Tooby and L. Cosmides, "Adaptation versus Phylogeny: The Role of Animal Psychology in the Study of Human Behavior," *International Journal of Comparative Psychology* 2 (1989): 105–18; J. Tooby, J. Barkow, and L. Cosmides, *The Adapted Mind: Evolutionary Psychology and the Generation of Culture* (Oxfordshire: Oxford University Press, 1995).

6. S. Pinker, *How the Mind Works* (New York: Norton, 1997), xii.

7. Wilson, *On Human Nature*, xii.

8. R. Andrew, "The Origin and Evolution of the Expressions of Primates, *Behavior* 20 (1963): 1–107; S. Chevalier-Skolnikoff, "Facial Expression in Non-human Primates," in *Darwin and Facial Expression: A Century of Research in Review*, ed. P. Ekman (New York: Academic Press, 1973); C. Darwin, *The Expression of Emotion in Man* (London: Murray, 1872); M. Gervais and D. Wilson, "The Evolution and Functions of Laughter and Humor: A Synthetic Approach," *Quarterly Reviews of Biology* 80 (2005): 39–430; W. Redican, "Facial Expressions in Non-human Primates," in *Primate Behavior: Developments in Field and Laboratory Research*, ed. L. Rosenblum (New York: Academic Press, 1975), 103–94; J. van Hoof, "Facial Expressions in Higher Primates" *Symposia of the Zoological Society of London* 8 (1962): 67–125.

9. M. Ross, M. Owren, and E. S. Zimmerman, "Reconstructing the Evolution of Laughter in Great Apes and Humans," *Current Biology* 19, no. 13 (2009): 2–6.

10. S. J. Gould, *Ontogeny and Phylogeny* (Cambridge, MA: Belknap Press, 1977), ix.

11. J. Maynard Smith and E. Szathmáry, *The Origins of Life: From the Birth of Life to the Origin of Language* (Oxford: Oxford University Press, 2000).

12. Tooby and Cosmides, "Adaptation versus Phylogeny"; J. Tooby and L. Cosmides, "The Past Explains the Present: Emotional Adaptations and the Structure of Ancestral Environments," *Ethology and Sociobiology* 11 (1990): 375–424; J. Tooby and L. Cosmides, "On the Universality of Human Nature and the Uniqueness of the Individual: The Role of Genetics and Adaptation," *Journal of Personality* 58 (1990): 17–67.

13. Lorenz, *On Aggression* (London: Methuen, 1966), xiii.

14. Dawkins, *The Selfish Gene* (Oxford: Oxford University Press, 1976), xii.

15. C. van Schaik et al., "Orangutan Cultures and the Evolution of Material Culture," *Science* 299 (2003): 102–5; R. W. Wrangham and the Chicago Academy of Sciences, *Chimpanzee Cultures* (Cambridge, MA: Harvard University Press in cooperation with the Chicago Academy of Sciences, 1994), xxiii.

16. P. K. Smith, H. Cowie, and M. Blades, *Understanding Children's Development*, 4th ed. (Malden, MA: Blackwell, 2003), xxvii; U. Bronfenbrenner, *The Ecology of Human Development: Experiments by Nature and Design* (Cambridge, MA: Harvard University Press, 1979), xv; E. H. Erikson, *Identity, Youth, and Crisis* (New York: W. W. Norton, 1968).

17. L. Schultz and R. Lore, "Communal Reproductive Success in Rats (*Rattus norvegicus*): Effects of Group Composition and Prior Social Experience," *Journal of Comparative Psychology* 107 (1993): 216–22; J. Moore, "Population Density, Social Pathology, and Behavioral Ecology," *Primates* 40 (1999): 5–26.

18. Lorenz, *On Aggression*, xiii.

19. Ibid.

20. R. D. Masters, *The Nature of Politics* (New Haven: Yale University Press, 1989), xvii.

21. Lorenz, *On Aggression*, xiii.

22. Wilson, *On Human Nature*, 28.

23. Erikson, *Identity, Youth, and Crisis*.

24. G. M. Fredrickson, *Racism: A Short History* (Princeton, NJ: Princeton University Press, 2002).

25. S. Wells, *The Journey of Man: A Genetic Odyssey* (New York: Random House, 2002), xvi; R. C. Lewontin, *The Genetic Basis of Evolutionary Change* (New York: Columbia University Press, 1974), xiii.

26. J. Haldane, "Population Genetics," *New Biology* 18 (1955): 34–51.

27. W. Hamilton, "The Genetic Evolution of Human Behavior I and II," *Journal of Theoretical Biology* 7 (1964): 1–52.

28. R. Trivers, "The Evolution of Reciprocal Altruism," *Quarterly Review of Biology* 46 (1971): 35–57.

29. J. Gore, H. Youk, and A. van Oudenaarden, "Snowdrift Game Dynamics and Facultative Cheating in Yeast," *Nature* 459 (2009): 253–56.

30. J. McDermott, "Biologists Begin Eavesdropping on 'Talking' Trees," *Smithsonian* 15 (1984): 84–86.

31. J. Nash, "Equilibrium Points in N-Person Games," *Proceedings of the National Academy of Sciences* 36 (1950): 48–49.

32. J. Maynard Smith, *Evolution and the Theory of Games* (Cambridge: Cambridge University Press, 1982), viii.

33. R. Dawkins, *The Selfish Gene* (Oxford: Oxford University Press, 1976).

34. Ibid.

35. R. M. Axelrod, *The Evolution of Cooperation* (New York: Basic Books, 1984).

36. E. W. Said, *Orientalism* (New York: Pantheon Books, 1978), xi.

Lessons: Who Starves and Why?

1. L. A. Clarkson and E. Margaret Crawford, *Feast and Famine: Food and Nutrition in Ireland 1500–1920* (Oxford: Oxford University Press, 2001), 61–66.

2. Oatmeal, or porridge, "the food of the people." In the medieval period, what came with the oatmeal signaled class distinctions: the wealthy put honey and fresh milk into their stirabout; the gentry added butter and milk; the laborers ate their oatmeal with buttermilk or water. See http://www.irish-society.org/Hedgemaster%20Archives/irish_table.htm.

3. Coarse bread made with several grains.

4. Clarkson and Crawford, *Feast and Famine*, 64.

5. Ibid., 68.

6. Ibid., 70.

7. Cormac Ó Gráda. *The Great Irish Famine* (Cambridge: Cambridge University Press, 1997), 68.

8. Melinda Smale and Thom Jayne, "Maize in Eastern and Southern Africa: 'Seeds' of Success in Retrospect," EPTD Discussion Paper No. 97, International Food Policy Research Institute, January 2003, 2–3.

9. William C. Maclean, Guillermo Lopez de Romaña, Robert P. Placko and George G. Graham, "Protein Quality and Digestibility of Sorghum in Preschool Children: Balance Studies and Plasma Free Amino Acids," *Journal of Nutrition* 111 (November 1981), 1928–36.

10. Liz Young, "Spaces for Famine: A Comparative Geographical Analysis of Famine in Ireland and the Highlands in the 1840s," *Transactions of the Institute of British Geographers* 21, no. 4 (December 1996): 672.

11. Ibid., 673.

12. Ibid., 671.

12. The Right to Food

1. Peter Rosset, "US Opposes Right to Food at World Summit," *World Editorial and International Law*, June 30, 2002, 1.

2. Xiaorong Li, "Making Sense of the Right to Food," in William Aiken and Hugh LaFollette, eds., *World Hunger and Morality*, 2nd ed. (Upper Saddle River, NJ: Prentice Hall, 1996), 153.

3. Xiaorong Li, "Making Sense of the Right to Food," 154.

4. "Food as a Human Right," Interview with Asbjorn Eide, *News & Views* (Washington, DC: International Food Policy Research Institute, April 2001), 5.

5. United Nations, General Assembly, *Universal Declaration of Human Rights*, Article 25, December 10, 1948.

6. Onora O'Neill, "The Dark Side of Human Rights," *International Affairs* 81, no. 2 (2005): 429.

7. Ellen Messer and Marc J. Cohen, "The Human Right to Food as a US Nutrition Concern," IFPRI Discussion Paper 00731 (Washington, DC: International Food Policy Research Institute, December 2007), 5. See also Philip Alston, "International Law and the Right to Food," in Asbjorn Eide, Wenche Barth Eide, Susanthe Goonatilake, Joan Gussow, and Omawale, eds., *Food as a Human Right* (Tokyo: The United Nations University Press, 1984), 165.

8. O'Neill, "The Dark Side of Human Rights," 429.

9. "The Right to Food in Theory and Practice," FAO Corporate Document Repository (Rome: Office of Director-General, FAO, 1998), 2.

10. The Conventions form the foundation for international humanitarian law and call for "the availability of food in cases of armed conflict"; two Protocols call for the right to food and state that "the starvation of civilians as a method of combat is prohibited." See Smita Narula, "The Right to Food: Holding Global Actors Accountable under International Law," Center for Human Rights and Global Justice Working Paper Number 7 (New York: New York University School of Law, 2006), 71–72.

11. The Right to Food, UN GAOR, 57th Session, Suppl. No. 49, UN Doc. A/RES/57/226 (203), 2.

12. For example, the constitutions of the Congo (Article 34), Ecuador (Article 19), Haiti (Article 22), Nicaragua (Article 63), South Africa (Article 27), Uganda (Article 14), and Ukraine (Article 18) recognize explicitly the right to adequate food as set out in ICESCR. The constitutions of Bangladesh (Article 15), Ethiopia (Article 90), Guatemala (Article 99), India (Article 47), the Islamic Republic of Iran (Articles 3 and 43), Malawi (Article 13), Nigeria (Article 16), Pakistan (Article 38), the Seychelles (Preamble), and Sri Lanka (Article 27) set the achievement of these goals as responsibilities of the state, while the constitutions of Brazil (Article 227), Guatemala (Article 51), Paraguay (Article 53), Peru (Article 6), and South Africa (Article 28) recognize the right of children to adequate food and nutrition.

13. Messer and Cohen, "The Human Right to Food," 17.

14. Narula, "The Right to Food," 76–77.

15. Ibid., 77, 79.

16. Thomas Poggee, "Unjust Social Rules, Killing and Causing Pain," 35th Annual Francis W. Gramlich Memorial Lecture, Dartmouth College, March 3, 2009.

17. Narula, "The Right to Food," 65.

18. Messer and Cohen. "The Human Right to Food," vi.

19. World Food Programme, "2007 Food Aid Flows," June 2008, Table 5, "Summary of Food Aid Deliveries in 2007 by Donor," 17.

20. Philip Alston, "International Law and the Right to Food," in Asbjorn Eide, Wenche Barth Eide, Susanthe Goonatilake, Joan Gussow, and Omawale, eds., *Food as a Human Right* (Tokyo: The United Nations University Press, 1984), 162.

21. Messer and Cohen, "The Human Right to Food," 1.

22. Alston, "International Law and the Right to Food," 163.

23. Messer and Cohen, "The Human Right to Food," 2.

24. "Rome Talks on Hunger Are Belittled by Britain," *New York Times*, June 12, 2002, A10. See also Peter Rosset, "US Opposes Right to Food at World Summit," *World Editorial and International Law*, June 30, 2002.

25. Rosset, "US Opposes Right to Food at World Summit," 2. It is indicative of the low priority given to these conferences that the United States sent only its secretary of agriculture to lead its delegation rather than a higher-ranking official.

26. Rosset, "US Opposes Right to Food at World Summit," 2.

27. *The Economist*, January 2, 1847, 3b; and January 30, 1847, 4a.

28. Rosset, "US Opposes Right to Food at World Summit," 2–3.

29. Ibid., 3.

30. Nasir Islam, "Food Aid: Conscience, Morality, and Politics," *International Journal* 36, no. 2 (Spring, 1981), 353.

31. Ibid.

32. Willy Brandt, *North-South: A Programme for Survival, Report of the Independent Commission on International Development Issues* (Cambridge, MA: The MIT Press, 1980), 90.

33. Centre for Global Negotiations, "The Brandt Equation: 21st Century Blueprint for the New Global Economy," http://www.brandt21forum.info.

34. Garrett Hardin, "Lifeboat Ethics: The Case Against Helping the Poor," *Psychology Today*, September 1974, 337.

35. Ibid., 339–340.

36. American Association for the Advancement of Science, http://atlas.aaas.org/index.php?part=2.

37. http://research.stlouisfed.org/fred2/data/EXUSUK.txt.

38. Peter Singer, "Famine, Affluence and Morality," in William Aiken and Hugh LaFollette, eds., *World Hunger and Morality*, 2nd ed. (Upper Saddle River, NJ: Prentice Hall, 1996), 26–27.

39. Ibid., 27. To spread the blame: Australia's aid to East Bengal was one-twelfth what it spent on a new opera house in Sydney. See also Islam, "Food Aid: Conscience, Morality, and Politics," 353.

40. Singer, "Famine, Affluence and Morality," 26–27.

41. Lester Brown, "Ethanol Could Leave the World Hungry," *Fortune*, August 16, 2006.

42. Singer, "Famine, Affluence and Morality," 27, 28, 29, 31.

43. Onora O'Neill, "Ending World Hunger," in William Aiken and Hugh LaFollette, eds., *World Hunger and Morality*, 2nd ed. (Upper Saddle River, NJ: Prentice Hall, 1996), 94. See also Onora O'Neill, "The Dark Side of Human Rights"; and Onora O'Neill, *A Question of Trust* (Cambridge: Cambridge University Press, 2002).

44. O'Neill, "Ending World Hunger," 94.

45. Ibid., 95, 107, 109.

46. John Rawls, *A Theory of Justice* (Oxford: Oxford University Press, 1971), 303. See also: Rawls, *Justice as Fairness: A Restatement* (Cambridge, MA: The Belknap Press of Harvard University, 2001).

47. Ibid., 109.

48. Ibid., 28.

49. Ibid., 109.

50. Islam, "Food Aid," 370.

51. "Plowshares into Swords: The Political Uses of Food," *QQ—Report from the Center for Philosophy and Public Policy*, 2, no. 4 (Fall 1982): 2.

52. Ibid., 4.

53. Ibid., 3.

54. Singer, "Famine, Affluence and Morality," 28.

55. "Plowshares into Swords," 4.

56. O'Neill, "Ending World Hunger," 109.

57. Stephen Devereux, *Theories of Famine* (London: Harvester/Wheatshaft, 1993), 167–168.

58. Nigel Dower, "Global Hunger: Moral Dilemmas," in Ben Mepham, ed., *Food Ethics* (London: Routledge, 1996), 9.

59. Sam Porter. "Confronting Famine: The Case of the Irish Great Hunger," *Nursing Inquiry* 5 (1998): 114.

13. Best Practices

1. John Dixon and Aidan Gulliver with David Gibbon, *Farming Systems and Poverty* (Rome: FAO, 2001), iii.

2. International Food Policy Research Institute, *Ending Hunger in Africa: Only the Small Farmer can Do It* (Washington, DC: IFPRI, 2002), 2; and, Dixon and Gulliver, *Farming Systems and Poverty*, 8.

3. Parliamentary Business, Item 573, at www.parliament.uk, July 30, 2009. Italics added.

4. Derek Byerlee and Carl K. Eicher, eds., *Africa's Emerging Maize Revolution* (Boulder, CO: Lynne Reiner, 1997), 18–19.

5. Aline Sullivan, "4 Emerging Tigers: Far-flung and Individualistic," *International Herald Tribune*, August 16–17, 1997, 15.

6. Byerlee and Eicher, *Africa's Emerging Maize Revolution*, 31. The prize was awarded by The Hunger Project, which withdrew it in 2001. See http://www.thp.org/what_we_do/key_initiatives/honoring_africa_leadership/laureate_list/zimbabwe_statement.

7. C. Ford Runge, Benjamin Senauer, Philip G. Pardey, and Mark W. Rosegrant, *Ending Hunger by 2050* (Washington, DC: IFPRI, 2003), 3.

8. International Food Policy Research Institute, *Ending Hunger in Africa: Only the Small Farmer Can Do It* (Washington, DC: IFPRI, 2002), 4.

9. Byerlee and Eicher, *Africa's Emerging Maize Revolution*, 4, 21.

10. "A Better Way to Fight Poverty," *New York Times*, May 5, 2005, A26.

11. David Siriri, et al., "Community-led School Meals Program in the Millennium Villages of Sauri, Kenya, and Ruhiira, Uganda," The Millennium Villages Project, paper presented at the 35th International Conference of the Global Health Council, May 27–31, 2008, Washington, DC. See also http://www.yara.com/sustainability/africa_program/millennium_villages/sauri_kenya.

12. Speech, Arthur G. O. Mutambara, "Rethinking the Africans Economic Model," May 25, 2008, Harare, Zimbabwe.

13. Per Pinstrup-Andersen, Rajul Pandya-Lorch, and Mark W. Rosegrant, *World Food Prospects: Critical Issues for the Early Twenty-first Century* (Washington, DC: International Food Policy Research Institute, October 1999), 20.

14. Goldman Sachs, "Women Hold Up Half the Sky," Global Economics Paper No. 164, March 4, 2008, 10.

15. ActionAid, *Hit or Miss: Women's Rights and the Millennium Development Goals* (London: ActionAid, 2009), 2; available at www.actionaid.org.uk.

16. Ibid., 2.

17. The Camfed Model, at http://uk.camfed.org.

18. World Health Organization, "Primary Health Care: Now More Than Ever," in *The World Health Report 2008* (Geneva: WHO Press, 2008).

19. Population Action International, "A Measure of Survival," October 15, 2007, available at http://www.populationaction.org/Publications/Fact_Sheets/FS36/Summary.shtml.

20. "An Agenda for Progress at a Time of Global Crisis: A Call for African Leadership," Annual Report of the Africa Progress Panel, 2009, 16; available at http://africaprogresspanel.socialmediarelease.co.za.

21. Margaret Chan, Director-General of the World Health Organization, "Primary Health Care—Now More Than Ever," speech Almaty, Kazakhstan, October 14, 2008.

22. World Health Organization, "Primary Health Care," 6.

23. Ibid., xii.

24. Ibid., 7.

25. "WHO Slams Global Health Care, Calls for Universal Coverage," available at http://www.cnn.com/2008/HEALTH/conditions/10/14/world.health.report/index.html.

26. "Insecticide Treated Bed Nets to Prevent Malaria," *British Medical Journal* 322 (2001): 249–250; see also World Health Organization, "Primary Health Care," 64.

27. "Deworming," *Kennedy School Bulletin*, Spring (2008), 14.

28. UNICEF, "A World Fit for Children, Statistical Review," *Progress for Children*, no. 6, December 2007, 8, 9.

29. Tom Kalil, chairman, The Clinton Global Initiative Global Health Working Group, at http://www.cnn.com/2008/POLITICS/09/23/kalil.newborns/index.html.

30. World Health Organization, "Primary Health Care," 51.

31. Chan, speech Almaty, Kazakhstan, October 14, 2008.

32. UN FAO, "Impact of Armed Conflict on the Nutritional Situation of Children," in *Study on the Impact of Armed Conflicts on the Nutritional Situation of Children* (Rome: FAO, 1996), 22.

33. Africa Progress Panel, *An Agenda for Progress at a Time of Global Crisis: A Call for African Leadership*, Annual Report of the Africa Progress Panel, 2009; available at http://africaprogresspanel.socialmediarelease.co.za.

34. Pinstrup-Andersen, Pandya-Lorch, and Rosegrant, *World Food Prospects*, 20–21.

35. United States Institute of Peace, *PeaceWatch*, July 2009, 4–7; see also http://www.usip.org/resources/united-states-institute-peace-teaches-international-security-personnel-resolve-conflicts.

36. "If the World Were Food, Nobody Would Go Hungry," *The Economist* November 21, 2009, 63.

37. Ibid., 72.

38. William Neuman, "A Growing Discontent," *New York Times*, March 12, 2010, B1, B5.

39. "Genetically Modified Food: The Attack of the Really Quite Likeable Tomatoes," *The Economist*, February 27, 2010, 16.

40. Interview, James Morris, World Food Programme, *IFPRI Forum*, June 2003.

41. Neuman, "A Growing Discontent," B5.

42. House of Commons, International Development Committee, "The Humanitarian Crisis in Southern Africa," Third report of Session 200–2003, *Vol. I: Report and Proceedings of the Committee*, HC 116–1, March 4, 2003, 166.

43. Ibid., 169–173.

44. *Economist*, November 21, 2009, 73.

14. Prescription for Change

1. Bob Dylan, "Like a Rolling Stone," *Highway 61 Revisited*, 1965.

2. Nigel Dower, "Global Hunger: Moral Dilemmas," in Ben Mepham, ed., *Food Ethics* (London: Routledge, 1996), 9–10.

3. James Grant, United National Children's Fund, *The State of the World's Children, 1987* (Oxford: Oxford University Press, 1987), 9.

Index

alpha-amylase, 81, 82

abiotic changes, 101–2

Abraham, Solomon, 3

absorption of nutrients, 80, 86–89

access to food. *See* food, access to

acetyl coenzyme A/acetyl CoA, 63

active transport, 88

acts of God theories. *See* food availability decline (FAD) theory

acts of man theories. *See* food entitlement decline (FED) theory

adenosine triphosphate (ATP), 62, 86, 87, 93, 174

adhesins, 214–15

aerobic metabolism, 64–65

Africa: agricultural challenges in, 268–72; conflicts in, 22, 190–92, 197, 278; democratization in, 23–24; disease prevention measures and challenges, 20–21, 22, 272, 293n46; education of girls, 273–74; ESAPs in, 132; female mortality in pregnancy and childbirth, 275; foreign land ownership in, 278–79; and genetically modified/engineered organisms, 260, 282, 283; and Internet, 281; maize in, 248–49, 269–70, 271, 283; and microfinance institutions, 280–81; moral economy, 128–29; natural resources in post-colonial, 190–98, 262; nutritional transition to maize, 248; population growth, 202; regional institutions, 279; and wealth paradox, 21–24, 189, 190–98. *See also* starvation and famine in Africa; Sub-Saharan Africa

African Peace and Security Architecture (APSA), 278

aggression and bond formation, 231–240; appeasement gestures, 239; cooperation, 240–45; functions of aggression, 232;

functions of pair bonding, 233; human plasticity, 234; individual bonds, 237–38; militant enthusiasm, 238–39; social organization without love, 236–37; synopsis, 245–46

agribusiness in U.S., 150–51, 282, 283

Agricultural Act (1949), 147, 149

Agricultural Trade Development and Assistance Act (1954), 147

agriculture: cash crops, 128–29, 131, 183–84, 197; challenges in Africa, 268–72; in China, 204, 205, 206, 207; commoditization of, by colonial powers, 128–29, 183–84, 248; and divergence of evolution, 99–101; early warning systems for crop failures, 14; famine as result of, 98; and Great Irish Famine, 44, 45, 49; and human divergence, 99–101; industrialization and energy use, 101; labor shortage effect of HIV/AIDS pandemic, 32; monoculture, 32, 44, 45, 105, 110, 154–55, 269; El Niño/La Niña effects on rain-fed, 200; origins of, 96–99, 100, 102; revolutions in, 101–7; and tragedy of the commons, 107–9. *See also* food production

alpha-linolenic acid, 68

allergies, 216

amino acids, 66, 69, 80-83, 90-93, 95, 157, 159-160, 164, 166–67

amphipathic compounds, 85

anabolic state, 90–91, 159–60

anabolism, defined, 61

anaerobic metabolism, 62–63

anatomy of nutrition, 78–80

anemia, 177

animal behavior, 230–31, 234, 235–38

anonymity of the flock, 235–36

anorexigenic hormones, 163

women's education impact on health, 272–73. *See also* mortality of children

China: demand challenges from rapid development, 202–11; environmental problems, 204, 205–6; as food donor, 142–43; and food insecurity, 204, 206; foreign land purchases, 278, 279; and grain prices, 189–90, 206, 207; industrialization, 204–5; nutritional transition in, 205–6; population growth, 202; precolonial food reserves, 128; urbanization, 204

chloroplasts, 61

Choctaw Nation, 185–86

cholera, 33, 118, 196, 198, 213, 219–20

chronic hunger, 4, 5, 16, 17, 22, 28–30, 35, 38, 40, 41, 123, 124–26, 136, 179, 256, 260, 285

chronic malnutrition, 29, 55, 165–66, 171, 212, 214–23

civilization as enabled by agriculture, 96, 97, 100, 102

civil wars, 192–93

Clarkson, L. A., 247

class structure and Great Irish Famine, 112

climate change, 101, 189, 198–202, 205, 311n53

Cold War politics, 153

collagen, 83

Collier, Paul, 189, 191, 192–93

colon, 80

colonialism: commodity agriculture, 128–29, 183–84, 248; divisions and dependencies, 182–83; maize, 248; and moral economy, 128–29; natural resources extraction, 183–84, 194

col-tan, 189, 194, 195

commensalism, 216

commodity production, 128–29, 131, 183–84, 197

communism and food relief, 152

compassion fatigue, 19–21, 33

compromised hosts at risk for infection, 217

condensation, 80–81

conditionalities for financial aid eligibility, 131, 265–67

conflicts: as cause of hunger and malnutrition, 31, 190–92, 277; and challenges of providing developmental assistance, 21; disease toll during, 197, 213, 218,

222; efforts to end African, 197, 277–78; and food insecurity, 190, 277; mortality during, 197, 212–13, 218, 222; natural resources as precipitators of, 189, 191, 192–97; scale of African, 22; in Sub-Saharan Africa (1950–2000), 191; and weapons sales, 288

conformation of a protein, 69

Congo. *See* Democratic Republic of the Congo

conservation of energy, 61, 62

consumption rationing as response to food shortage, 126

Continental Early Warning System (CEWS), 278

Convention on the Elimination of All Forms of Discrimination Against Women, 256

cooperative behaviors, 240–45

coping strategies for chronic hunger, 5, 40, 124–26, 136

core-periphery disparity in Great Irish Famine, 50–51

corn: in Africa, 248–49, 269–70, 271, 283; for biofuel (ethanol), 263, 279; nutritional deficits, 306n31; U.S. subsidies for production of, 151

Corn Laws, 48, 49–50

Corrigan, Sr. Brigid, 55

Cosmides, Lena, 229

Costa Rica, 131

Cotton, Ann, 273–74

Crawford, E. Margaret, 247

Cromwell, Henry, 180

Cromwell, Oliver, 180

culture as enabled by agriculture, 96, 97, 100, 102

cytokines, 216

Daly, Mary, 45

Dam, Carl Peter Henrik, 169

Darfur, 24, 126–27, 197, 277

dark reaction vs. light reaction in photosynthesis, 61

Davis, Mike, 128, 189, 198, 200

Dawkins, Sir Richard, 242, 243, 244–45

deaths. *See* mortality

debt relief, 281

enclosure, 104

endocrine glands, 91

endocytosis, 89

energy: biofuels, 17, 18–19, 263, 279–80;
   conservation of, 61, 62; dependence of
   agriculture on, 101; living organism's
   metabolic processing of, 68, 75–76;
   photosynthesis as original life, 60–61, 64;
   protein-energy malnutrition, 157, 163–68,
   217, 225; storage in humans, 93, 163–64;
   use by wealthy countries, 201–2

entropy, living organisms' subversion of,
   75–76

environmental causes of hunger: climate
   change, 101, 189, 198–202, 205, 311n53;
   pollution, 11, 201–2, 204, 205, 262

environmental evolution, 99

environmental exploitation and evolution,
   232

enzyme prosthetic group (B$_1$), 65

enzymes, function of, 65, 81–85

Erikson, Erik, 239

ESAPS (economic structural adjustment
   programs), 8, 131–32, 133

esophagus, anatomy of, 79

ESS (evolutionary stable strategy), 241–42

An Essay on the Principle of Population
   (Malthus), 12, 35

essential amino acids, 69

essential fatty acids, 68

ethanol, 263, 279

ethical behavior, moral and human rights of,
   254. *See also* right to adequate food

Ethiopia case study, 3, 7, 11–12, 124–25, 153–55,
   191–92

eukaryotes, 59

European Commission (EC), 144

ever-normal granaries, 128–29, 134, 138, 140,
   301n21

evolution: and development of agriculture,
   97, 99–101; and exploitation of environment, 232

Evolution and The Theory of Games (Smith,
   John Maynard), 241–42

evolutionary/intentionality theory of
   development of agriculture, 97

evolutionary psychology, 230–31

evolutionary stable strategy (ESS), 241–42

The Evolution of Cooperation (Axelrod), 244

exotoxins, 214, 220

facial expression recognition, 229–30

facilitated diffusion, 88–89

FAD (food availability decline) theory.
   See food availability decline (FAD) theory

famine: agricultural practices as cause of, 98;
   artificial, 123, 295n3, 300–301n2; biblical
   references to, 56, 106; catalytic causes of,
   27, 31–33, 43–51, 111–14 , 123–24, 130, 136;
   definitions of, 29–30, 41, 126, 127; diseases
   of, 25, 218–23; as economic and social
   phenomenon, 301n3; historical background, 55–56; lack of scientific study on
   biology of, 56–60; medieval period, 35;
   mortality, 26, 41, 117, 119, 155, 213, 218–23,
   295n3; physiology of starvation in, 57;
   predisposing causes of, 27, 30–31, 31–33,
   111. *See also* Great Irish Famine case
   study; starvation and famine in Africa

Famine Early Warning System (FEWS), 14,
   140, 191

famine food, 127, 131

Famine Pot, 116

FAO (Food and Agricultural Organization),
   140

farming. *See* agriculture

fasting state, 91–92

fats, 65–66, 68, 83–84, 93–94, 164

fat-soluble vitamins, 71

fatty acids, 65, 68

feasting hypothesis of development of
   agriculture, 97

fed state, 90–91, 159–60

FED (food entitlement decline) theory, 34,
   39–40, 43–46, 146, 286

FEWS. *See* Famine Early Warning System

Field, John, 29, 125

First World Food Conference (1974), 140

fixed capital, types of, 100

flavin adenine dinucleotide (FAD) (B$_2$), 64

floods, 198, 199

food, access to: affordability, 130; as definer
   of starvation, 127; and land purchases
   by foreign countries, 278–79; as moral

responsibility, 108. *See also* right to adequate food

Food and Agricultural Organization (FAO), 19, 140, 141, 255, 277

food availability decline (FAD) theory: and Great Irish Famine causes, 43, 44–45, 46–49, 110; synergy with FED in producing hunger, 286; theoretical discussion, 34, 36–37

food entitlement decline (FED) theory, 34, 39–40, 43–46, 146, 286

Food First/Institute for Food and Development Policy, 15

Food for Education and Child Nutrition, 149

Food for Peace Act (1954), 147, 305n17

Food for Progress Act (1985), 147, 149

food-for-work projects, 115, 143, 146

food insecurity: and childhood mortality, 277; in China, 204, 206; and conflict, 190, 277; demand for vs. supply of food, 37; and farm size, 268–72; government policies' exacerbation of, 137, 138; with hunger, 5, 22, 28

food prices: and biofuels, 17, 18–19, 263, 279–80; and emergency food relief, 146; international focus on (1970s), 13; seasonality of, 132; spikes in, 18–19, 46, 48, 131, 279. *See also* grain prices

food production: in China, 204, 206, 207; and climate change, 205; commodity production, 128–29, 131, 183–84, 197; and conflict, 197; and emergency food relief, 146; and hunger, 106; land purchases by foreign countries, 278–79; measuring, 140; El Niño/La Niña impact on, 199; percent that is food aid, 142; and population growth, 105; subsidies for, 131, 132, 151; surpluses, 209

food reserves, 14, 128–29, 134, 138, 140, 301n21

food seeking behavior, 3, 55, 56, 157–63

food supply: and food insecurity, 37; grain reserves, 8, 128–29, 132–34, 301n21; need for increase in, 13, 17; and poorest of the poor's access to grain, 203; as predisposing cause of starvation and famine, 31; Soviet disruption of grain supplies (1970s) , 12, 13. *See also* food production

Foreign Assistance Act (1948), 152

Four Horsemen of the Apocalypse, 212, 214

Frederickson, George, 239

free market economics: and colonialism, 128–29; and genetically modified/engineered organisms, 282, 283; and Great Irish Famine, 112–13, 115; and international financial institutions, 123, 131, 184; and Internet, 281; as response to hunger, 123; and right to adequate food, 257–60; and starvation, 134, 136–37; theoretical considerations, 8. *See also* *laissez-faire* economics

free will, existence of, 227–28

fuel-food crisis (2007–2008), 18–19

Funk, Casimir, 169

game theory, 241–45

gastrointestinal system, 78

Gaud, William, 105

genetically modified/engineered organisms (GMO/GEO), 249, 260, 282–84

genetics in human behavior, 227–31

Geneva Conventions of 1948 and Protocols of 1977, 255–56, 318n10

Gerald of Wales, 182

Ghana, 131, 274

girls, education of, 272–75

global climate change, 101, 189, 198–202, 205, 311n53

Global Information and Early Warning System (GIEWS), 14, 140

glucagon, 160

gluconeogenesis, 66, 92, 160

glucose: levels, 90, 91–92, 159, 160–61; metabolism, 62, 66, 81–82, 88, 90, 93–95

glycolysis, 62

GMO/GEO. *See* genetically modified/engineered organisms

God and creation of humans, 227–28

governments: food aid as instrument of foreign policy, 151–56, 258, 265–67, 306n34; and food insecurity, 137, 138; foreign land purchases by, 278–79; as leading donor, 142–43; responsibility for protecting right to food, 14–15, 254, 258–60, 318n12; U.S. role in food aid, 147–51; weakness and corruptions as catalytic causes of starvation, 31. *See also* politics of food/starvation; responding to hunger

grain prices: and amount of food aid, 150; biofuels impact on, 18–19; and Chinese demand, 189–90, 206, 207; effect of dumping, 134; increase in urban populations, 203; price and production, 135; Soviet impact on (1970s), 12, 208–9, 313–14n113

grain reserves, 8, 128–29, 132–34, 138, 140, 301n21. *See also* corn

Grameen Bank, 280

Grant, James P., 24, 25, 289

Great Britain, 179, 180–81. *See also* Great Irish Famine case study

Great Depression, 36

"The Great Grain Robbery," 208–9, 210, 313–14n113

Great Hunger: Ireland 1845–1849 (Woodham-Smith), 49

Great Irish Famine case study: age and death by starvation, 117, 119; catalytic causes, 111–14; and causes of starvation, 41–51; effect of evictions, 249; and *laissez-faire* economics, 259; Malthusian theory applied to, 36; moral economy and British settlement, 129; mortality, 48–49, 51, 117–20, 213, 247–50; nutritional lessons, 110–11, 247–48; overview, 7–8; population enslavement, 180–81; prejudice, 179–86; racism, 182; relief operations, 7, 114–17; and slave trade, 180–81; and Sub-Saharan Africa famine, 182–83

Green Revolution, 102, 105

GTP (guanosine triphosphate), 64

Guns, Germs, and Steel (Diamond), 96–97

Haile Selassie I, Emperor of Ethiopia, 3, 153, 306n36

Haiti, 131–32

Haldane, J. B. S., 240

Hamilton, W. D., 240

Hardin, Garrett, 107, 261, 262

Haworth, Walter, 169

health care, 21, 275–77

Heavily Indebted Poor Countries (HIPCS), 281

Hegel, Georg Wilhelm Friedrich, 228

heme proteins, 176

heterotrophs, 60

Higden, Ranulf, 181

Hill, Archibald, 62

HIPCS. See Heavily Indebted Poor Countries

Hippocrates, 168–69

HIV/AIDS, 21, 22, 32, 273, 293n46

Hobbes, Thomas, 96

Hochschild, Adam, 184–85, 194

Hopkins, Frederick Gowland, 169

hormones, 91, 159, 162

How the Mind Works (Pinker), 229

human behavior/nature: cooperative, 240–45; ethical, 254; food seeking, 3, 55, 56, 157–63; genetic basis for, 227–31; plasticity in, 234. *See also* political behavior

human capital, 45, 100–101

Human Development Index, 22

human divergence and development of agriculture, 99–101

humanitarian aid. *See* relief operations; responding to hunger

human plasticity, 234

human rights, 10, 15–16, 152, 254, 256, 275. *See also* right to adequate food

humoral immunity, 216

hunger: as creation of politics, 155; defined, 28, 157–58; early 21st-century increase in, 17; and gender, 273; global reduction in (1996–2000), 16–17, 260; physiology of food-seeking behavior, 157–63; regulation and control of, 162–63. *See also* famine; responding to hunger; starvation

hunger artists, 57

hungry season, 129

hunter-gatherer societies, 97, 98, 103, 106

Hurricane Katrina, 200, 311n53

hydrochloric acid, 82

hydrogen bonds, 84

ICIHI. *See* Independent Commission on International Humanitarian Issues

IMF. *See* International Monetary Fund

immediate hypersensitivity, 216

immigration. *See* emigration

immunity against disease, 216–17
income and urbanization, 203
indentured servitude, 181
Independent Commission on International Humanitarian Issues (ICIHI), 39
India, 202, 210, 224, 283
industrialization, 101, 204–5
inequality, socioeconomic: as basis of hunger problem, 37; food distribution, 5, 38–39, 48–50, 198, 261, 265; and Great Irish Famine, 47; and nutritional crisis vs. nutritional transition, 17–18; wealth paradox, 21–24, 190–98; wealthy class's justification for poor's starvation, 35–36; widening gap, 17–24, 46. *See also* poverty
insecurity, food. *See* food insecurity
insider vs. outsider definitions of starvation, 29–30, 103, 124–30
insulin, 90–91, 92, 159–60
internal homeostasis, 89–90, 161
International Convention on the Rights of the Child (UN), 255
International Covenant on Economic, Social and Cultural Rights (UN), 255, 257
international humanitarian response. *See* relief operations; responding to hunger
International Monetary Fund (IMF), 123, 131–32, 133
Internet, 281
iodine deficiency, 175
Irish Famine. *See* Great Irish Famine case study
Irish Relief Association, 116
iron, 175–77
iron-sulfur proteins, 176
islets of Langerhaus, 91

Jackson, Andrew, 185
Japan, foreign land purchases by, 278, 279
jatropha, 279–80

Kabila, Laurent-Désiré, 195, 196
Kant, Immanuel, 264
Karrer, Paul, 169
Kennedy, Gordon, 162
Kenya, 271–72, 276–77, 281

ketogenesis, 92–95
Keynes, John Maynard, 36
Keys, Ansel, 56–57
kinetic energy, defined, 61
King Leopold's Ghost (Hochschild), 194
Kingsley, Charles, 182
Kissinger, Henry, 14
Klare, Michael, 192
Krebs, Hans Adolph, 63
Krebs citric acid cycle, 63–64
Kühn, Friedrich Wilhelm, 65
kwashiorkor, 32, 164–65, 166–68

labor, forced movement of, 183
lactic acid, 63
laissez-faire economics: in Africa, 184; and Great Irish Famine causes, 7, 47–51, 184, 259; and Malawi famine response, 123; social cost of, 42–43
Lake, Lucy, 274
land, arable, 205, 207
"land grabbing," 278–79
land tenancy system, 154
large intestine, anatomy of, 80
Leakey, R. E., 103
lecithin, 84–85
Leopold II, King of Belgium, 194
leptin, 162
Levanzin, Agostino, 57
Leviathan (Hobbes), 96
Lewin, R., 103
"Lifeboat Ethics" (Hardin), 261
life from scientific perspective, 74–76
light reaction vs. dark reaction in photo-synthesis, 61
linoleic acid, 68
Lipmann, Fritz Albert, 63
lipostat theory, 162
Live Aid rock concerts, 11
Li Xiaorong, 253–54
Lloyd, W. F., 107
Lomonosov-Lavoisier law of the conserva-tion of mass, 62
long-term development vs. short-term relief assistance, 13. *See also* Millennium Development Goals (MDGs)
Lorenz, Konrad, 231–34, 235, 237–39

loss of entitlement concept, 106
loud emergencies vs. silent emergencies, 24–25, 29–30
Luttrell, Clifton, 210

Maathai, Wangari Muta, 109
Mabbs-Zeno, Carl, 29
macromolecules, 80. *See also* proteins; triglycerides
macronutrient deficiency (protein-energy malnutrition), 32, 65, 157, 163–68, 217, 225
macronutrients, types and functions of, 66–70
maize. *See* corn
maize revolution, 248, 269–270
maja'a concept, 127
malaria, 5, 20–21, 225, 271, 272, 275
Malawi case study, 7–8, 123, 129–35
Mali case study, 123, 128, 135–38, 303n62
Mallon, Mary, 220
malnutrition: chronic, 29, 214–23; and conflicts, 191, 277; and death of children, 223, 225; defined, 29; and education of women, 272–73; and end of moral economy, 132; and food seeking behavior physiology, 157–63; macronutrient deficiency, 32, 65, 157, 163–68, 217, 225; micronutrient deficiency, 168–77, 225; and nutritional transition, 203; pathophysiology of starvation, 157; protein-energy, 157, 163–68, 217, 225; in Sub-Saharan Africa, 202; summary, 177–78
Malthus, Thomas, 12, 35, 212, 214, 249
Malthusian theory, Great Irish Famine as case study for, 42, 110. *See also* food availability decline (FAD) theory
marasmus, 164–66, 167
Markandaya, Kamala, 158
market economy. *See* free market economics
Marshall Plan (1948), 152
Maslow, Abraham, 158
McAfee, Kathy, 149, 150
MDGs (Millennium Development Goals), 19–21, 73–74, 114, 225, 256, 293n33
mechanization, 104
Médecins Sans Frontières (MSF), 15, 136–37
media impact on awareness of starvation, 11

medieval period, famine in, 35
MEND (Movement for the Emancipation of the Niger Delta), 193
Mengistu Haile Mariam, 153, 191–92, 306nn36–37
Messer, Ellen, 191
metabolic states, 90–91, 159–60
metabolism, 61–66, 159, 162–63
Mexico, 131
Meyerhof, Otto, 62
micelles, 85
microfinance institutions, 280–81
micronutrient deficiency, 168–77, 225
micronutrients, types and functions of, 65, 70–71
militant enthusiasm, 238–39
militarization, 191–92
Millennium Declaration, 20, 256
Millennium Development Goals (MDGs), 19–21, 73–74, 114, 225, 256, 293n33
Millennium Villages, 271–72, 283
minerals, dietary, 71, 174–77
Minkowski, Oscar, 159
Minnesota Starvation Experiment, 57–58
Minot, George, 169
mitochondrial respiration, 64
Mobutu, Joseph, 194–95
monoculture, 32, 44, 45, 105, 110, 154–55, 269
monosaccharides, 67
Monsanto, 282, 283
moral economy, 128–29, 132, 138
moral imperative in providing food, 6–7, 108, 260–65. *See also* right to adequate food
moral judgments on the poor, 13, 35–36, 48, 267
moral legitimacy, 266
Morris, James T., 32, 143, 155, 198
mortality: and banality of death, 223–25; and chronic hunger, 30; from chronic malnutrition complications, 214–17; during conflicts, 197, 212–13, 218, 222; from diseases, 26, 33, 117–19, 197, 212–25; as driver of policy responses, 126; and famine, 26, 41, 117, 119, 155, 213, 218–23, 295n3; in Great Irish Famine, 48–49, 51, 117–20, 213, 247–50; introduction, 212–14;

orexigenic hormones, 162

organelles, 61

Origins (Lewin and Leakey), 103

Osler, Sir William, 212, 214

osmosis, 86

"otherness" paradigm, 103, 179, 236, 237, 239–40, 245–46

outsider vs. insider perspectives on experience, 29–30, 103, 124–30

ownership conflicts, 192

oxidative phosphorylation, 64

oxyntic cells, 82

pancreas, 91

paradox of wealth, 21–24, 190–98

parasitism, 216

Pareto equilibrium, 243

parietal cells, 82

Pastoral Activities and Services for people with aids, Dar es Salaam Archdiocese (PASADA), 55

pathogens, 214

pathophysiology of starvation, 157–68

Pauling, Linus, 84

Peel, Sir Robert, 47–48, 114

Peet, Richard, 129

PEM (protein-energy malnutrition), 32, 65, 157, 163–68, 217, 225

pepsin, 83

peptide bond, 69

peptide chains, 82

peristalsis, 79

personal ownership and development of agriculture, 103

pestilence, 218–23

phagocytosis, 217

Philippines, 131

photosynthesis as original energy of life, 60–61, 64

phylogeny, 230–31

pica, 177

Pinker, Stephen, 228, 229

Pogge, Thomas, 16

political behavior, biological basis for: aggression and bond formation, 231–46; genetics in human behavior, 227–31; introduction, 226–27

politics of food/starvation: and catalytic causes of starvation/famine, 31, 33; commonalities, 179; conditionalities, 265–66; economic theories, 8; Ethiopian impact, 11; food aid as political instrument, 151–56, 258, 265–67, 306n34; and Great Irish Famine, 42, 46–50; and lack of will to end hunger, 3, 19, 20; in Malawi, 135; and threats to food reserves, 14

Pollan, Michael, 101, 151

pollution, 11, 201–2, 204, 205, 262

polypeptide chains, 69–70

polysaccharides, 67

poorest of the poor population: "bottom billion" composition, 6, 17–19; climate change impact on, 200; as consistent recipients of food aid, 143; and global grain supply, 203; increase in, 5; Irish of 19th century as, 7, 50

population factor: and China, 202; and emigration, 110; and food production, 105; in Great Irish Famine, 44–45, 180–81; international concerns over growth (1970s), 13; limits in hunter-gatherer societies, 98; and natural resources, 192; and poverty, 261; as predisposing cause of starvation/famine, 31; and pressure on food supplies, 5, 13–14; starvation as "positive check" on overpopulation, 12, 35–36; urbanization, 202–4

positive check concept in population theory of starvation, 12, 35–36

potato factor in Great Irish Famine, 44–45, 48, 111–14

potential energy, defined, 61

poverty: as basis of hunger problem, 3–6, 12–13, 16, 31, 34, 37, 38–40, 286–87; and child mortality, 276; children in, 179; and chronic hunger, 28–29; and climate change, 200–201, 311n53; and conflict, 197; and food aid's disruption of local communities, 146; and gender, 273; in Great Irish Famine, 45–47, 50–51; and lack of investment in human capital, 101; Millennium Development Goals on, 20; moral judgments on the poor, 13, 35–36, 48, 267; and population growth, 261; of

Sub-Saharan Africa, 22. *See also* poorest of the poor population

predisposing causes of starvation/famine, 27, 30–31, 43–51, 111. *See also* food supply; population factor; poverty

prices. *See* food prices

primary commodities. *See* natural resources

primary energy deficiency, 164–66, 167

primary protein deficiency, 164–65, 166–68

Principles of Political Economy (Malthus), 12, 110

"Prisoner's Dilemma, the," 242–44

private voluntary organizations (PVOs), 144, 148, 150

program aid, 142, 259

project food aid, 142, 259

prokaryotes, 59, 66

prolonged semistarvation vs. total fasting starvation, 57, 58

protein-energy malnutrition (PEM), 32, 65, 157, 163–68, 217, 225

proteins, 66, 69–70, 82–83, 163, 176, 214–17

proximate causes of death during famine, 27, 33, 117–20

pseudospeciation, 239

Public Law 480, 147, 148

Pumpelly, Raphael, 97

PVOs (private voluntary organizations), 144, 148, 150

pyruvate, 62–63

Quakers, 116, 117

racism, 181–82, 184–86, 240

Rapoport, Anatol, 244

rationing of consumption, 40, 126

Ravenholt, Albert, 206

Reagan, Ronald, 155

reciprocal altruism, 240–41

regional cooperation in Sub-Saharan Africa, 24, 269, 280, 289

regional food stockpiles, international call for, 140

relief camps, conditions and consequences, 32–33, 146, 149–50

relief operations: food quality issue, 33; Great Irish Famine, 7, 114–17; vs. long-term development aid, 37; media's role in jump-starting, 11; Niger, 137; reliance on FAD theory, 37. *See also* emergency food relief

resource wars, 189, 191, 192–97

respiration in metabolism, 61–66

responding to hunger: biofuels issue, 279–80; conflict resolution to reduce violence, 277–78; debt relief, 281; distribution methods and agencies, 143–51; food aid definition, 141–42; food security and smallholder farming, 268–72; and genetically modified/engineered organisms, 282–84; health care, 275–77; insider vs. outsider definitions of, 124–28; Internet resources, 281; introduction, 268; land grabbing problem, 278–79; in Malawi, 123, 129–31, 132, 133–35; in Mali, 123, 135–36, 137; microfinancing of institutions, 280–81; necessary steps in, 287–89; in Niger, 123, 135–37; outsider vs. insider definitions of, 124–28; overview, 6; regional institution building, 280; summary, 285–87; women and education, 272–75. *See also* governments; nongovernmental organizations (NGOs); relief operations

revolutions in agriculture, 101–7

Rickettsia, 222

right to adequate food: attaching conditions to aiding others, 265–67; as basic human right, 14–16; developing consciousness of, 14–15; elements of, 253–54; government role, 14–15 , 254, 258–60, 318n12; international legal structure for, 254–56, 318nn10, 12; market effects on, 257–60; obligation of haves to have nots, 260–65; overview, 10; and *Universal Declaration of Human Rights*, 10, 15–16, 254, 256, 275

Right to Food Resolution, U.S., 14–15

Rindos, David, 97

risk-mapping, 140

Robinson, Mary, 185–86

Rosenfeld, Stephen S., 313–14n113

Rosset, Peter, 260

Rotstayn, Leon, 201–2

Russell, Lord John, 48, 114–15

Rwanda, 23, 195

saccharides, 81

SADC (Southern Africa Development Community), 24, 269, 280

safety in numbers survival concept, 235–37

salts, 174

sanitation, lack of access to, 73, 223, 224

Saro-Wiwa, Ken, 193

Sauer, C. O., 97

Scott, John Paul, 228

Scrimshaw, Nevin, 30, 124

scurvy, 114, 168–69

SEACOM, 281

Seaman, John, 145

seasonal hunger, 28, 119, 132, 138

seasonality of food prices, 132

self-determinism, existence of, 227–28

The Selfish Gene (Dawkins), 242, 243

semistarvation, 56–57, 58

Sen, Amartya: on causes of starvation, 12–13, 31, 34, 38–40, 42, 106; and enclosure process, 104; food prices and access to food problem, 132

Senegal, 132

Shaw, Timothy, 156

Sheeran, Josette, 5, 6, 17, 18–19, 26

Shell Oil, 193

Shepherd, Jack, 23, 125–26

Shigella, 218, 219

Sierra Leone, 224, 276

silent emergencies: as applied to Great Irish Famine, 43; defined, 5–6; Ethiopian-global context, 11–12; and food as human right, 14–16; and invisibility of rural poor, 50–51; vs. "loud emergencies," 24–25, 29–30; outsider vs. insider observations, 124–28; overview, 24–26; population growth food supply pressures, 13–14; poverty as basis of hunger problem, 3–6, 12–13, 16, 34, 37, 38–40, 286–87; safe drinking water access, 73; and socioeconomic inequality, 17–24

silent epidemics, 123–24

Singer, Peter, 262–63, 264, 266

single-crop agriculture, 32, 44, 45, 105, 110, 154–55, 269

slavery, 103, 179–82

smallholder farming and food security, 268–72

small intestine, anatomy of, 79–80

Smith, Adam, 100

Smith, Elizabeth, 267

Smith, John Maynard, 241–42

Snow, John, 219–20

social disintegration and starvation, 30, 124–26

Society of Friends, 116, 117

sociobiology, 228–31

Sociobiology: The New Synthesis (Wilson), 229

sociopolitical factors: African political developments, 23–24; colonial commodity agriculture, 128–29, 183–84, 248; cost of *laissez-faire* economics, 42–43; Great Irish famine, 46–50, 112, 179–86, 247–50; maize in Africa, 248–49; relationship to biological factors, 10; threat of unrest from the hungry, 17. *See also* inequality; political behavior; politics of food/starvation

sodium-potassium pump, 86–88

Soup Kitchen Act (1847), 116, 117

soup kitchens, 115–16, 117, 118

South Asia, 20, 224, 276

southern Africa 2003 case study, 145–46

Southern Africa Development Community (SADC), 24, 269, 280

Soviet Union and grain, 12, 112, 190, 208–9, 313–14n113

Stanley, Henry Morgan, 194

starches, 67

starvation: age and death by, 117, 119; biochemistry of, 89–95; definitions of, 29–30, 124–28; natural causes of, 31–32, 101, 189, 198–202, 205, 311n53; pathophysiology of, 157–68; predisposing causes, 27, 30–31, 43–51, 111; and social disintegration, 30, 124–26. *See also* catalytic causes of starvation/famine

starvation and famine in Africa, outside causes: climate change factor, 198–202; demand challenges from rapidly developing economies, 202–11; introduction, 189–90; wealth paradox, 190–98. *See also* food prices

starvation artists, 57

starvation wages and market economy, 115